Ear Diseases and CT

Zilong Yu
Editor

Ear Diseases and CT

PMPH PEOPLE'S MEDICAL PUBLISHING HOUSE

Springer

Editor
Zilong Yu
Otolarynology & Head and Neck Surgery
Beijing Tongren Hospital
Beijing, China

ISBN 978-981-99-7222-7 ISBN 978-981-99-7220-3 (eBook)
https://doi.org/10.1007/978-981-99-7220-3

This Springer imprint is published by the registered company Springer Nature Singapore Pte Ltd.
The registered company address is: 152 Beach Road, #21-01/04 Gateway East, Singapore 189721, Singapore

Paper in this product is recyclable.

Preface

Inflammation, trauma, tumors, and congenital malformation of the ear are common diseases that frequently occur in Otolaryngology and Head & Neck Surgery, and they are also long-term questions that otologists have to resolve. The ear mainly consists of the temporal bone, which not only houses the end organs of hearing and equilibrium, the smallest isolated bone (ossicle) and articulation in the human body, but also these organ are deeply embedded in the temporal bone, making it challenging to directly observe the condition of diseases and their relationships with the surrounding structures. Numerous cranial nerves, especially the facial nerve, and large blood vessels run through the temporal bone or surround it, making the temporal bone one of the most complex bones in the human body. A detailed study of the clinical anatomy and pathological radiology of the temporal bone will provide important information for the diagnosis of ear disease, the planning of surgical strategies, and the judgment of prognosis.

High-resolution computed tomography (HRCT) offers superior spatial resolution and contrast between bone, soft tissue, and air. It can precisely demonstrate the normal structure, anatomic variations, and pathological conditions of the temporal bone. Different directional scans (such as axial, coronal, and sagittal) have their distinguishing features and advantages for displaying specific structures in the temporal bone. Multi-direction observations and comprehensive analysis will be beneficial for fully recognizing diseases and making correct conclusions. Certainly, HRCT scanning has its drawbacks in displaying soft tissue diseases (including the tumor), otogenic intracranial complications, cerebrospinal fluid ear leakage, and others. In order to mitigate this disadvantage, other examination modalities, such as magnetic resonance imaging, were also used to diagnose related diseases, aiming to improve the practicality of this book. For instructions on how to operate these modalities, please refer to the related studies.

In order to easily understand the content of this book easily and enhance the ability to read radiographic images, a progressive approach, from easy to difficult, is adopted. First, we present the clinical anatomy of the temporal bone from multiple directions, highlighting important surgical structures and providing detailed explanations. Then, we compare the sectional anatomy of the temporal bone with its corresponding CT image in axial, coronal, and sagittal views, respectively. This self-contrast can help us recognize and remember the CT images easily. Finally, we showcase typical pathological radiologic images of ear diseases from the aforementioned viewing positions, and in some cases, intraoperative findings are used to identify those conditions with their corresponding images, aiming to verify them mutually. This approach is designed to enable a comprehensive understanding of the pathological radiologic imaging of the temporal bone and assist in making correct diagnoses and surgical treatment decisions for ear diseases.

We would like to express our thanks to our colleagues in the Department of Otolaryngology and Head & Neck Surgery, as well as the Department of Radiology at Beijing Tongren Hospital and Beijing Institute of Otolaryngology for their support. We also thank People's Medical Publishing House for publishing *Ear Disease and CT* in Chinese.

Beijing, China
March 2023

Zilong Yu

Conflict of Interest

The authors declare that there are no conflicts of interest regarding the publication of this book.

Contents

Editors and Contributors

Editor

Zilong Yu Department of Otolaryngology Head and Neck Surgery, Beijing Tongren Hospital, Capital Medical University, Beijing, China

Associate Editors

Bentao Yang Department of Radiology, Beijing Tongren Hospital, Capital Medical University, Beijing, China

Yong Li Department of Neurosurgery, Beijing Tongren Hospital, Capital Medical University, Beijing, China

Contributors

Shubin Chen Department of Otolaryngology Head and Neck Surgery, Beijing Tongren Hospital, Capital Medical University, Beijing, China

Haijiang Dai Department of Otolaryngology Head and Neck Surgery, Beijing Tongren Hospital, Capital Medical University, Beijing, China

Shusheng Gong Department of Otolaryngology Head and Neck Surgery, Beijing Friendship Hospital, Capital Medical University, Beijing, China

Xiping Li Department of Otolaryngology Head and Neck Surgery, Beijing Anzhen Hospital, Capital Medical University, Beijing, China

Yong Li Department of Neurosurgery, Beijing Tongren Hospital, Capital Medical University, Beijing, China

Jie Wang Department of Otolaryngology Head and Neck Surgery, Beijing Tongren Hospital, Capital Medical University, Beijing, China

Bentao Yang Department of Radiology, Beijing Tongren Hospital, Capital Medical University, Beijing, China

Zilong Yu Department of Otolaryngology Head and Neck Surgery, Beijing Tongren Hospital, Capital Medical University, Beijing, China

1 Clinical Anatomy of Ear

Zilong Yu

The ear is a peripheral organ for hearing and equilibrium, it consists of the external ear, middle ear, and inner ear. The bony portion of the external auditory canal, middle ear, inner ear, and internal acoustic meatus is located in the temporal bone.

1.1 Clinical Anatomy of Temporal Bone

The temporal bone is a compound bone, consists of the squamous, tympanic, mastoid, petrous, and styloid portion. It is located at the both sides of the head, inlays among the sphenoid bone, parietal bone, and occipital bone, and composes a part of the lateral skull base. Numerous cranial nerves, internal carotid artery, and internal jugular vein run through or pass by the temporal bone, the end organs of the hearing and equilibrium is embedded in it, so the temporal bone is one of the most complex bones in human body, and it has important clinical significance to understand the anatomy and the relationship with the adjacent structures of the temporal bone.

1.1.1 Squamous Portion of Temporal Bone

The squamous (scalelike) portion is located at the anterior-superior part of the temporal bone, and forms the outer wall of the middle cranial fossa, the roof of the external auditory canal (EAC), and contributes to the glenoid fossa of the temporomandibular joint. The lateral surface of this portion is smooth with slightly bulging, and the temporal muscle attaches on it. A curved bony ridge runs from the root of zygomatic arch to the top notch over the posterior-superior area of external auditory porus, is called temporal line, which can be regarded as a reference extracranial landmark of the middle cranial fossa base, the inferior edge of the temporal muscle attaches here.

The inner aspect of the squamous portion presents slight depressions for the convolutions of the temporal lobe of the brain, and a vertical groove for the middle meninge artery. The squamous portion is connected with the petrous portion by the petrosquamous fissure (Fig. 1.1).

1.1.2 Tympanic Portion of Temporal Bone

The tympanic portion is a flat-curved shape bone plate, is located under the squamous portion, in front of the mastoid portion, at the lateral aspect of the petrous apex. This portion composes the bony anterior wall, base wall, and a part of the posterior wall of the external auditory canal (Figs. 1.1 and 1.2). The tympanic portion is connected with the squamous portion by the tympanosquamous fissure in front of it. The anterosuperior ridge is located at the anterosuperior aspect of the external auditory canal. Sometimes this ridge needs to be removed because it overlays the field of vision during myringoplasty. The tympanic portion is also connected with the mastoid portion by tympanomastoid fissure posteriorly, the medial aspect of this fissure, it adjoins the mastoid (vertical) segment of the facial nerve.

At the medial aspect of the tympanic portion, it is connected with the petrous portion by the petrotympanic fissure, and composes the lateral-inferior bony wall of the eustachian tube. The anteroinferior part of the tympanic portion constitutes the posterior wall of the mandibular fossa. The posterosuperior part of the tympanic portion is absent, called Rivinus notch, where no fibro-annulus exists, but the pars flaccida of tympanic membrane attaches here. At the medial end of the tympanic portion, there is a small and shallow groove, called tympanic sulcus, the fibro-annulus at the edge of tympanic membrane fits in it. If the tympanic portion is not fully developed, the congenital stenosis of the external auditory canal will take place, and if this portion is not development at all, the atresia of the external auditory canal will occur.

Z. Yu (✉)
Department of Otolaryngology Head and Neck Surgery, Beijing Tongren Hospital, Capital Medical University, Beijing, China

Z. Yu (ed.), *Ear Diseases and CT*, https://doi.org/10.1007/978-981-99-7220-3_1

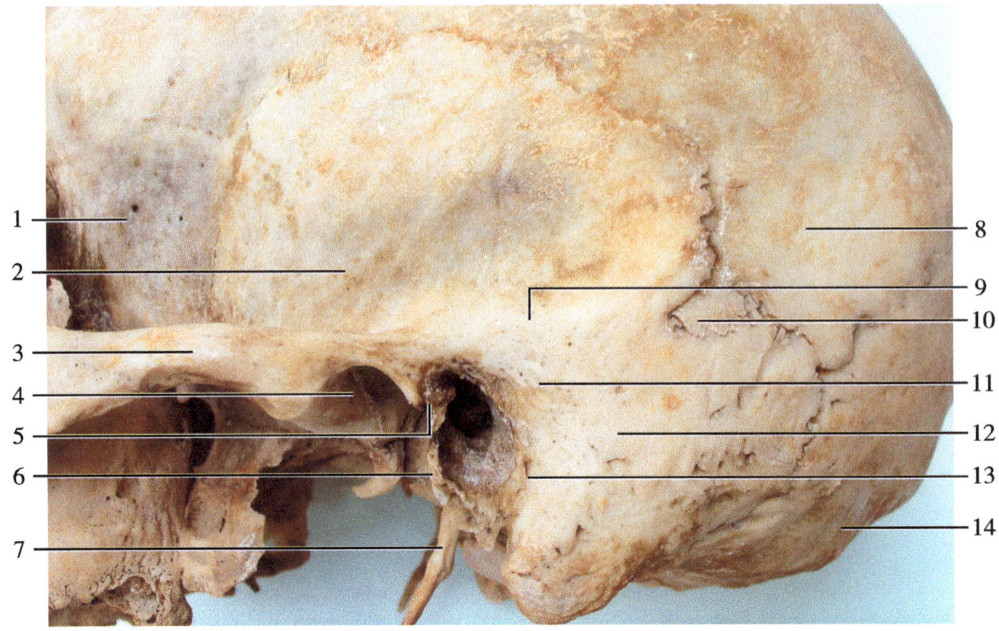

Fig. 1.1 Lateral view of temporal bone and its adjacent structures (left). (1) Sphenoid bone. (2) Squamous portion of temporal bone. (3) Zygomatic process of temporal bone. (4) Mandibular fossa. (5) Tympanosquamous fissure. (6) Tympanic portion of temporal bone. (7) Styloid process. (8) Parietal bone. (9) Temporal line. (10) Top notch. (11) Cribriform area. (12) Mastoid process. (13) Tympanomastoid fissure. (14) Occipital bone

1.1.3 Mastoid Portion of Temporal Bone

The mastoid portion is located under the squamous portion, looks like a pyramid process, the so-called mastoid process. It is connected with the petrous apex medially, and forms the tympanomastoid fissure anteriorly. The lateral surface of the mastoid portion is rough, at the anterosuperior aspect of this portion, that means the posterosuperior region of the external auditory canal has a bony ridge, called the suprameatal spine. At the posterosuperior region of this spine and below the temporal line, there is an area rich in small pores which calls the cribriform area, an important surface landmark of the tympanic antrum during the tympanomastoid surgery. The sternocleidomastoid muscle is attached to the lower part of the mastoid process, and there is always a mastoid foramen penetrating inside and outside the mastoid bone near the posterior edge, which is called mastoid conducting vessel (emissarium mastoideum). This vessel connects the extracranial vein with the sigmoid sinus through this foramen. Sigmoid sinus thrombophlebitis can affect the postauricular tissue through this foramen, and can result in the postauricular subperiosteal abscess. At the medial side of the mastoid tip, there is a deep groove, named the mastoid notch, or called digastric groove, digastric muscles attach here. When air cells in the tip of the mastoid develop very well, the medial wall of it will become very thin, the cholesteatoma in the mastoid cavity can destroy the wall, the pus accumulated in the mastoid can burst into this notch, and forms the abscess between the sternocleidomastoid muscle and the deep cervical fascia, named Bezold abscess. The stylomastoid foramen is located in front of the digastric groove and at the posterolateral side of the styloid process, this is the cranial exit of the facial nerve. The shallow groove on the medial side of the notch and accompanying it is called the occipital artery groove (Fig. 1.2), the occipital artery passes through here. When the mastoid process is well pneumatized, a corresponding arc-shaped bone ridge, called the digastric crest, can be seen on the inter-surface of the mastoid cavity of the digastric groove. The intersection of the ridge and the posterior wall of the external auditory canal and the line between the incudal fossa can be used as one of the landmarks of the vertical segment of the facial nerve when the bone of the posterior wall of the external auditory canal is removed. The deep part of this line is the vertical segment of the facial nerve, and the inner side of the front end of the ridge is the stylomastoid foramen. At the junction of the medial-posterior aspect of the mastoid process and the lateral-posterior aspect of the petrous portion, there is a deep zigzag groove called sigmoid sulcus. When the mastoid air cell is poorly developed, the bone plate of the sigmoid sinus is solid, and the distance from the posterior wall of the external auditory canal is short, or very close, there is only a thin layer of bone plate, which is called the anterior displacement of the sigmoid sinus; When the sigmoid sinus is very close to the lateral bone cortex of the mastoid process, it is called the lateral displacement of sigmoid sinus. In this case, the sigmoid sinus can be damaged and cause serious bleeding when mastoid surgery is performed via the retroauricular approach, which can hinder the operation, or air embolism may occur, endangering life. When the mastoid process is well pneumatized, partial bone absence of the anterior wall of the sigmoid sulus may occasionally occur. Some patients may have pulsatile tinnitus on the ipsilateral ear. Gently pressing the carotid artery at the same mandibular angle, the tinnitus can become weaker or temporarily disappear. The tegmen of the

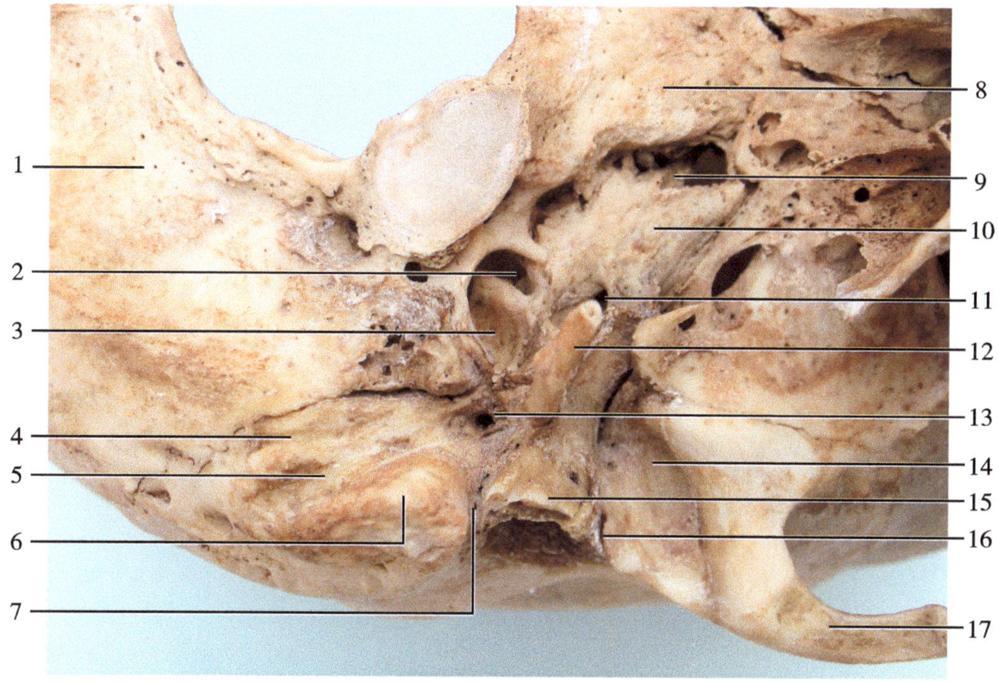

Fig. 1.2 Skull base view of temporal bone and its adjacent structures (left). (1) Occipital bone. (2) Nerve part of jugular foramen. (3) Vascular part of jugular foramen. (4) Occipital artery groove. (5) Digastric muscle groove. (6) Mastoid tip. (7) Tympanomastoid fissure. (8) Clivus. (9) Internal orifice of carotid artery canal and foramen lacerum. (10) Petrous apex. (11) External orifice of carotid artery canal. (12) Styloid process. (13) Stylomastoid foramen. (14) Mandibular fossa. (15) Tympanic portion of temporal bone. (16) Tympanosquamous fissure. (17) Zygomatic process of temporal bone

tympanic antrum and the bone plate of the sigmoid sinus meet to form a sinodural angle. During mastoid surgery, the tympanic antrum can be found forward along this angle.

In the development of temporal bone, if the squamous portion extends too far to the mastoid process, the mastoid air cells can be divided by a bony plate into two parts, the inner and outer parts, this bony plate is called Korner septum. This septum can be dense, and often meets it when opening part of the mastoid air cells. If it is not noticed, it is often mistaken for having reached the inner wall of the mastoid process so that the deep condition cannot be completely cleared.

The mastoid process of infants under 2 years of age is only rudimentary, and there is no mastoid process as a barrier at the stylomastoid foramen. When the infants under this age suffer from postauricular subperiosteal abscess, do not rashly use the adult postauricular incision (that means the vertical downward incision) to perform the operation, so as to avoid damaging the facial nerve.

1.1.4 Petrous Portion of Temporal Bone

The petrous portion is similar to a recumbent triangular pyramid, also known as petrous pyramid. It is located at the base of the lateral skull, embedded between the great wing of the sphenoid bone and the base of the occipital bone, and houses the hearing and balance organs. There are one bottom, one tip, three faces, and three edges. The bottom faces outward and merges with the squamous and mastoid portion; The tip is rough and slightly upward, and the internal orifice of the carotid artery canal is here, and forms the posterior outside of the foramen lacerum. The three faces of the petrous portion are descripted as follows:

Anterior surface: It composes the rear part of the middle cranial fossa, which is connected with the intracranial surface of the squamous portion through the petrosquamous fissure. From the inside out, there are the following important structures: the trigeminal semilunar ganglion impression near the petrous apex; two small grooves parallel to the long axis of the petrous portion at the posterolateral side of the impression. The medial groove is the greater petrosal nerve groove, and the lateral groove is the lesser petrosal nerve. The posterolateral end of the greater petrosal nerve groove is a hiatus of the facial nerve canal, through which the greater petrosal nerve penetrates. There is a large bulge on the outside of the impression, the arcuate eminence, below which the anterior semicircular canal is located. In recent years, anterior semicircular canal dehiscence syndrome has become one of the research hotspots in otology, and HRCT scan can show the location and length of the fissure. In front of the arcuate eminence, there is a shallow concave thin bone plate, which are anterior tympanic tegmen and posterior tympanic antrum tegmen, they separate the tympanic cavity and tympanic sinus from the middle cranial fossa (Fig. 1.3).

Posterior surface: It is also the anterior to the posterior cranial fossa, which is a triangular bone surface surrounded by the superior petrosal sinus, inferior petrosal sinus, and sigmoid sinus (Fig. 1.4). The medial part of this face is the internal acoustic porus, which leads to the internal acoustic meatus. There is a fissure located at the lateral-posterior aspect of the internal acoustic porus, covered by a thin bone

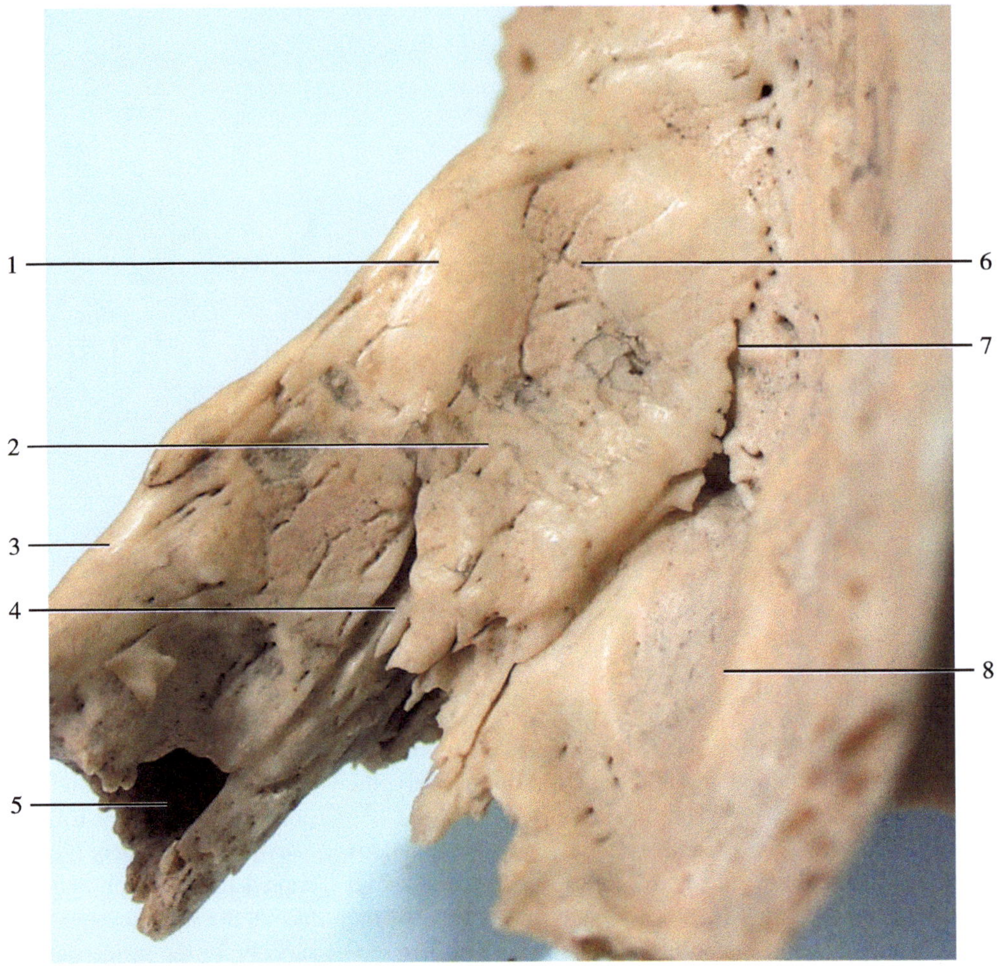

Fig. 1.3 Anterior view of petrous part of temporal bone (left). (1) Arcuate eminence. (2) Tympanic tegmen. (3) Trigeminal semilunar ganglion impression. (4) Superficial petrosal nerve groove. (5) Internal orifice of carotid artery canal. (6) Tegmen of tympanic antrum. (7) Petrosquamous fissure. (8) Squamous portion of temporal bone

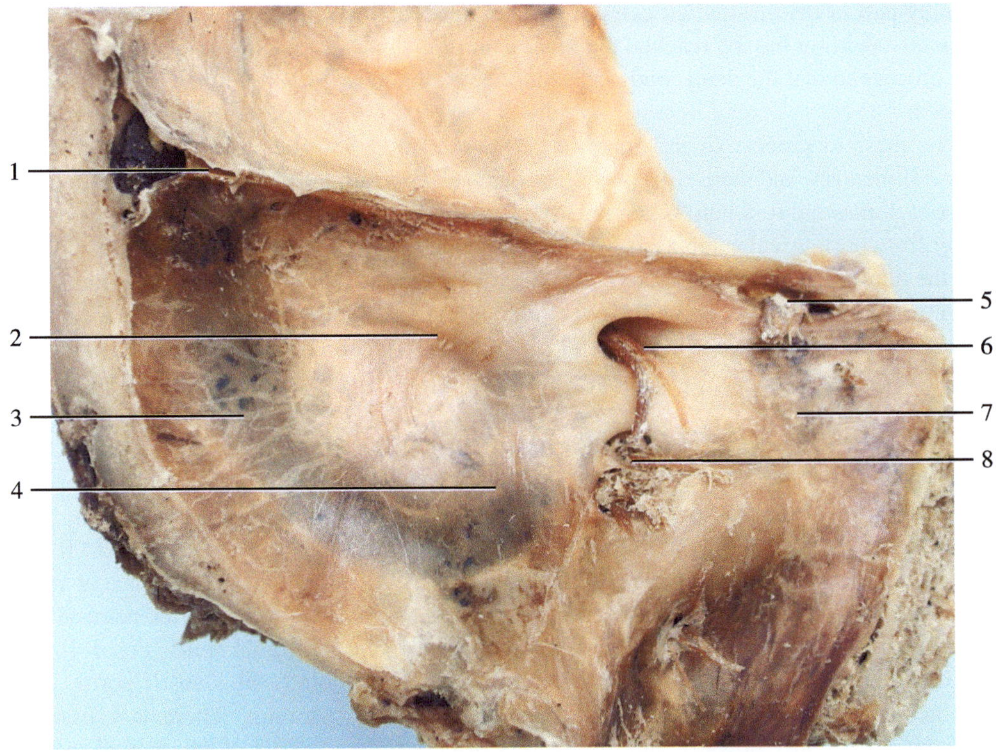

Fig. 1.4 Posterior view of petrous part of temporal bone (left, dura mater reserved). (1) Superior petrosal sinus. (2) Endolymphatic sac fissure. (3) Sigmoid sinus. (4) Vascular part of jugular foramen. (5) Trigeminal nerve semilunar impression. (6) Internal acoustic porus and vestibulocochlear nerve. (7) Inferior petrosal sinus. (8) Nerve part of jugular foramen

plate called the endolymphatic sac fissure (Fig. 1.5), which is the outer opening of the vestibular aqueduct. The latter leads to the vestibule of the bony labyrinth through the medial side of the common crus formed by the posterior and anterior semicircular canals, through which the endolymphatic duct passes. The upper part between the internal acoustic porus.

and the endolymphatic sac and near the upper edge of the petrous portion is the subarcuate fossa. Subarcuate artery and vein pass through the petromastoid duct and enter tympanic antrum under the anterior semicircular canal arch and above the lateral(horizontal)semicircular canal, and they are the only blood vessels that communicate the posterior cranial fossa and the tympanic antrum. They provide vascular supply to the otic capsule of the vestibule, semicircular canals, the mastoid antrum, and portions of the facial nerve canal (Akyol et al. 2011). The petromastoid canal is rarely of clinical importance other than serving as an anatomic landmark. Still, radiologists should be wary of confusing it for a fracture or other pathology (Benson and Lane 2022).

Inferior surface: It composes a part of the lateral skull base with uneven surface. The bone surface of the anterior medial part is rough, which is the attachment of the petrostaphylinus (levator veli palati muscle), tensor tympani muscle, and the cartilage of the eustachian tube. The posterior lateral part has two deep concaves adjacent to the anterior medial and the posterior lateral part. The anterior medial part is the external orifice of the carotid artery canal, through which the internal carotid artery and the carotid artery nerve plexus pass. The carotid artery canal first rises vertically along the anterior wall of the tympanic cavity, and then bends forward and runs horizontally in front of the cochlea, opening at the internal orifice of the carotid artery canal at the petrous apex. The posterior and outer part of the external carotid artery orifice is the jugular fossa, which is the top of the Glomus jugular (Figs. 1.2 and 1.6). The jugular foramen is the place where the internal jugular vein exits, it is composed of the jugular notch of the occipital bone and the petrous portion of the temporal bone and it is divided into the posterior external vascular area (Glomus jugular) and the anteromedial nerve area (glossopharyngeal nerve, vagus nerve, accessory nerve). The tumor in the jugular foramen area can cause the expansion of the foramen area and bone destruction. On the thin bone ridge between the external opening of the carotid artery canal and the jugular fossa, there is the inferior opening of the tympanic canaliculus, and the tympanic branch of the glossopharyngeal nerve-the Jacobson nerve, passes through. There is a triangular impression on the anteromedial side of the jugular fossa and close to the jugular interphysis (arteriovenous ridge), which is the location of the petroganglion of the glossopharyngeal nerve. There is a small hole at the bottom of the concave, which is the external aperture of the cochlear canaliculus. The cochlear canaliculus leads outward to the beginning of the scala tympani of the modiolus, containing the perilymph.

Three margins of petrous portion: The upper margin of the petrous part is the longest, with a superior petrosal groove containing the superior petrosal sinus; At the medial part of the inferior margin of the petrous portion, there is a

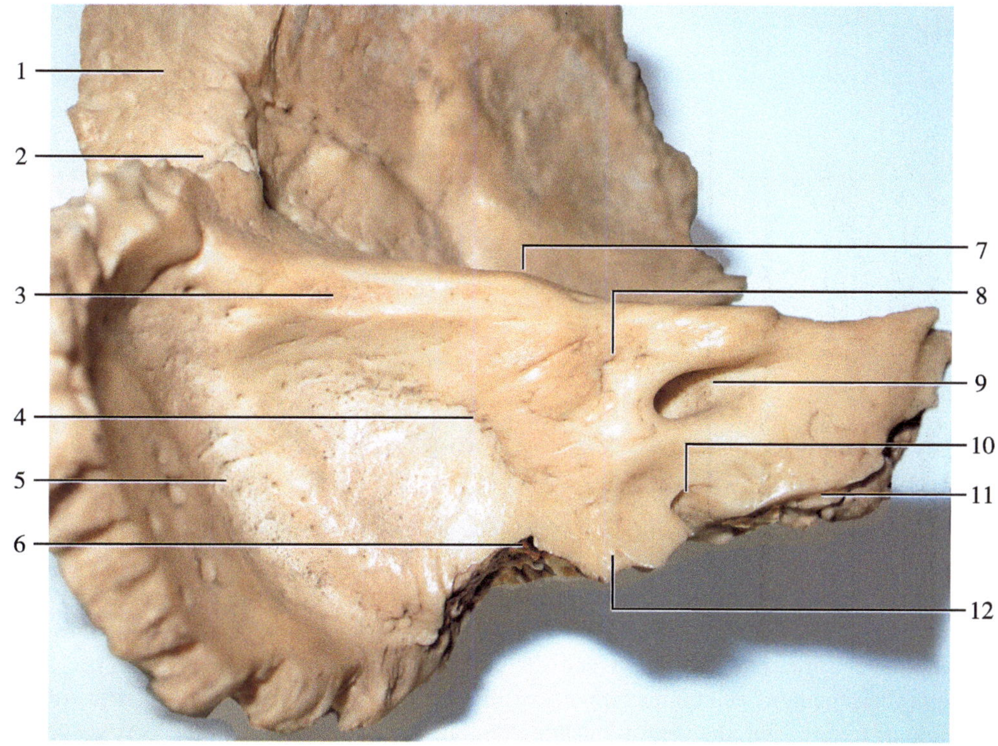

Fig. 1.5 Posterior view of petrous part of temporal bone (left). (1) Squamous portion of temporal bone. (2) Top notch. (3) Superior petrosal groove. (4) Fissure of endolymphatic sac. (5) Sigmoid sulus. (6) Vascular part of jugular foramen. (7) Arcuate eminence. (8) Subarcuate fossa (outer opening of petrolacteal canal). (9) Internal acoustic porus. (10) Nerve part of jugular foramen and external opening of cochlear canaliculus. (11) Inferior petrosal sinus. (12) Jugular interphysis

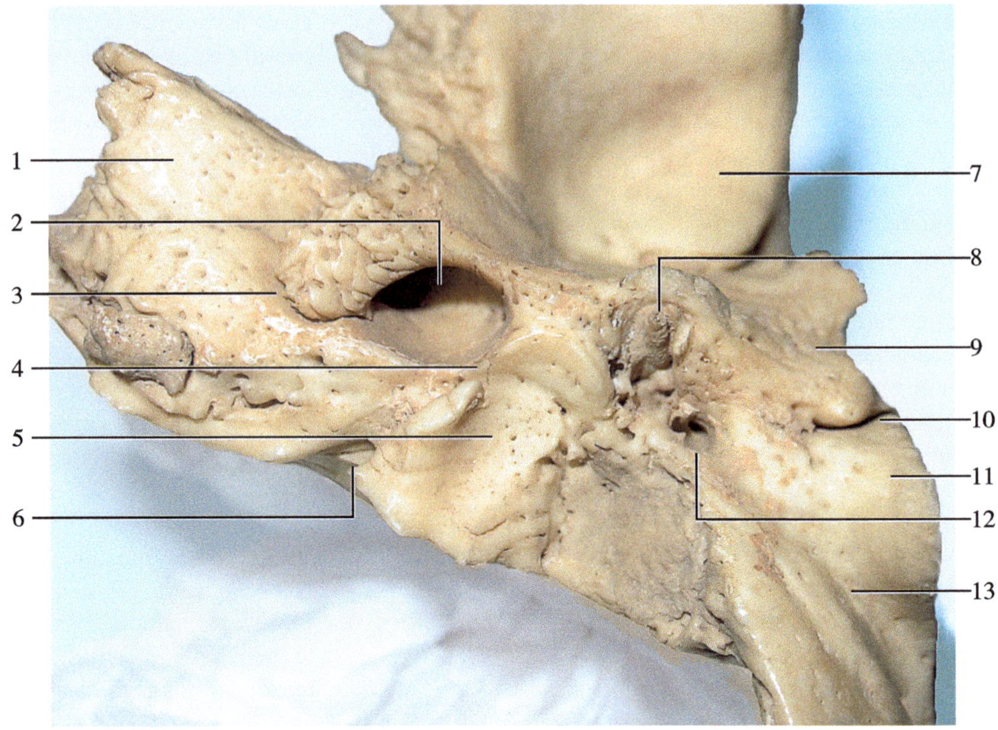

Fig. 1.6 Inferior view of petrous portion of temporal bone (left). (1) Attachment part of levator veli palatine muscle. (2) External orifice of carotid artery canal. (3) Petrotympanic fissure. (4) Arteriovenous ridge. (5) Jugular fossa. (6) Nerve area of jugular foramen (external opening of cochlear canaliculus). (7) Mandibular fossa. (8) Styloid process. (9) Tympanic portion of temporal bone. (10) Tympanomastoid fissure. (11) Mastoid process. (12) Stylomastoid foramen. (13) Digastric groove

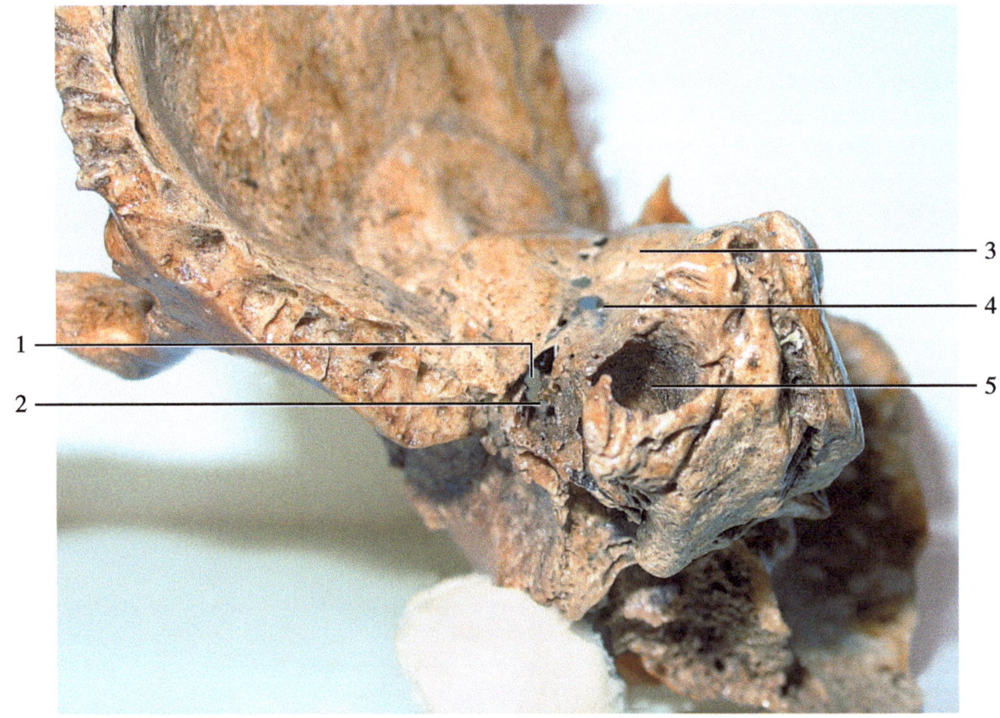

Fig. 1.7 Petrous apex view of petrous portion of temporal bone (right). (1) Semicanal of tensor tympani muscle. (2) Eustachian tube. (3) Arcuate eminence. (4) Hiatus of facial nerve. (5) Internal opening of carotid artery canal

petrosal groove containing the inferior petrosal sinus; its lateral end is located nearby the jugular foramen. The inner part of the front edge of the petrous portion is connected with the great wing of the sphenoid bone to form the petrosphenoidal fissure. The outer part and the corresponding parts of the squamous and tympanic portion form the petrosquamous fissure and the petrotympanic fissure, respectively. Between the petrous portion and the squamous portion, there are two bony canals parallel up and down that enter the tympanic cavity. The upper part is the semicanal of the tensor tympanic muscle, and the lower part is the eustachian tube (Fig. 1.7).

Internal acoustic meatus: Internal acoustic meatus is located in the petrous portion of the temporal bone, it is a bony canal containing the facial nerve, the vestibular nerve, the cochlear nerve, and the labyrinthine artery and vein. The internal acoustic porus in the medial part of the back of the petrous part is oblate, the rear edge is sharp and protruding, and the front edge is flat without obvious edge. The average length of the internal acoustic meatus is about 10 mm, and its lateral end is closed by a vertical osseous plate with a cribriform hole. This plate is the fundus of internal acoustic meatus, which constitutes the majority of the inner wall of the vestibule and the cochlea, and this fundus is divided into two areas with different sizes by a transverse crest (Fig. 1.8). The superior area is small and is divided into two parts by a vertical crest (Bill's bar), which is usually located on the lateral side of the transverse crest; Therefore, the fundus is divided into four quadrants: anterosuperior, posterosuperior, anteroinferior, and posteroinferior quadrant. The anterosuperior quadrant is a small hole, called the facial nerve area, that is, the entrance of the facial nerve canal, which is the narrowest part of the facial nerve bone canal in the temporal bone; From then on, the facial nerve enters the bone canal (fallopian canal) as a labyrinthine segment and reaches the geniculate ganglion forward and outward; the posterosuperior quadrant, called the superior vestibular area, has a larger hole that pass through the upper terminal branch of the vestibular nerve. The anteroinferior quadrant is the cochlear area, a relatively large area compared with the others, numerous small spiralis foraminosus arrange in this quadrant, it is the place where the cochlear nerve fibers pass through. The length of the cochlear nerve canal is about 1–2 mm. It moves forward and outward, as a result, when observing from the internal acoustic porus, the cochlear area cannot be seen completely due to the obstruction of the anterior wall of the internal acoustic meatus. The vestibular end of the basal turn of the cochlea is close to the inferior vestibular area (Fig. 1.9), therefore, the cochlear nerve foramen and the fine holes (cribriform) of the cochlear nerve fibers around the basal turn of the cochlea occupy most of the area below the transverse crest; behind the cochlear quadrant is the inferior vestibular area in posteroinferior quadrant, with several small holes, which are passed by the inferior terminal branch of the vestibular nerve that innervates the saccule. There is a singular foramen in the posterior part of the inferior vestibular quadrant and the posterior inferior wall of the internal acoustic meatus, through which the posterior ampullary nerve (also called the singular foramen nerve) passes, which is the terminal branch of the inferior vestibular nerve. The singular canal is rarely of radiologic interest, though it does serve as a landmark during some procedures (Agirdir et al. 2001). Sometimes a small foramen can be seen at the posterior part of the transverse crest, known as the transverse crest foramen, whose significance is still unclear (Kozerska and Skrzat 2015; Schart-Moren et al. 2018).

The internal acoustic meatus is the thin part of the temporal bone. Transverse fractures of the temporal bone can often penetrate the internal acoustic meatus, causing damage to the inner ear and the facial nerve.

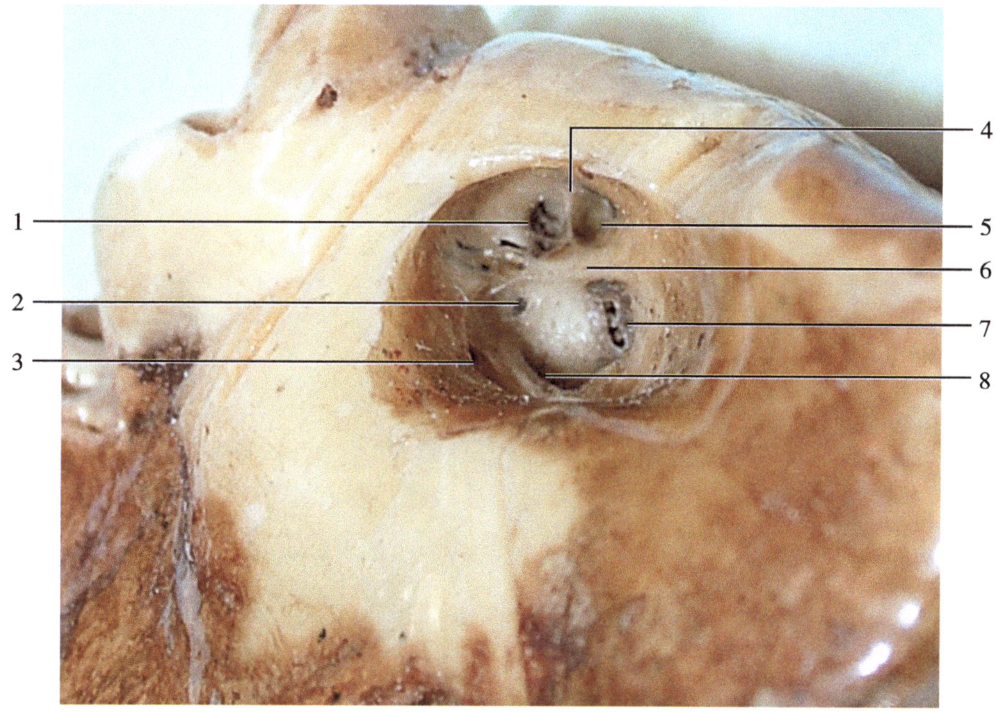

Fig. 1.8 Fundus of internal acoustic meatus (left). (1) Superior vestibular nerve foramen area. (2) Inferior vestibular nerve foramen area. (3) Singular foramen. (4) Bill's crest. (5) Facial nerve foramen area. (6) Transverse crest. (7) Cochlear nerve foramen area. (8) Cochlear nerve fiber (vestibular end) foramen area of base turn of cochlea

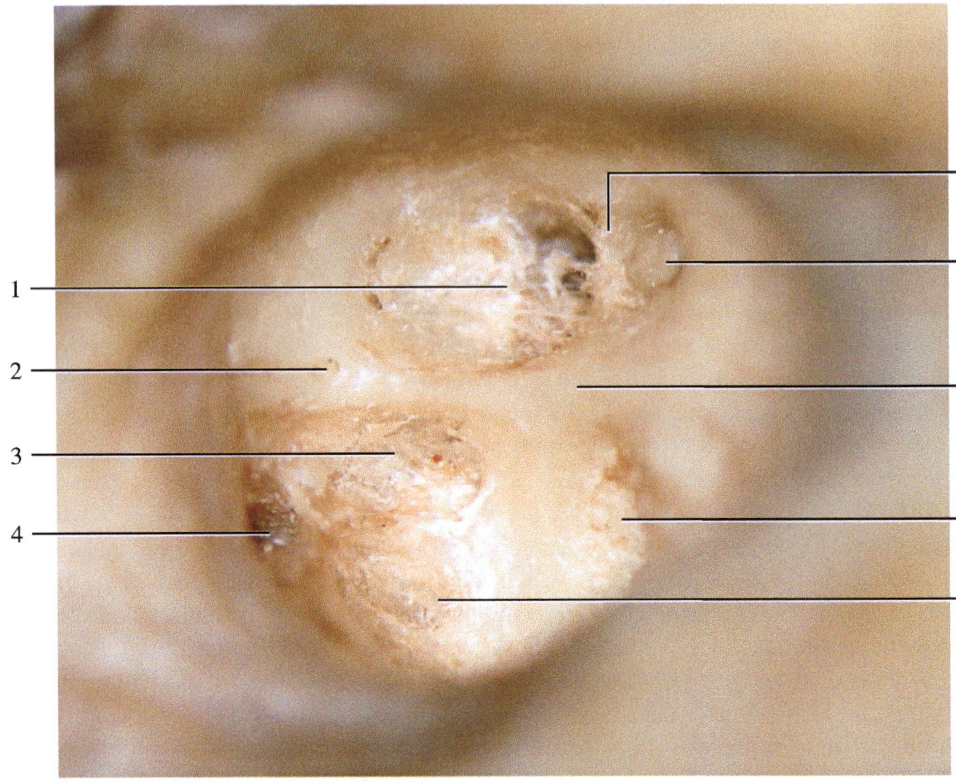

Fig. 1.9 Fundus of internal acoustic meatus (left, attaching soft tissue). (1) Superior vestibular foramen area. (2) Transverse crest foramen. (3) Inferior vestibular foramen area. (4) Singular foramen. (5) Bill's crest. (6) Facial nerve foramen area. (7) Transverse crest. (8) Cochlear nerve foramen area. (9) Cochlear nerve fiber (vestibular end) foramen area of base turn of cochlea

1.1.5 Styloid Process

The styloid process originates from the lower part of the tympanic portion of the temporal bone and extends forward and downward. It is a thin and long bone with average length about 25 mm; The stylopharyngeus, styloglossus, stylohyoideus, et al. attach at the distal end of the styloid process. There is a stylomastoid foramen (Fig. 1.2) between the styloid process and the mastoid process, which is the inferior opening of the facial nerve canal, that is, the cranial exit of the facial nerve.

1.2 Anatomy of External Ear

The external ear includes the auricle and the external auditory canal.

1.2.1 Auricle

The auricle is attached to both sides of the skull with the aid of auricle cartilage, muscles, ligaments, and skin, with an angle of 30–45° to the squamous portion of temporal bone. The auricle is mainly composed of auricle cartilage. The surface is covered with skin. The front skin is directly connected with the perichondrium, there is less subcutaneous connective tissue, which is prone to frostbite, and the subcutaneous hematoma is not easy to absorb during trauma. Auricular trauma or cartilage injury during surgery can cause perichondritis, cartilage necrosis, and easily lead to auricle deformation. The part of the lobule is composed of fat and connective tissue, without cartilage. The outer edge of the auricle is a convoluted ear ring (helix), and the antihelix is located the medial side of the helix and parallels with the helix. The fossa between the helix and the antihelix is called scaphoid fossa or scapha, the upper end of the antihelix is divided into two crura, between the two crura is a triangular fossa, and the front of the antihelix is a deep concave concha, which is the most common site of pseudocyst of the auricle. The concha is divided into the upper cymba concha and the lower cavum concha by the crus of helix (Fig. 1.10). In front of the concha cavity is the external auditory canal opening. The protrusion in front of the external auditory canal is the tragus, which contains cartilage to partially overlap the external auditory canal opening. The depression between the tragus and the crus of the helix is the incisura anterior auris (Figs. 1.11 and 1.12), where there is no cartilage, and the incision here can directly reach the bone of the external auditory canal. Auricular cartilage is continuous with that of external audi-

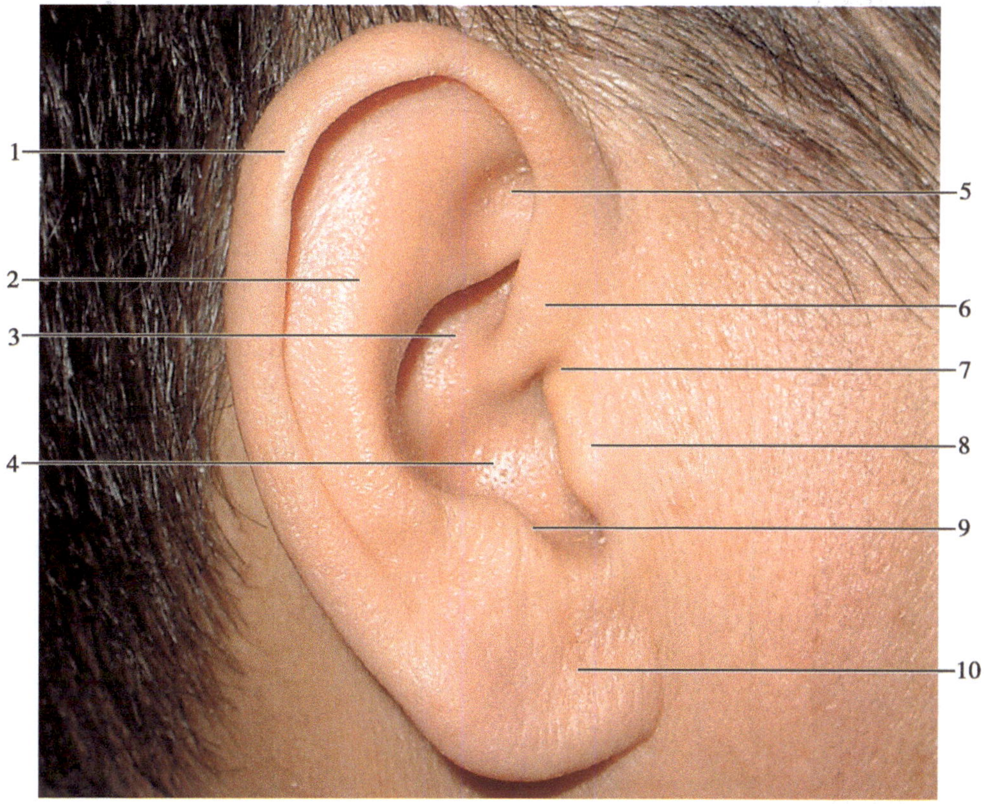

Fig. 1.10 Surface landmark of auricle (right). (1) Helix. (2) Antihelix. (3) Cymba conchae. (4) Cavum conchae. (5) Triangular fossa. (6) Helix crus. (7) Incisura anterior auris. (8) Tragus. (9) Antitragus. (10) Lobule

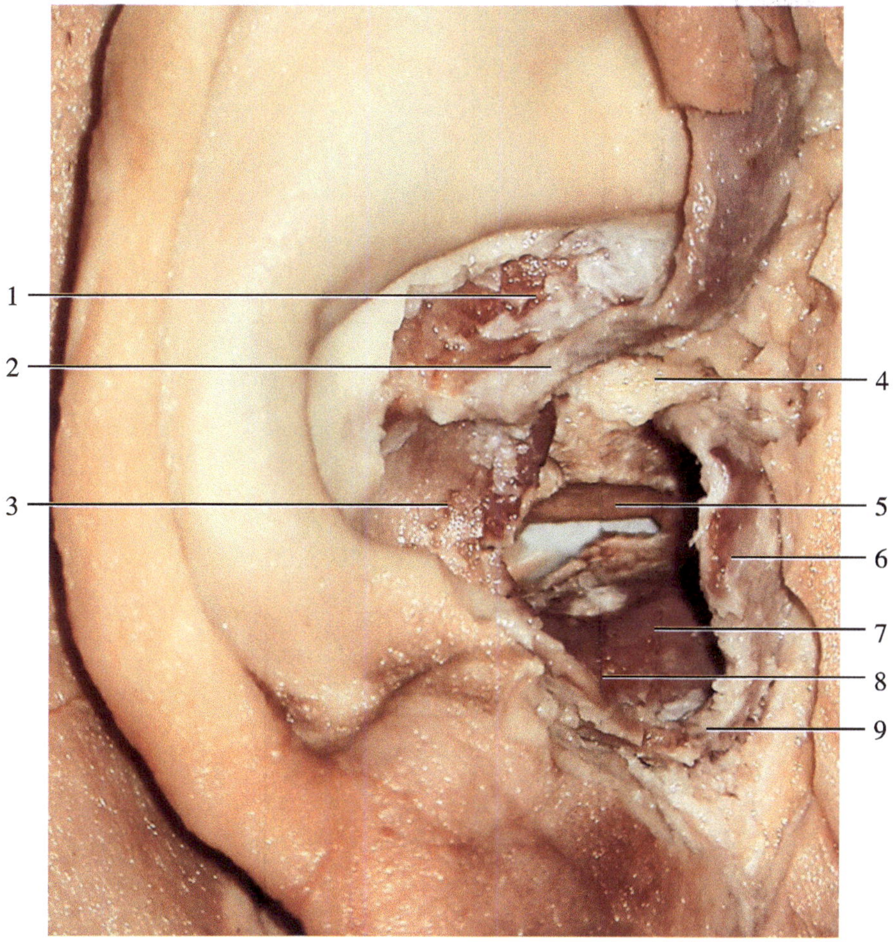

Fig. 1.11 Anatomy of concha and external auditory canal opening (right). (1) Cymba conchae. (2) Helix crus. (3) Cavum conchae. (4) Incisura anterior auris. (5) Skin of external auditory canal. (6) Auricular cartilage. (7) External auditory canal cartilage. (8) Cartilage of antitragus. (9) Intertragic notch

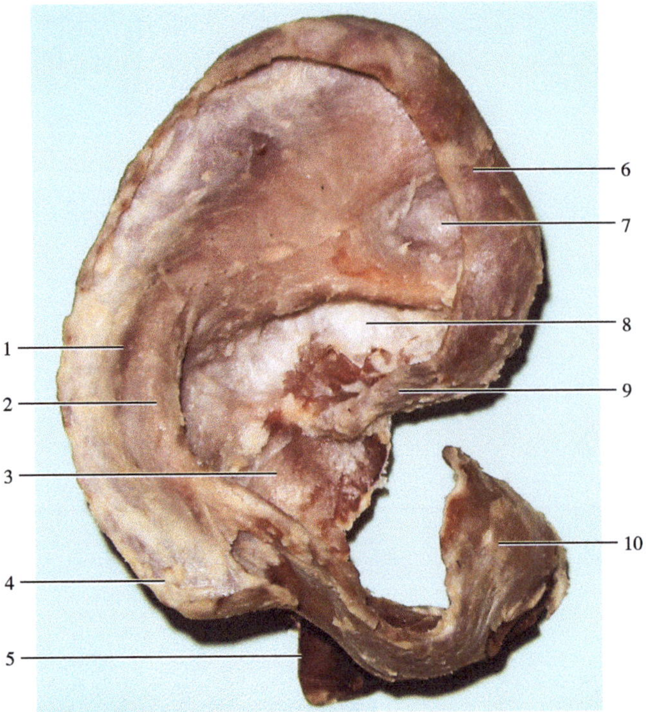

Fig. 1.12 Anterior view of external ear cartilage (right). (1) Scaphoid fossa (2) Antihelix. (3) Concha. (4) Free edge of helix. (5) Posterior wall cartilage of external auditory canal. (6) Helix. (7) Triangular fossa. (8) Cymba conchae. (9) Helix crus. (10) Tragus

tory canal (Figs. 1.12 and 1.13). One site infection can cause the entire external ear cartilage infection.

1.2.2 External Auditory Canal

The external auditory canal starts from the bottom of the concha cavity and reaches the tympanic membrane inwards. It is a slightly S-shaped blind tube with a length of 2.5–3.5 cm, outer 1/3 of the external auditory canal is cartilage and the inner 2/3 is bony (Fig. 1.14). There are two constrictions in external auditory canal, one is the junction of cartilage and bone, the other is about 0.5 cm far away from the tympanic membrane, the latter is called isthmus. The skin of cartilaginous part contains cerumen glands similar to sweat glands, which can secrete cerumen, and is rich in hair follicles and sebaceous glands. It is a common site of furuncle. The bony external auditory canal is composed of the tympanic portion of temporal bone, the lower edge of the squamous portion of the temporal bone and the anterior upper part of the mastoid process. The lower position of the middle cranial fossa is common when the upper wall of the external auditory canal is poorly developed, and the cholesteatoma of the external auditory canal is common in the bony part of this canal.

Fig. 1.13 Posterior view of external ear cartilage (right). (1) Triangular fossa. (2) Concha. (3) Tragus. (4) Inferior wall cartilage of external auditory canal. (5) Posterior wall Cartilage of external auditory canal. (6) Helix

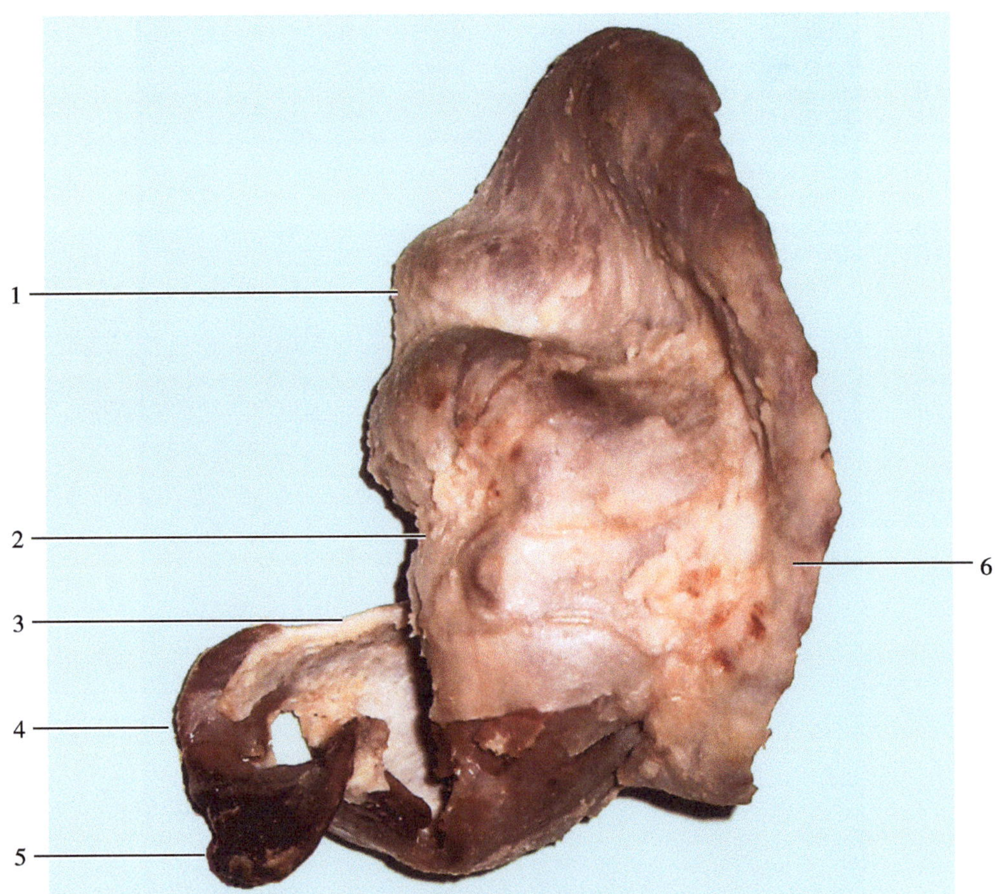

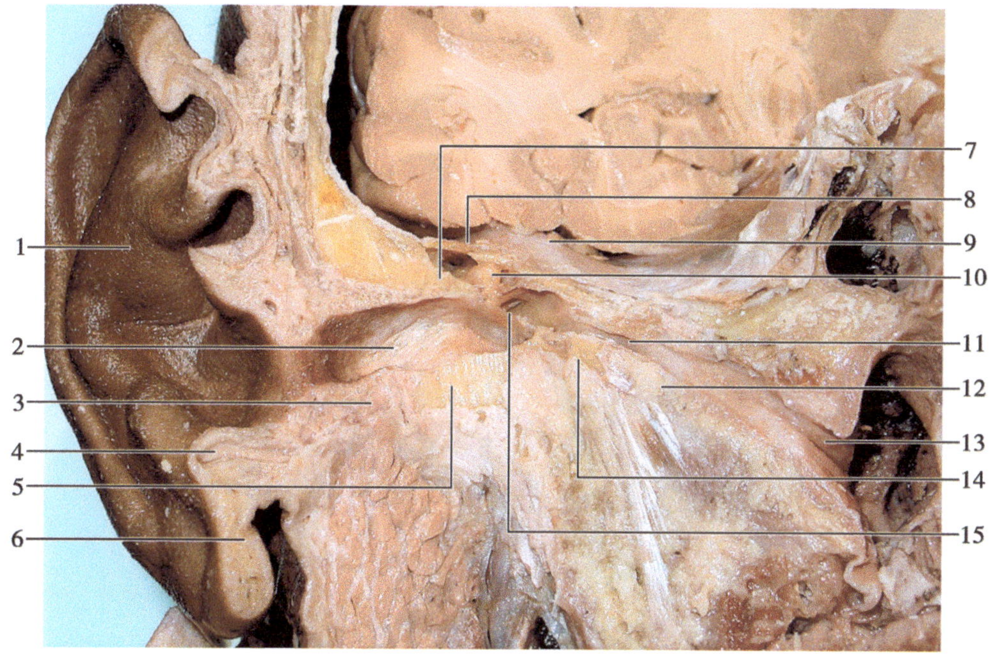

Fig. 1.14 Anatomy of ear in coronal view (right). (1) Auricle. (2) External auditory canal. (3) Cartilaginous part of external auditory canal. (4) Concha cartilage. (5) Bony part of external auditory canal. (6) Lobule. (7) Tympanic scutum. (8) Tegmen tympani. (9) Arcuate eminence. (10) Malleus. (11) Isthmus of eustachian tube. (12) Cartilaginous part of eustachian tube. (13) Pharyngeal orifice of eustachian tube. (14) Bony part of eustachian tube. (15) Tympanic membrane

1.3 Anatomy of Middle Ear

The middle ear consists of four parts: tympanic cavity, eustachian tube, tympanic antrum, and mastoid process (Figs. 1.14 and 1.15).

1.3.1 Tympanic Cavity

The tympanic cavity (or tympanum) is an **air-containing** space lined with the mucosa, most of which is located between the tympanic membrane and the lateral wall of the inner ear. It is connected with the downward and medial nasopharynx through the eustachian tube anteriorly (Fig. 1.14), and the tympanic cavity is also connected with the tympanic antrum and the mastoid cavity through the entrance of the tympanic antrum (aditus ad antrum) (Fig. 1.15). The tympanic cavity can be divided into three parts according to the upper and lower margins of the pars tensa of the tympanic membrane: (1) The epitympanum, or the attic, is the tympanic cavity located above the level of the upper margin of the pars tensa; (2) The mesotympanum is located between the upper and lower edge level of pars tensa, that means the tympanic cavity is located between the pars tensa of tympanic membrane and the inner wall of the tympanic cavity; (3) Hypotympanum, a small part of the middle ear, lies below the level of the lower margin of the pars tensa of the tympanic membrane, reaches the tympanic floor. The upper and lower length of the tympanic cavity is about 15 mm, and the anterior and posterior length is about 13 mm; The inner and outer length is about 6 mm in the epitympanum and about 4 mm in the hypotympanum. The distance between the mesotympanum and the promontory is the shortest, only about 2 mm. There are ossicles, nerves, muscles and ligaments in the tympanic cavity.

1.3.1.1 Six Walls of Tympanic Cavity

The tympanic cavity is like a roughly oblong space with six walls: lateral, medial, anterior, posterior, top, and bottom wall.

Lateral wall is composed of bone and membrane. The bony part is small, which is the lateral wall of the attic above the tympanic membrane, also known as the tympanic scutum (Fig. 1.14). The bony part is composed of the squamous portion of the temporal bone and the medial part of the tympanic portion. The obtuse or disappearance of the tympanic scutum is one of the characteristic changes of the epitympanic cholesteatoma on the CT image of the temporal bone. The membrane part is large, that is tympanic membrane. The tympanic membrane is between the tympanic cavity and the external auditory canal, which is an inward concave, elliptical, and translucent membrane (Fig. 1.16); the tympanic membrane is about 9 mm high, 8 mm wide, and 0.1 mm thick. The front and lower part of the tympanic membrane inclines inward and forms an angle of 45–50° with the bottom of the external auditory canal. Therefore, the anterior inferior wall of the external auditory canal is longer than the posterior-superior wall. The edge of the tympanic membrane is slightly thick, most of them are embedded in the tympanic sulcus by fibrocartilage annulus, which is the pars tensa. At the tympanic notch where the upper tympanic sulcus is absent, the tympanic membrane is directly attached to the temporal bone, which is relatively loose, and is called the pars flaccida. The main signs of the tympanic membrane are the short process

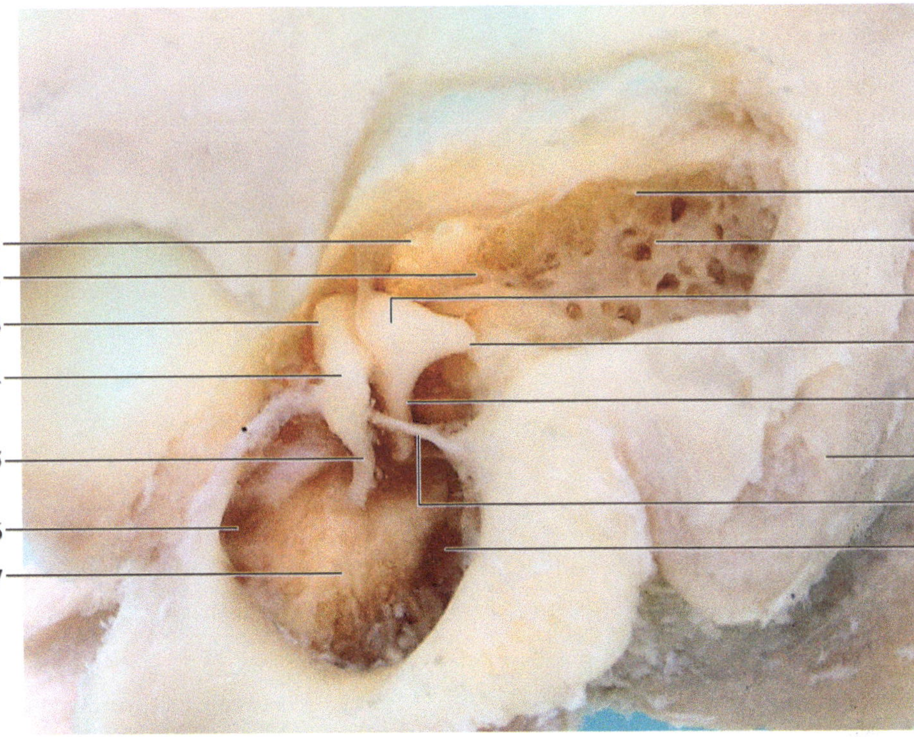

Fig. 1.15 Eustachian tube, tympanic cavity, tympanic antrum and mastoid process (left). (1) Tegmen tympani. (2) Aditus ad antrum. (3) Head of malleus. (4) Neck of malleus. (5) Manubrium. (6) Tympanic orifice of eustachian tube. (7) Promontory. (8) Tegmen tympanic sinus. (9) Tympanic antrum. (10) Body of incus. (11) Short crus of incus. (12) Long crus of incus. (13) Mastoid process. (14) Chorda tympani. (15) Cochlear window niche

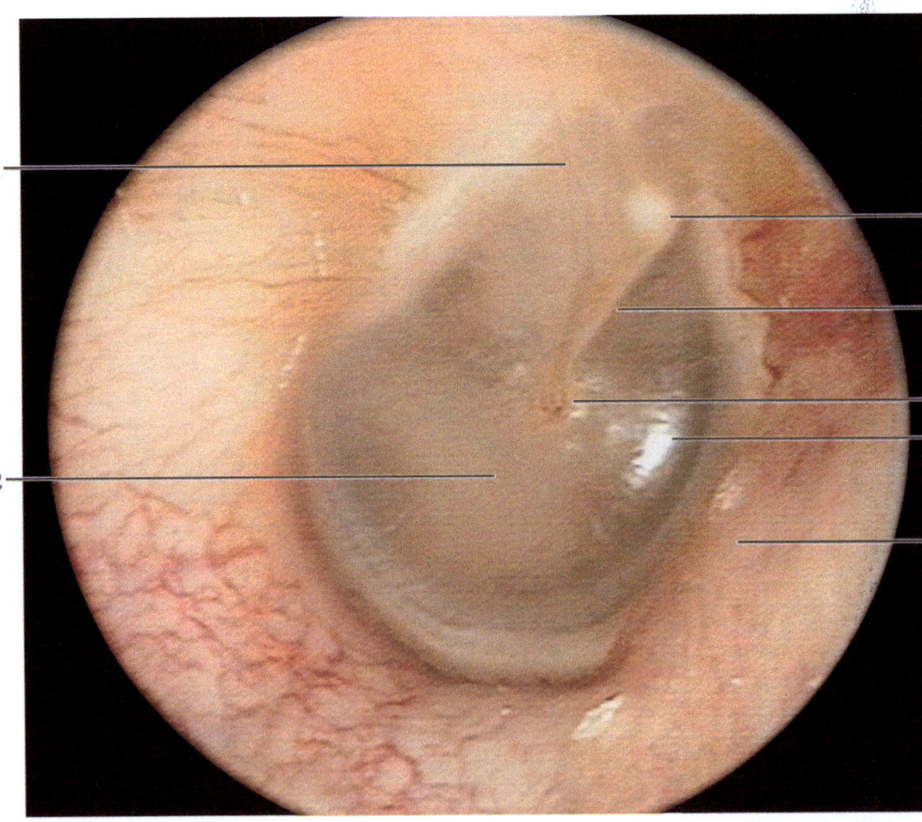

Fig. 1.16 Surface landmark of tympanic membrane (right). (1) Pars flaccida. (2) Pars tensa. (3) Short process of malleus. (4) Manubrium. (5) Umbo. (6) Cone of light. (7) Anterior inferior wall of external auditory canal

of the malleus located at the upper front, the light cone is located at the anteroinferior part of the tympanic membrane and the malleus handle is located between the two. The structure of the tympanic membrane can be divided into three layers: the outer layer is the epithelial layer, which is a stratified squamous epithelium continuous with the skin of the external auditory canal; The middle is the fibrous layer, which contains the shallow radial fibers and the deep annular fibers. The malleus handle is attached to the middle of the fibrous layer, and the pars flaccida does not have this layer; The inner layer is mucosa, which is continuous with the tympanic mucosa.

Medial wall is the lateral wall of the inner ear, which has multiple prominences and pits. The larger domelike prominence in the center of the inner wall is the promontory, which is the basal turn of the cochlea. Vestibular window, located in the small niche (vestibular window niche) at the posterosuperior part of the promontory, with an area of about 3.2 mm^2, is fitted by the footplate of stapes and the surrounding annular ligaments, and leads inward to the vestibule of the inner ear. Cochlear window niche is located in the small niche behind the promontory, which is closed by the cochlear window membrane, with an area of about 2 mm^2, and passes through the scala tympani of the cochlea inwards. The horizontal (tympanic) segment of the facial nerve canal is located above the vestibular window. The lateral semicircular canal is located at the posterosuperior part of the facial nerve canal and the medial-inferior wall of the aditus ad antrum, where labyrinthine fistula often occurs. The processus cochleariformis is located slightly anterosuperior aspect of the vestibular window and is formed by the outward bending of the semicanal of the tensor tympani; The tendon of the tensor tympani muscle protrudes from the processus cochleariformis and ends outward at the medial side of the neck of the malleus (Fig. 1.17).

Anterior wall The medial-inferior part of the anterior wall is separated from the internal carotid artery by a very thin bone plate; There are two openings in the upper part of the anterior wall: the upper is the opening of the semicanal of the tensor tympani muscle, which contains the tensor tympani muscle and the lower is the tympanic opening of the Eustachian tube (Fig. 1.18).

Posterior wall is wide above and narrow below, and the vertical (mastoid) segment of facial nerve passes through the medial side of this wall. There is a small hole in the upper part of the posterior wall, called aditus ad antrum, through which the tympanic antrum communicates with the epitympanum (Fig. 1.15). At the bottom of the aditus ad antrum and on the outside of the junction of the horizontal and vertical segments of the facial nerve canal (also known as the second genu of the facial nerve), there is a small fossa containing the short crus of the incus, called the incudal fossa, which is important landmarks of the facial nerve and the lateral semicircular canal during the middle ear surgery. In the medial-inferior aspect of the posterior wall, which is equal to the height of the vestibular window, there is a small eminence, called pyramidal eminence, which is located in the inner front of the vertical segment of the facial nerve (Yu et al. 2021). There is a small canal (containing the stapedius muscle branch of the facial nerve) inside, and the tendon of stapedius muscle is emitted from the pyramidal eminence and attaches to the back of the stapes neck. The chorda tympani nerve is a branch of facial nerve within the temporal bone, which is equivalent to the pyramidal eminence, passes anterosuperiorly in the posterior canaliculus and enters the middle ear (McManus et al. 2012).

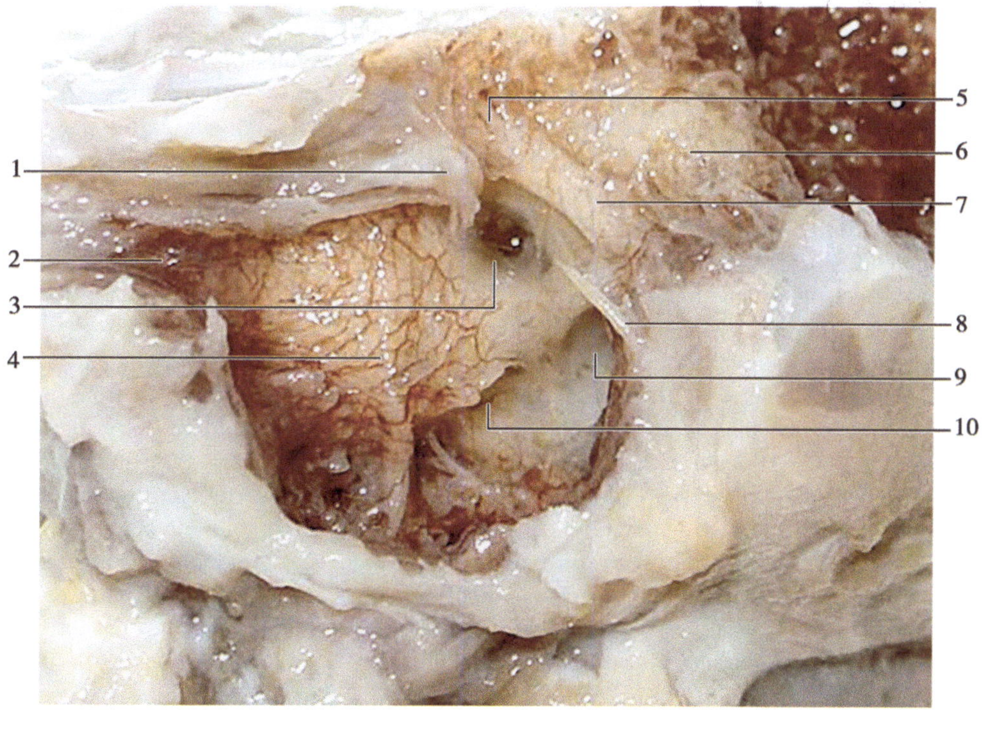

Fig. 1.17 Lateral wall of tympanic cavity (left). (1) Tensor tympani. (2) Eustachian tube. (3) Vestibular window. (4) Jacobson's nerve on promontory. (5) Geniculate ganglion. (6) Lateral semicircular canal. (7) Horizontal segment of facial nerve. (8) Chorda tympanic nerve. (9) Tympanic antrum. (10) Cochlear window niche

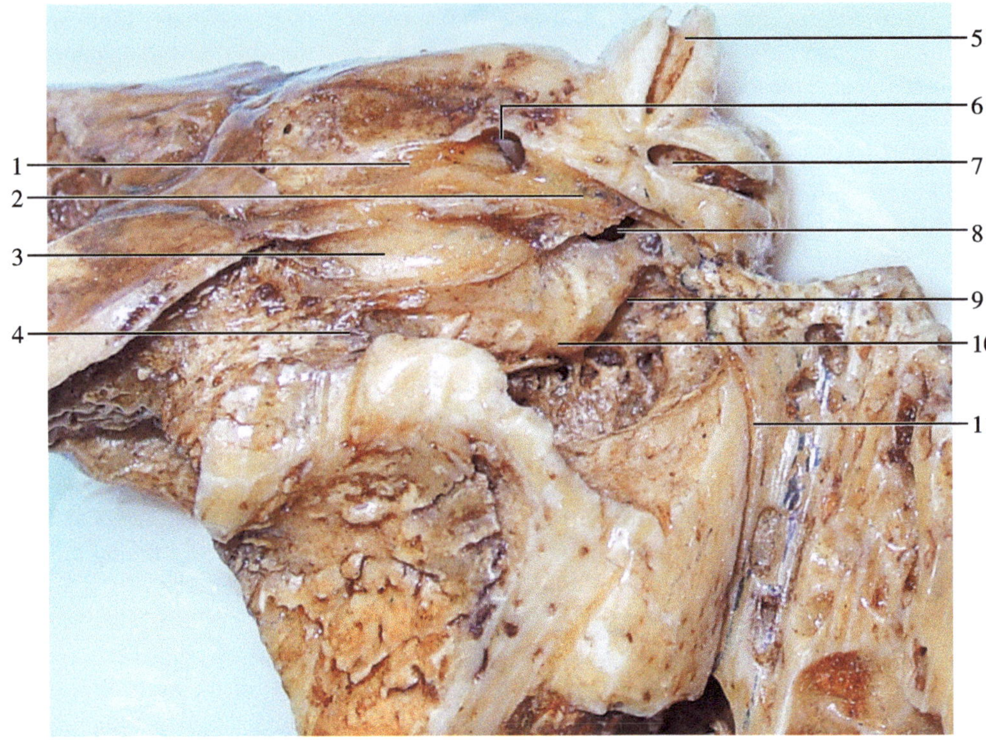

Fig. 1.18 Bony structure of medial wall of tympanic cavity (left). (1) Hiatus of facial nerve canal. (2) Bony canal of facial nerve. (3) Semicanal of tensor tympani muscle. (4) Eustachian tube. (5). Anterior semicircular canal. (6) Geniculate ganglion. (7) Lateral semicircular canal. (8) Vestibular window. (9) Cochlear window niche. (10) Promontory. (11) Nerve canal of chorda tympani

In the temporal bone, there are two muscles located in the bone canal, one is stapedius muscle and another is tensor tympani muscle.

The retro-tympanum is located behind the posterior margin of the tympanic membrane, with tympanic sinus and facial recess. Tympanic sinus referred to the space between vestibular window, cochlear window, and posterior wall of tympanum (Figs. 1.17 and 1.19), is located in the inferior part of the retro-tympanum and the medial-inferior part of the pyramidal eminence, its posterior side is adjacent to the vertical segment of the facial nerve, and the lateral side is bounded by the pyramidal eminence and the stapedius tendon. The shape and size of the tympanic sinus vary with the degree of pneumatization of the temporal bone and is often the place where the concealed condition is located. CT scan of the temporal bone has a certain suggestive effect on the judgment of its pre-operative status. Facial recess: the outer edge is the posterolateral wall of the retro-tympanum and chorda tympani nerve, the inner edge is the vertical segment of the facial nerve, and the upper edge is the incudal fossa (Fig. 1.20). From the transverse view of the retro-tympanum, the tympanic sinus is located at the medial side of the pyramidal eminence, and the facial nerve recess is located at the lateral side of the pyramidal eminence. The exploration of the retro-tympanum through the incision of the facial recess, the pyramidal eminence, the suprastapedial structure, the vestibular window, the cochlear window, the long crus of the incus, and the stapes can be observed.

Prussak space also called the superior recess of the tympanic membrane is located between the pars flaccida of the tympanic membrane and the neck of the malleus. The upper boundary is the lateral ligament of the malleus, and the lower boundary is the short process of the malleus. This space may play a role in the formation of attic cholesteatoma.

Anterior recess of epitympanum: that is, the anterior recess of the malleus head. A vertical bone plate originated from the tegmen tympani (anterior plate of the epitympanum) in front of the malleus head is also known as the cog ridge. In front of this plate, a larger cavity can be formed, also known as the anterior recess of the epitympanum or supratubal (eustachian tube) recess. The cog ridge is located at the upper part of the processus cochleariforms. After removing this ridge, the supratubal recess can connect the epitympanum. The geniculate ganglion of the facial nerve is located in the front of the bone plate and the inner side of the supratubal recess.

Superior wall, also known as the tegmen tympani, is composed of the front of the petrous portion of the temporal bone, and the posterior part of the wall is connected with the tegmen of tympanic antrum (Figs. 1.14 and 1.15). The tympanic cavity is separated from the temporal lobe of the brain in the middle cranial fossa by this wall. The petrosquamous fissure on this wall is not closed at the time of the baby. The small blood vessels of the dural meninges are connected with the tympanic cavity through this fissure, which can become one of the ways for otitis media infection to enter the intracranial.

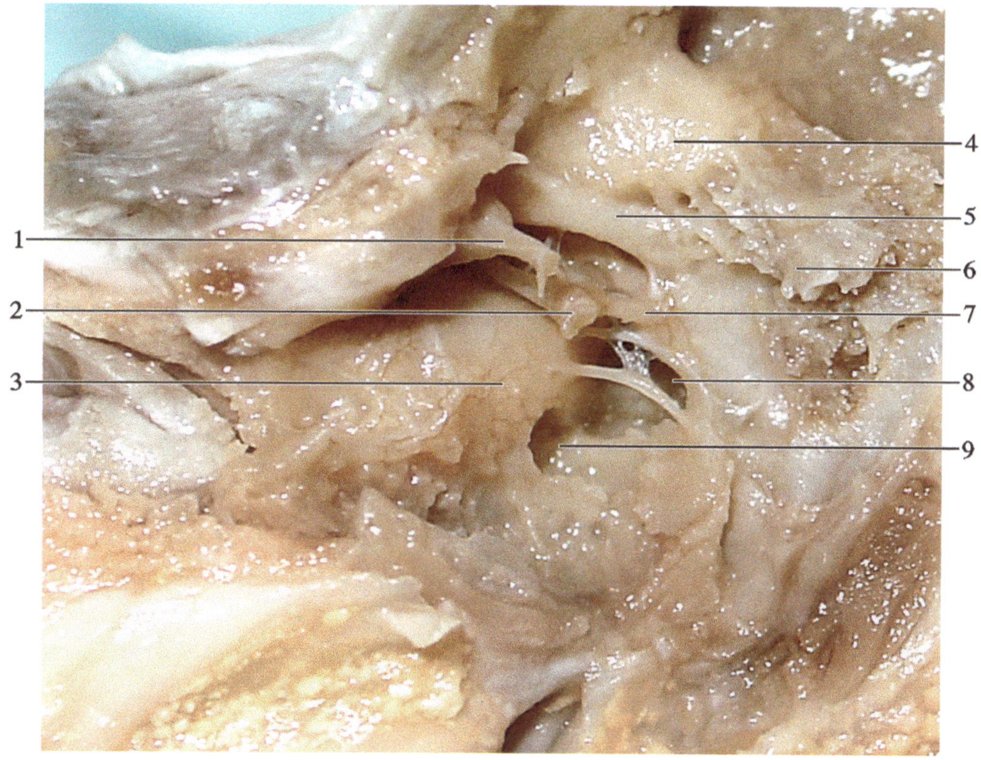

Fig. 1.19 Anatomy of retro-tympanic cavity (left). (1) Tensor tympani. (2) Stapes. (3) Promontory. (4) Lateral semicircular canal. (5) Horizontal segment of facial nerve. (6) Facial recess. (7) Pyramidal eminence and stapedial muscle. (8) Tympanic sinus. (9) Cochlear window niche

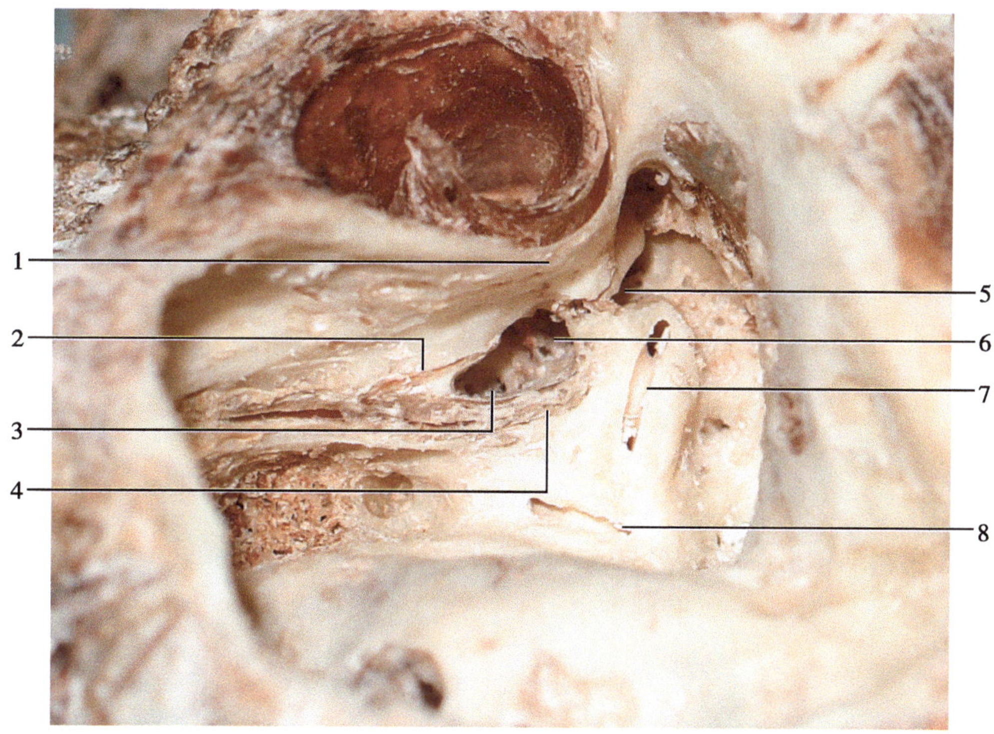

Fig. 1.20 Facial recess (left). (1) Posterior wall of external auditory canal. (2) Chorda tympani. (3) Cochlear window niche. (4) Facial nerve. (5) Short crus of incus. (6) Stapes. (7) Lateral semicircular canal (opened). (8) Posterior semicircular canal (opened)

Inferior wall is a bone plate narrower than the superior wall. Sometimes, if the bony floor of the hypotympanum is dehiscent, the dome of the Glomus jugular may protrude upward into the posteroinferior part of tympanic cavity and be seen through the tympanic membrane, which is called higher position of glomus jugular, this condition can be found on the right side more frequently. Attention should be paid when operating in the post-hypotympanum. The posterior wall of the carotid artery composes the anteromedial inferior wall of hypotympanum.

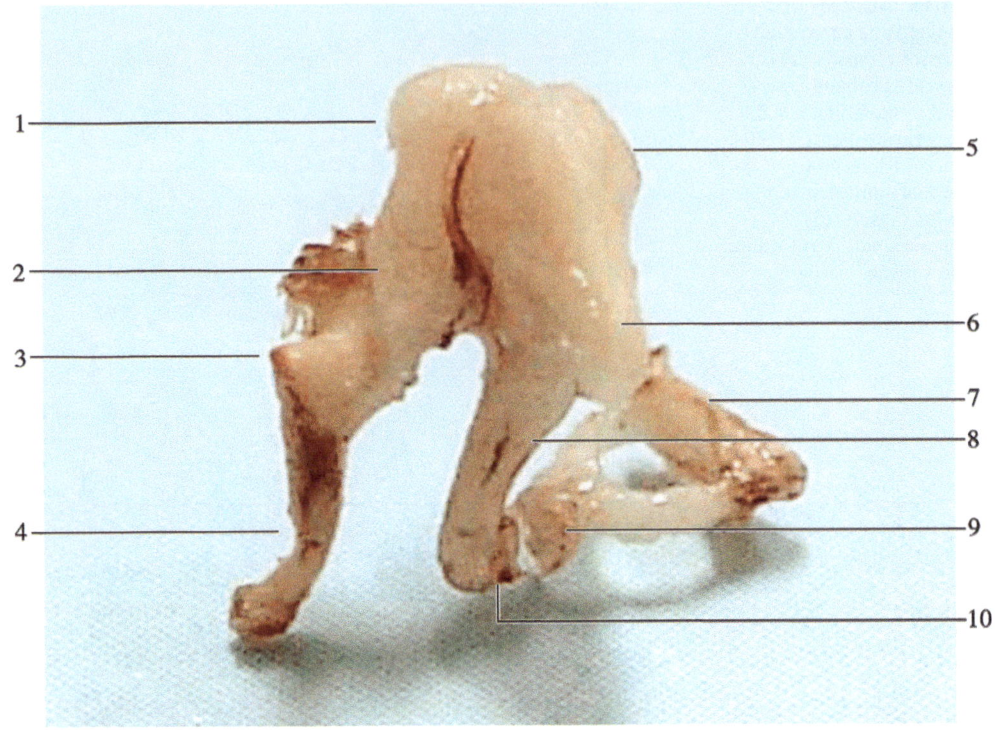

Fig. 1.21 Ossicular chain (left). (1) Head of malleus. (2) Neck of malleus. (3) Short process of malleus. (4) Manubrium. (5) Body of incus. (6) Short crus of incus. (7) Footplate of stapes. (8) Long crus of incus. (9) Head of staple. (10) Lenticular process

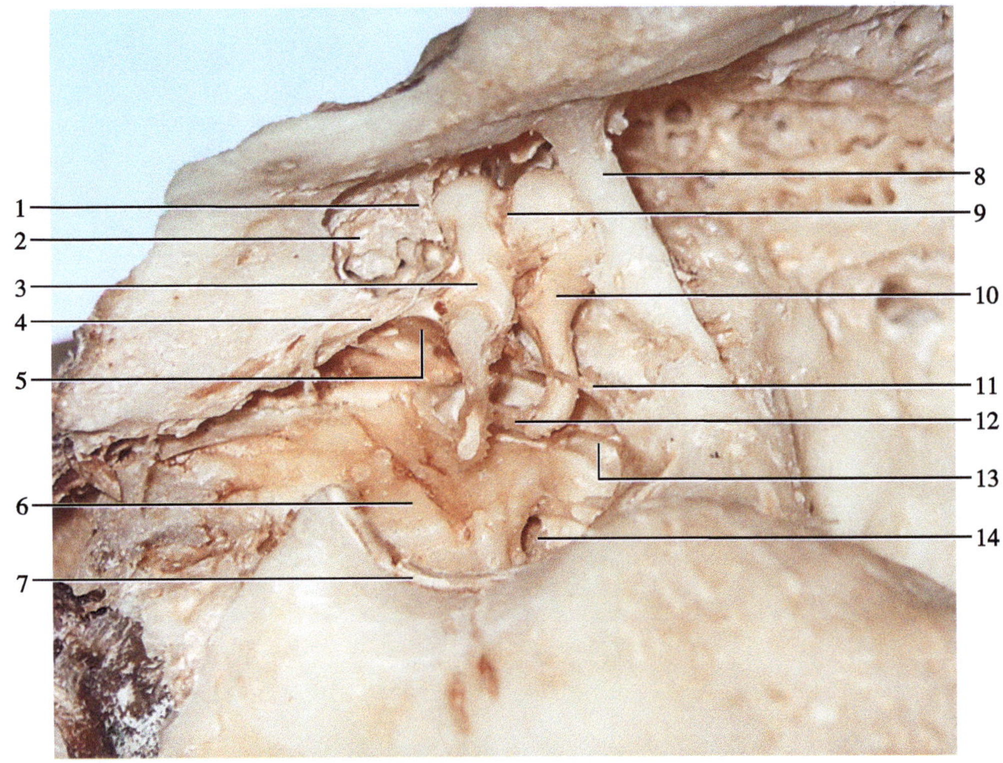

Fig. 1.22 Contents of tympanic cavity (left). (1) Cog's ridge. (2) Anterior recess of epitympanum. (3) Malleus. (4) Tensor tympani muscle. (5) Tympanic diaphragm. (6) Promontory. (7) Fibrous annulus of tympanic membrane. (8) Lateral wall of aditus ad antrum. (9) Incudomalleolar articulation. (10) Incus. (11) Chorda tympani nerve. (12) Stapes. (13) Stapes tendon. (14) Cochlear window niche

1.3.1.2 Contents of Tympanic Cavity

Auditory ossicles are the smallest group of isolated bones in the human body, which consists of the malleus, incus, and stapes to form an ossicular chain (Figs. 1.21, 1.22, 1.23, and 1.24). These delicate bones are entirely covered with the middle ear mucosa. They are connected the tympanic membrane with the vestibular window, represent the normal pathway of sound transmission across the tympanic cavity.

The malleus has a small head, neck, short process (lateral process), long process (anterior process), and handle (manu-

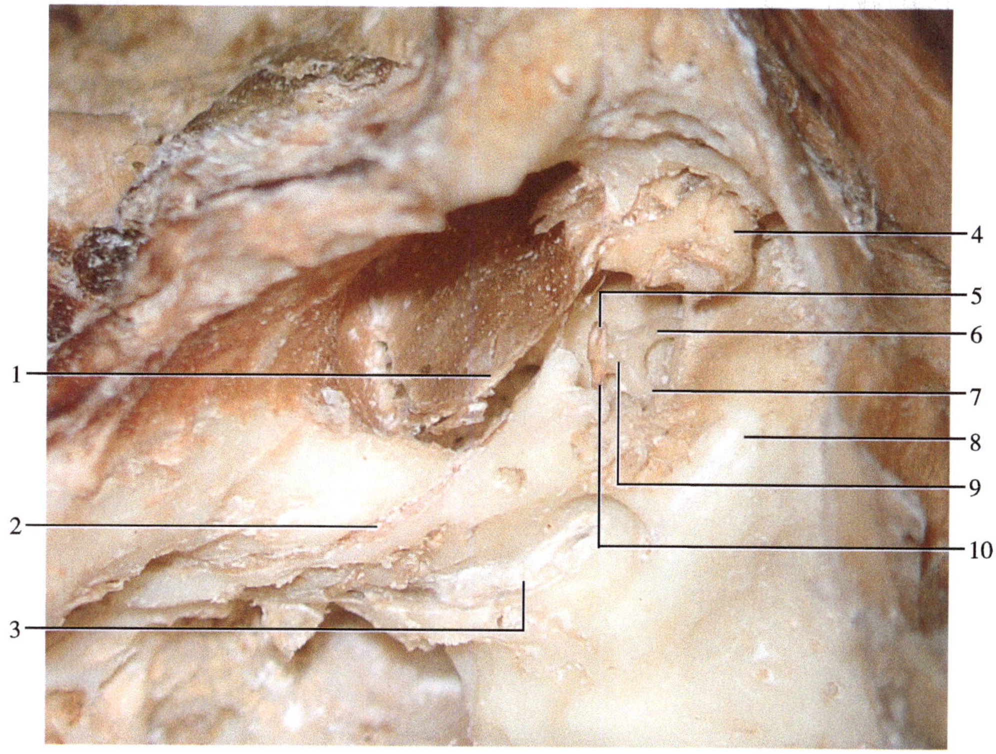

Fig. 1.23 View of malleus and Stapes after incus removal (left). (1) Tympanic membrane. (2) Chorda tympani nerve. (3) Second genu of facial nerve. (4) Head of malleus. (5) Head of stapes. (6) Anterior crus of stapes. (7) Inferior crus of stapes. (8) Lateral semicircular canal. (9) Neck of stapes. (10) Stapedial muscle

brium). The malleus handle and the short process are embedded between the mucous membrane layer and the fibrous layer of the tympanic membrane. The head and neck extend above the upper margin of the tympanic membrane into the epitympanum. There is a concave surface in the back of the small head of the malleus, which forms a joint with the incus body; the incus is divided into body, long crus and short crus. The incus body is located at the rear of the epitympanum, and its anterior and medial side slightly is connected with the small head of the malleus to form the incudomalleolar articulation. The short crus is located in the incudial fossa at the bottom of the aditus ad antrum, and the long crus is located behind the handle of the malleus, and the end is slightly enlarged to the medial side, called lenticular process, which forms the incudostapedial articulation with the small head of the stapes; the stapes is divided into small head, neck, anterior crus, posterior crus, and footplate. Head, neck, and crura—form the "superstructure" of the stapes (Benson and Lane 2022). The oval footplate closes the vestibular window. An annular ligament is connected with the vestibular window and the footplate. The small head is connected with the lenticular process of the long crus of the incus, and the neck is very short (Figs. 1.21 and 1.24).

Ossicular ligament is composed of supramalleal ligament, anterior malleus ligament, lateral malleus ligament, superior incus ligament, posterior incus ligament and stapes annular ligament. The ossicular is fixed in the tympanic cavity by those ligaments (Figs. 1.25 and 1.26).

Tympanic diaphragm: The transition between the meso- and epitympanum is divided by the facial nerve canal, the long crus of incus, the stapes head, the pyramid eminence, the stapes tendon, and the mucosal fold covering them, which is called tympanic diaphragm. There is a small hole in the front and back of the tympanic diaphragm to connect the meso- and epitympanum, which are, respectively, called the anterior and posterior tympanic isthmus, which also are the checkpoints for ventilation or drainage of the tympanic cavity (Fig. 1.22).

Tympanic muscle: (1) *The tensor tympani muscle* starts from the cartilage of the eustachian tube, the greater wing of the sphenoid bone and the wall of the tensor tympani muscle canal (Figs. 1.17 and 1.19), and its tendon bypasses the processus cochleariformis backward and terminates at the neck of the malleus at a right angle outward, and is driven by a small branch of the mandibular branch of the trigeminal nerve. When the muscle contracts, it pulls the manubrium inward to increase the tension of the tympanic membrane, so as to prevent the tympanic membrane from being broken or hurting the inner ear; (2) *The stapedius muscle*, which is the smallest muscle in human body, starts from the pyramidal eminence of the posterior wall of the tympanum and ends at the back of the neck of the stapes (Figs. 1.23 and 1.25). Its movement is controlled by the stapedius muscle branch of the facial nerve; When this muscle contracts, it can pull the small head of the stapes backward, so that the rear edge of the stapes footplate is the fulcrum, and the front edge rises outward to reduce the pressure of the inner ear.

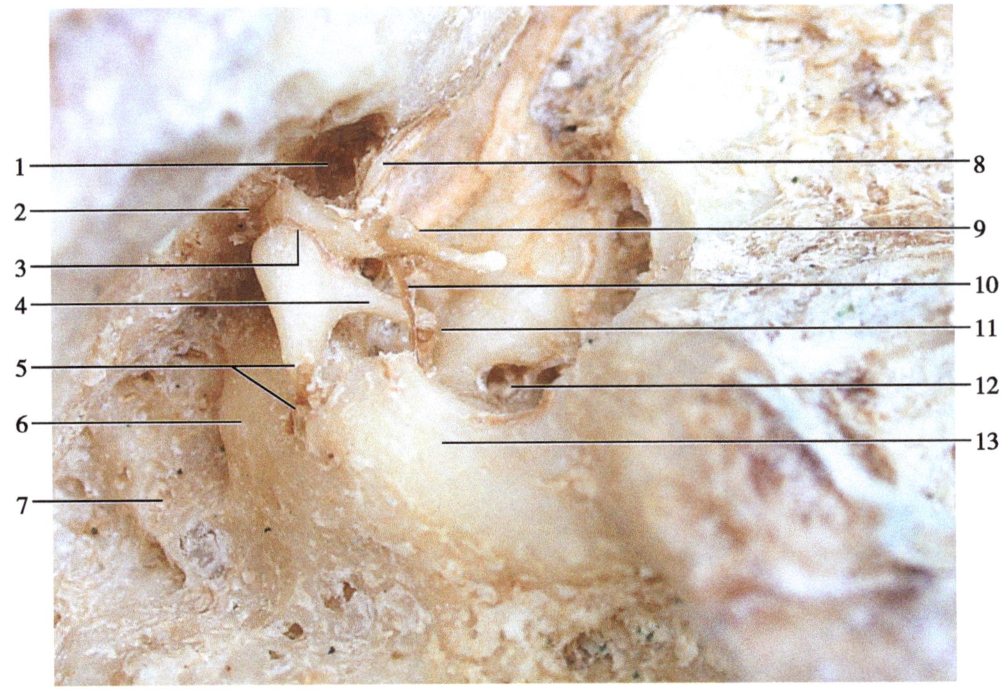

Fig. 1.24 Mastoid cavity view of tympanic contents (right). (1) Anterior recess of epitympanum. (2) Malleus and supramalleal ligament. (3) Incudomalleolar articulation. (4) Long crus of incus. (5) Short crus of incus and its ligaments. (6) Lateral semicircular canal. (7) Tympanic antrum. (8) Anterior ligament of the malleus. (9) Short process of malleus. (10) Chorda tympani. (11) Incudostapedial articulation. (12) Cochlear window niche. (13) Facial nerve ridge (the lateral bone wall of vertical segment of facial nerve)

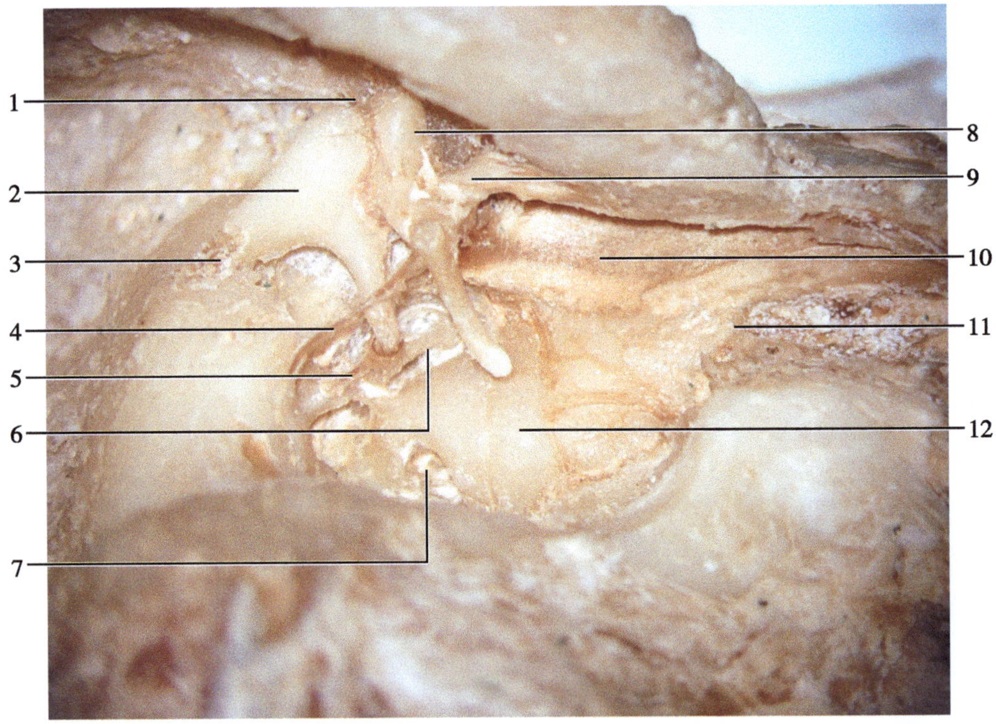

Fig. 1.25 External auditory canal view of tympanic contents (right). (1) Supramalleal ligament. (2) Incus. (3) Incudal fossa (ligament). (4) Chorda tympani nerve. (5) Stapedial muscle. (6) Stapes. (7) Cochlear window niche. (8) Tegmen tympani. (9) Anterior ligament of malleus. (10) Tensor tympani muscle. (11) Eustachian tube. (12) Promontory

Chorda tympani nerve is separated from the vertical segment of the facial nerve, and enters the tympanic cavity inwards and forwards in the small foramen (iter chordae posterius), at the level of the pyramid eminence, and adjacent to the inner side of the tympanic membrane. It passes through the tympanic cavity between the neck of the malleus and the long crus of the incus, and enter the petrotympanic fissure (iter chordae anterius) forward and downward (Figs. 1.15, 1.18, 1.22 and 1.24), and finally joins with the lingual nerve to sense the taste of the front 2/3 part of the tongue and allocate the sublingual and submaxillary salivary gland.

Jacobson's nerve is the eponym given to the tympanic branch of the glossopharyngeal nerve which is the first branch of the glossopharyngeal nerve and arises from the inferior ganglion of cranial nerve IX just below the jugular foramen outlet. First, this nerve enters the temporal bone via

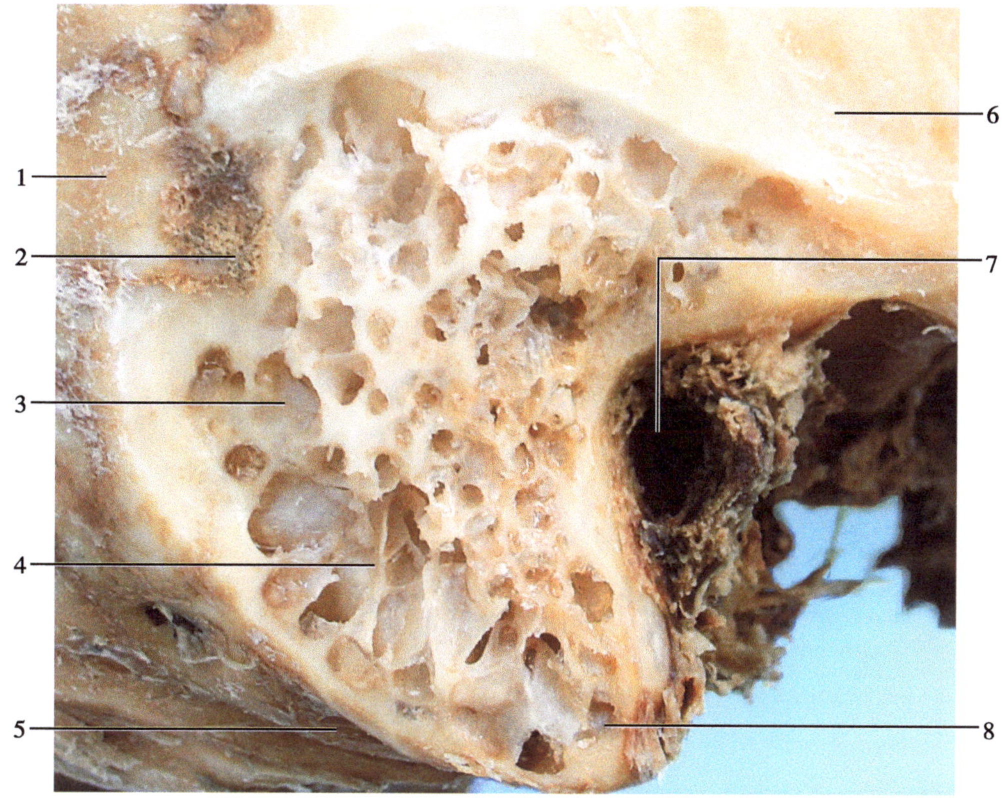

Fig. 1.26 Pneumatic type of mastoid process (right). (1) Parietal bone. (2) Top notch. (3) Mastoid air cells. (4) Air cell septum. (5) Digastric groove. (6) Squamous portion of temporal bone. (7) External auditory canal. (8) Mastoid tip

tympanic canaliculus at the bottom of tympanic cavity (also known as Jacobson's canal), then, this nerve splays over the promontory as tympanic plexus, is usually located in submucosal grooves (Fig. 1.17) on the bone. Last, the parasympathetic fibers of the nerve exit tympanic cavity as a contributor to the lesser petrosal nerve. Clinically, Jacobson's nerve is best known for its association with paragangliomas, which are benign but locally destructive tumors.

1.3.2 Eustachian Tube

The eustachian tube, commonly known as the pharyngotympanic tube, is the tube connecting the tympanic cavity and the nasopharynx (Fig. 1.14). The bony eustachian tube consists of the semicanal of the tensor tympanic muscle and the semicanal of the eustachian tube (Figs. 1.7, 1.17 and 1.18). The tympanic orifice at the outer end of the tube is located at the lower part of the upper half of the anterior wall of the tympanic cavity (Fig. 1.17); The pharyngeal orifice at the medial end is located at the lateral wall of the nasopharynx and at the posterior and lower part of the posterior end of the inferior turbinate. The eustachian tube is inward, forward, and downward to the nasopharynx, so the eustachian tube forms an angle of about 40° with the horizontal plane and 45° with the sagittal plane. The adult has a total length of about 35 mm, and the outer 1/3 is the bone part, which is located at the junction of the tympanic portion and the petrous portion of the temporal bone, and at the anterolateral side of the internal carotid artery canal. Only a thin bone plate is separated from the tensor tympani muscle above, and the inferior wall is thick, often with pneumatization; The inner 2/3 is composed of cartilage and fibrous membrane. The widest inner diameter is the tympanic orifice, which is narrower inwards. The junction between bone part and cartilage part is the narrowest, called isthmus (Fig. 1.14), with an inner diameter of about 1–2 mm; The cartilage part is gradually widened from the isthmus to the nasopharynx. The mucosa of the cartilage part is like a fold and has the function of valve. The eustachian tube, which is normally passively closed, has the function of preventing the pharyngeal fluid from entering the tympanic cavity. The tensor veli palati, levator veli palati, and pharyngeal muscle of eustachian tube originate from the cartilage and connective tissue membrane (the first two end at the soft palate, and the latter ends at the posterior wall of the pharynx), when opening, swallowing, and yawning, the pharyngeal orifice of eustachian tube can be opened with the help of the contraction of the above three muscles to regulate the pressure of the tympanic cavity, so as to maintain the balance between the internal and external pressure of the tympanic membrane.

1.3.3 Tympanic Antrum

The tympanic antrum is the air-containing cavity at the posterosuperior part of the tympanic cavity. The tympanic antrum is connected with the epitympanum through the aditus ad antrum forward, and the mastoid air cell is connected with the lower part of tympanic antrum backward; The upper part is separated from the middle cranial fossa by the tegmen tympani antrum. The horizontal (lateral) semicircular canal convexities and facial nerve canal (see Fig. 1.17) locate at the front and lower part of the inner wall of the aditus ad antrum. The posterior wall is separated from the posterior cranial fossa by the mastoid air cell and the bone plate of the sigmoid sinus. The outer wall is the cribriform area of the mastoid cortex.

1.3.4 Mastoid Process

The mastoid process can be divided into four types according to the degree of air cell development: (1) Pneumatic type (Fig. 1.26): the mastoid process is completely pneumatized, the air cell is large and the bone wall of the interval is thin, accounting for about 80%. (2) Diploic type: the mastoid process is poorly pneumatized, and the air cell is small and numerous, which is shaped like the skull. (3) Sclerotic type (Fig. 1.27): the mastoid process is not pneumatized and the bone is dense. (4) Mixed type: both or all of the above three types exist at the same time (Fig. 1.28).

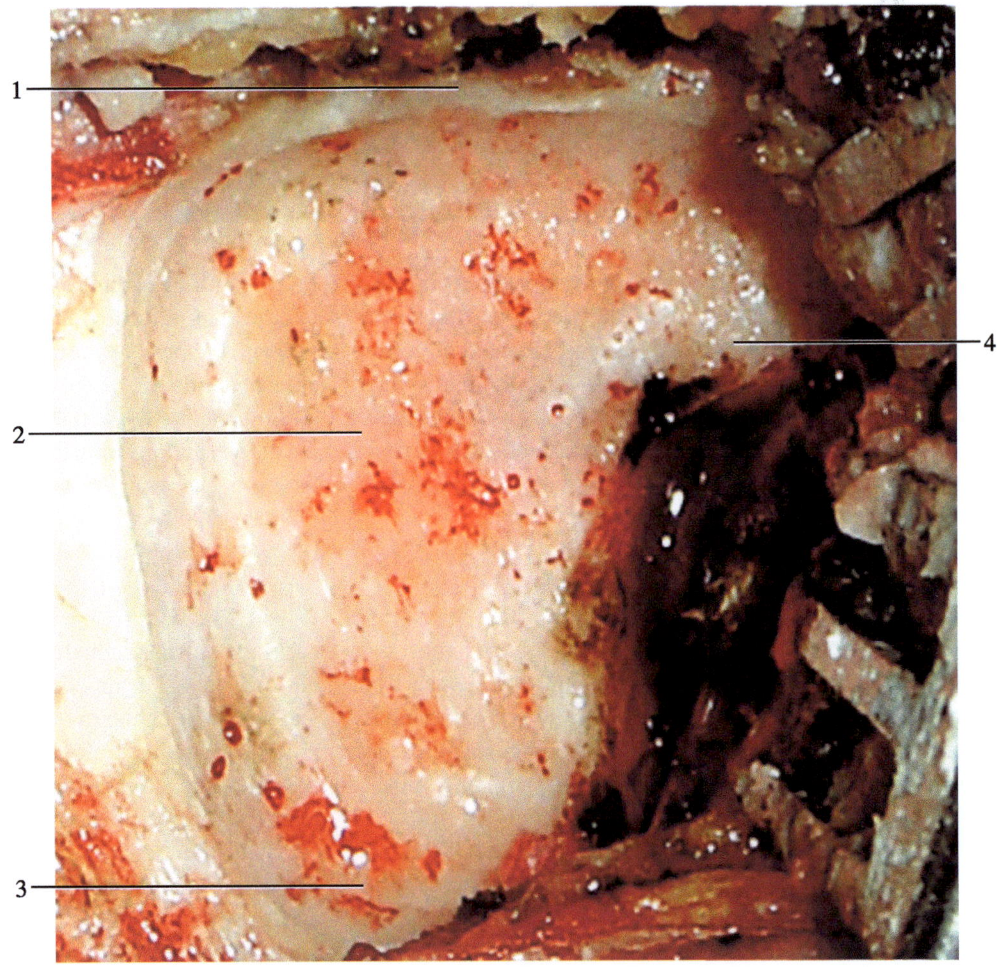

Fig. 1.27 Sclerotic type of mastoid process (right). (1) Temporal line. (2) Sclerotic mastoid. (3) Mastoid tip. (4) Superior wall of external auditory canal

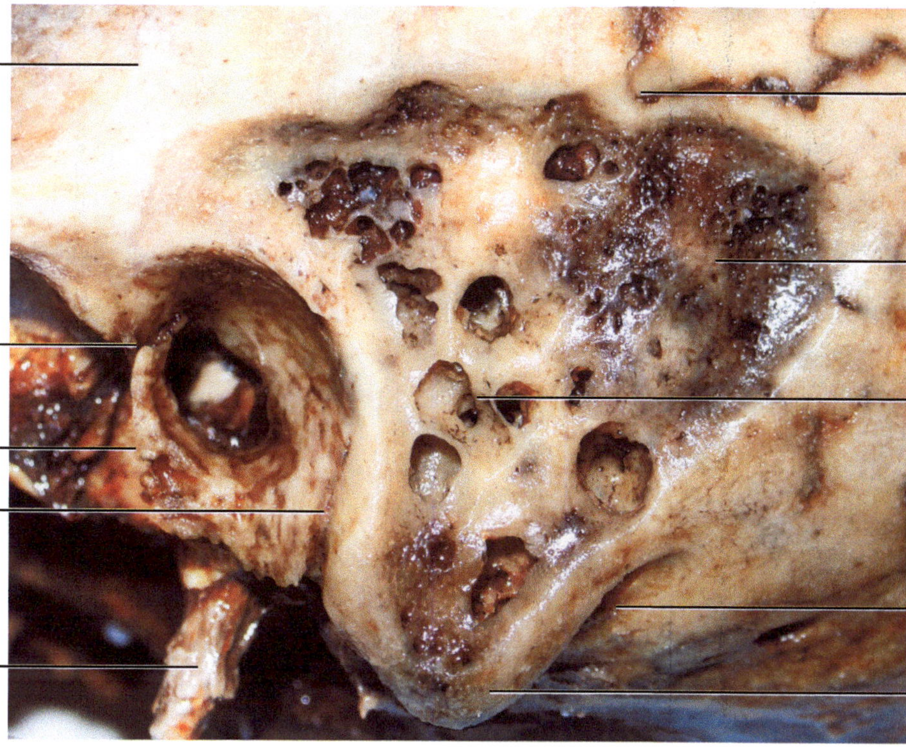

Fig. 1.28 Mixed type of mastoid process (left). (1) Squamous portion of temporal bone. (2) Tympanosquamous fissure. (3) Tympanic portion of temporal bone. (3) Tympanomastoid fissure. (5) Styloid process. (6) Top notch. (7) Diploid bone. (8) Mastoid air cells. (9) Digastric groove. (10) Mastoid tip

1.4 Anatomy of Inner Ear

The inner ear, also known as the labyrinth, is the location of the auditory and balance sensory receptors, located in the petrous part of the temporal bone. The anterolateral part of the inner ear is the middle ear cavity, the anteromedial part is the internal carotid artery, the posteromedial part is the posterior cranial fossa (cerebellopontine angle area), and the posterolateral part is the tympanic antrum and mastoid cavity (Fig. 1.29). The inner ear is divided into osseous labyrinth (also known as the otic capsule) (Benson and Lane 2022) and membranous labyrinth, which are similar in shape. The membranous labyrinth is fixed in the osseous labyrinth by means of fiber bundles. The membranous labyrinth contains endolymph. The perilymph is located between the membranous labyrinth and the osseous labyrinth. The membranous labyrinth is a continuous closed system, but perilymphatic fluid surrounding the membranous labyrinth is continuous with the subarachnoid space through the cochlear canaliculus, which provides direct exchange of fluid with the spinal fluid. Only the osseous labyrinth is described in this book.

The osseous labyrinth is composed of the most compact bone in the body, which can be divided into vestibule, semicircular canal, and cochlea (Fig. 1.30).

1.4.1 Vestibule

The vestibule is located between the cochlea and the semicircular canal, is slightly elliptical (Fig. 1.31), slightly narrow at the anteroinferior part. An oval small hole on the lateral surface of the vestibule leads into the scala vestibuli of the cochlea; The posterosuperior part of the vestibule is slightly wider and connects with five openings of three semicircular canals.

The outer wall of the vestibule is a part of the medial wall of the tympanum, which has a vestibular window and is closed by the footplate of the stapes; The medial wall is a part of the fundus of the internal acoustic meatus, and the labyrinthine segment of the facial nerve passes through the bone of the upper wall; the lower wall is bone wall. The inner surface of the vestibule is relatively complex. There is an oblique bone ridge that bends from top to bottom, called the vestibule crest. The front of the crest is a spherical recess, containing the saccule. There are several small holes in the wall of the recess, called the middle cribriform spot (saccule cribriform area); Behind the crest is the elliptical recess, which contains the utricle. There are several small holes in the wall of this recess and the anterior upper end of the vestibular crest, called the upper cribriform spot (the ampullary

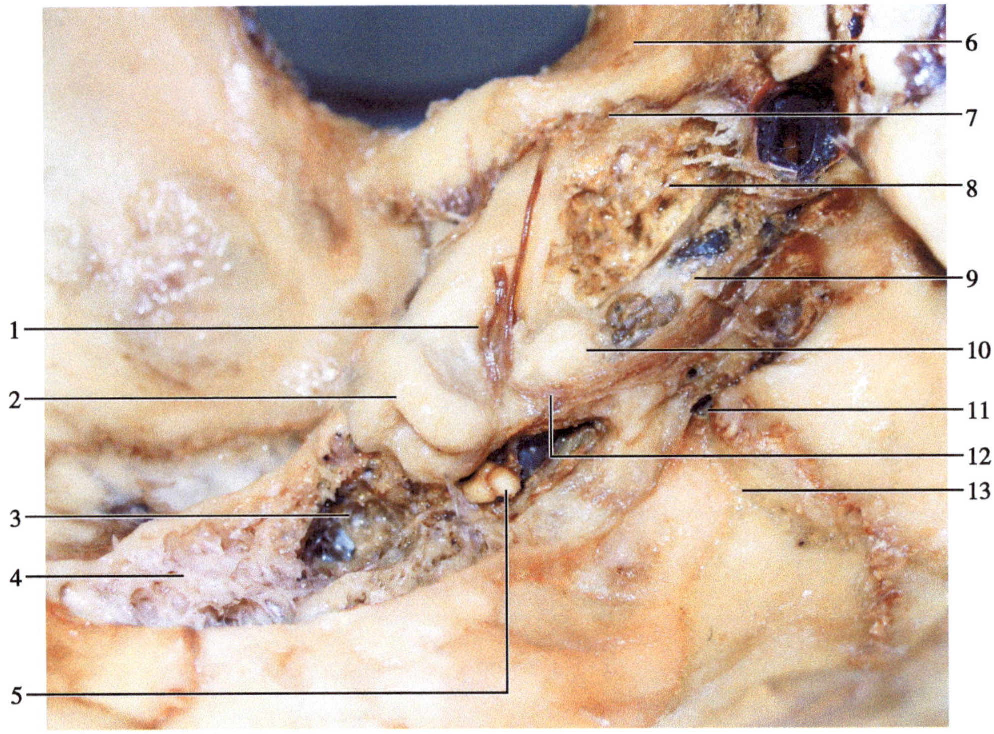

Fig. 1.29 Inner ear and adjacent structures (right). (1) Vestibulocochlear nerve in internal acoustic meatus. (2) Semicircular canal. (3) Tympanic antrum. (4) Mastoid cells. (5) Ossicle. (6) Clivus. (7) Petrooccipital fissure (inferior petrosal sinus). (8) Petrous apex cells. (9) Carotid artery canal. (10) Cochlea. (11) Spinous foramen. (12) Geniculate ganglion. (13) Groove of middle meningeal artery

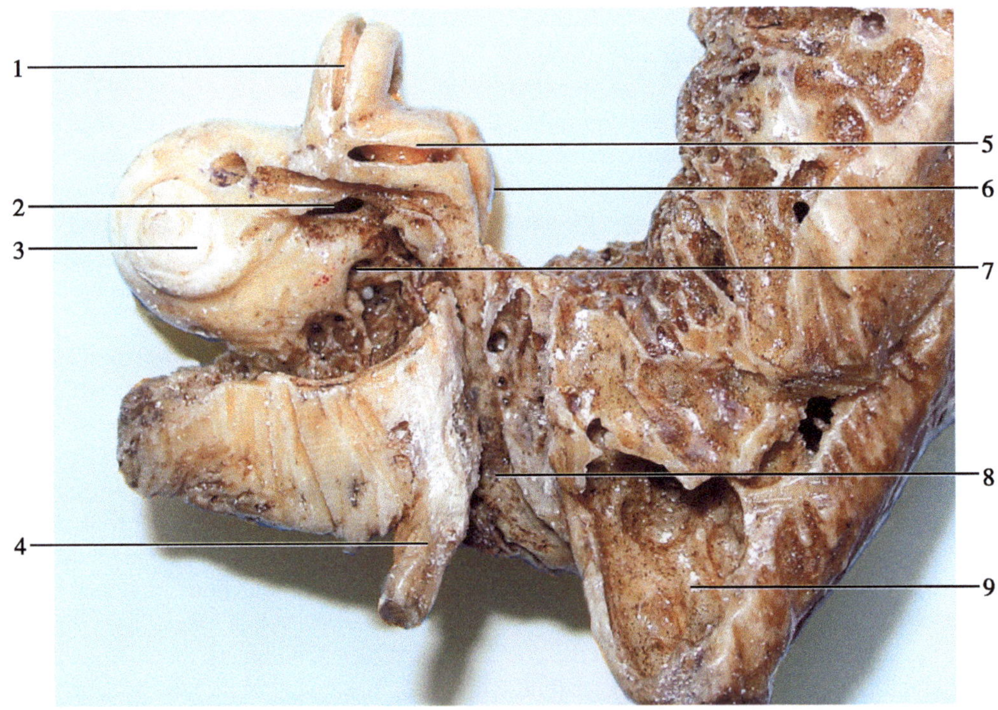

Fig. 1.30 Osseous labyrinth (left). (1) Anterior semicircular canal. (2) Vestibule. (3) Cochlea. (4) Styloid process. (5) Lateral semicircular canal. (6) Posterior semicircular canal. (7) Cochlear window niche. (8) Stylomastoid foramen. (9) Mastoid cells

cribriform area of the utricle sac). There is a vestibular aqueduct (containing endolymphatic duct) at the front and lower part of the utricle recess (Fig. 1.31); the vestibular aqueduct walks backward and outward at the medial side of the common crus of the semicircular canal, and its outer opening is located at the fissure of the endolymphatic sac behind the petrous part of the temporal bone (Fig. 1.32). Enlargement of vestibular aqueduct is one of the most common malformations of the inner ear. On temporal bone CT, the inner diameter of the middle segment of vestibular aqueduct is larger than 1.5 mm. The posteroinferior end of the vestibular crest is bifurcated, with cochlear recess, the area between this crest and the ampulla of the posterior semicircular canal calls the inferior cribriform spot (ampullary cribriform area).

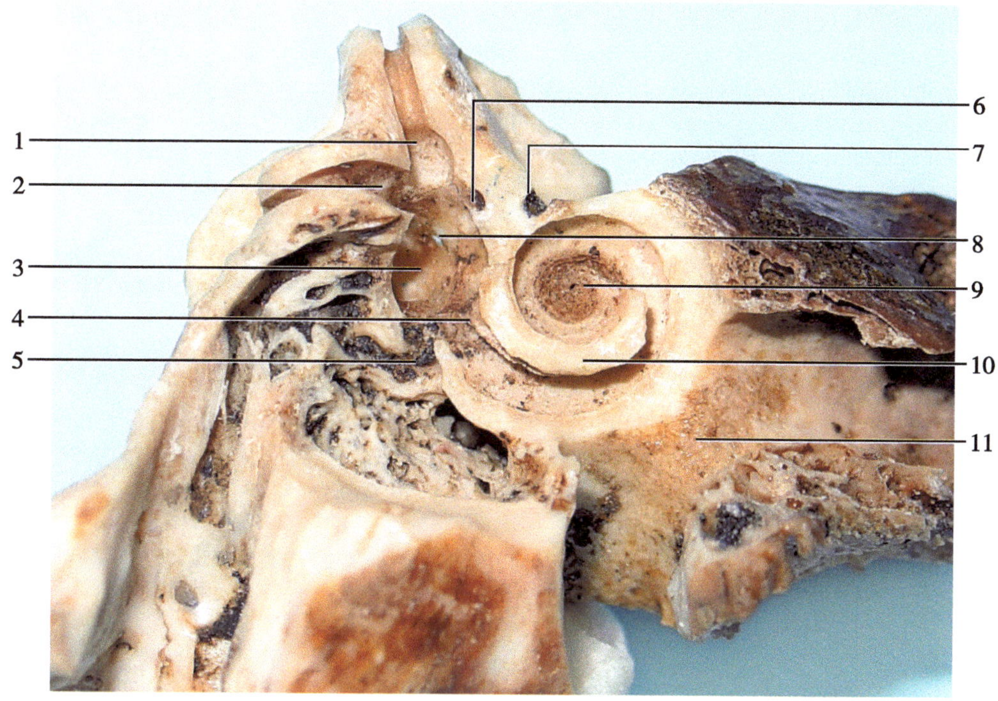

Fig. 1.31 Profile of osseous labyrinth (right). (1) Ampulla of anterior semicircular canal. (2) Ampulla of lateral semicircular canal. (3) Vestibule. (4) Spiral osseous plate. (5) Cochlear window niche. (6) Superior vestibular nerve. (7) Labyrinthine segment of facial nerve. (8) Internal orifice of vestibular aqueduct (endolymphatic duct). (9) Modiolus. (10) Osseous cochlear duct. (11) Carotid artery canal

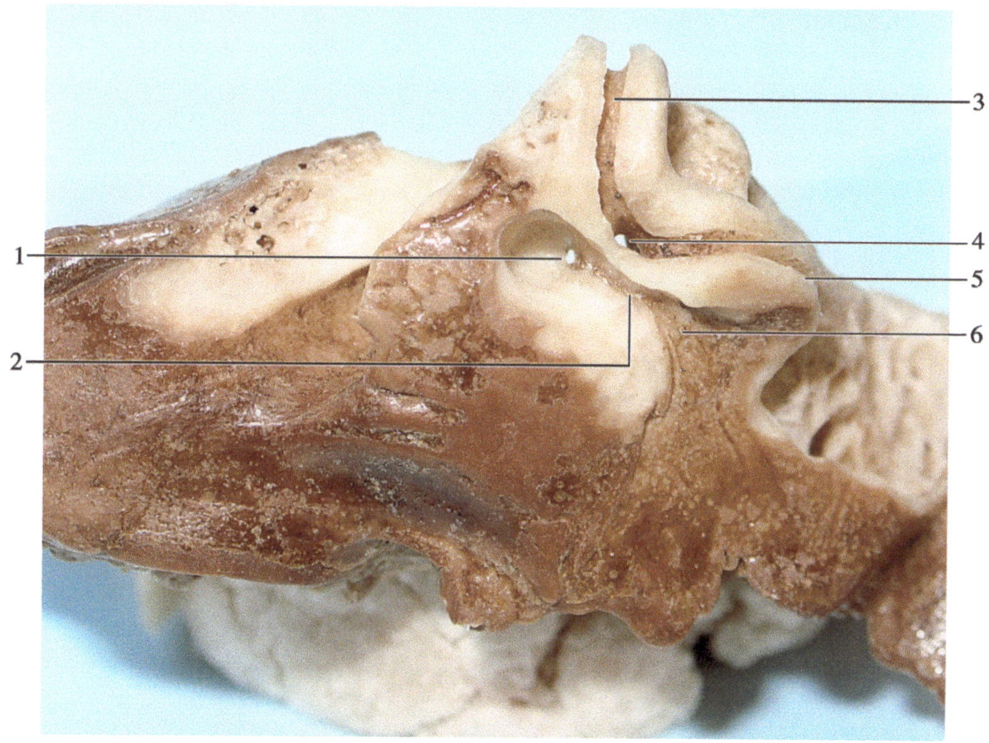

Fig. 1.32 Vestibular aqueduct course viewed from posterior cranial fossa (right). (1) Internal orifice of vestibular aqueduct. (2) Vestibular aqueduct. (3) Anterior semicircular canal. (4) Common crus. (5) Posterior semicircular canal. (6) Endolymphatic sac fissure

The vestibular aqueduct opens at the vestibule (internal opening), first moves inward and then moves backward, bypasses the medial side of the common crus of the semicircular canal, and then expands backward and outward to form the endolymphatic sac, which is similar to the shape of ginkgo biloba.

1.4.2 Semicircular Canals

The osseous semicircular canals are located at the posterosuperior part of the vestibule and there are three arched bone canals. According to their position, they are called lateral (horizontal), anterior and posterior semicircular canal. Both ends of each semicircular canal open in the vestibule, and its enlarged end is ampulla, with an inner diameter of about twice the lumen. The inner end of the anterior semicircular canal and the upper end of the posterior semicircular canal form a common crus, so the three semicircular canals have five openings in total to enter the vestibule. The lateral semicircular canals on both sides of the head are on the same plane and form an angle of 24–30° with the horizontal plane (Benson and Lane 2022). The plane of the anterior semicircular canals on both sides of the head extends backward and is perpendicular to each other, and also perpendicular to the long axis of the petrous portion on the same side. The plane of the posterior semicircular canals on both sides extends forward and is also perpendicular to each other, but parallel to the petrosal long axis on the same side; the plane of the anterior semicircular canal on one side and the posterior semicircular canal on the other side are parallel to each other (Figs. 1.33, 1.34, 1.35, 1.36, and 1.37), so the three semicircular canals can sense the head angular acceleration stimulation in any direction.

1.4.3 Cochlea

The cochlea is located in front of the vestibule, coiled upon itself like a snail shell (Figs. 1.30 and 1.38). It mainly consists of the central modiolus and the surrounding bony cochlear duct (Fig. 1.31). Cochlear duct spirals around the modiolus 2½–2¾ turns, the basal turn is equivalent to the promontory. The cochlear base is backward and inward, forming the fundus of the internal acoustic meatus. The top of the cochlea is outward and forward, close to the tympanic orifice of the eustachian tube. The shape of the modiolus is like a cone, containing cochlear nerve and spiral ganglion cells. The bony spiral plate extending from the modiolus also rotates in the osseous cochlear duct. The shape of the cochlear nerve fibers is like scattered cables distributed in the modiolus (Fig. 1.39). The basilar membrane extends from the bony spiral plate to the outer wall of the osseous cochlear duct, and divides the osseous cochlear duct into upper and lower compartments (for the convenience of describing the internal structure of the cochlea, the cochlea is generally rotated upward by about 90° from its natural anatomical position, making the cochlea top up and the cochlea bottom down, then described). The vestibular membrane also divides the upper compartment into two compartments, so the osseous cochlear duct owns three compartments: the upper one is scala vestibuli, which starts from the vestibule and contains the perilymph; The middle is the scala media, namely the membrane-cochlear duct-the membranous labyrinth, and contains the endolymph; the lower part is scala tympani, which starts from the cochlear window and is sealed by the

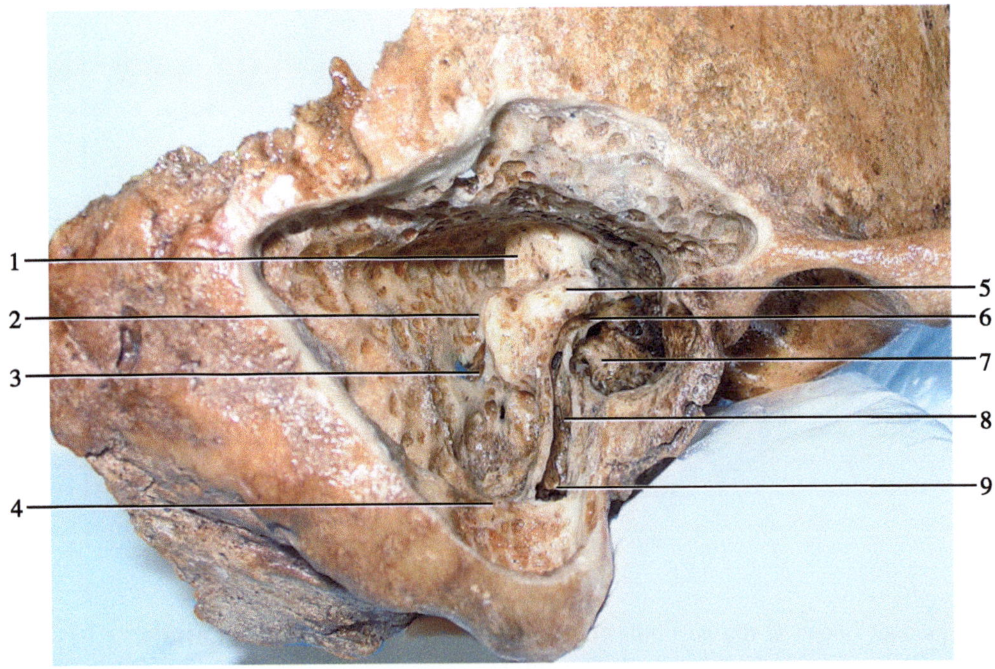

Fig. 1.33 Relationship between semicircular canal and endolymphatic sac fissure (right). (1) Anterior semicircular canal. (2) Posterior semicircular canal. (3) Endolymphatic sac fissure. (4) Digastric crest. (5) Lateral semicircular canal. (6) Horizontal segment of facial nerve canal. (7) Promontory. (8) Vertical segment of facial nerve canal. (9) Stylomastoid foramen. In addition, the figure shows what is seen when the cells in the pneumatized mastoid process are cleared out(skeletonization): the spatial relationship of semicircular canal, endolymphatic sac and facial nerve. The endolymphatic sac is located behind the posterior semicircular canal and below the extension line of the plane of the lateral semicircular canal

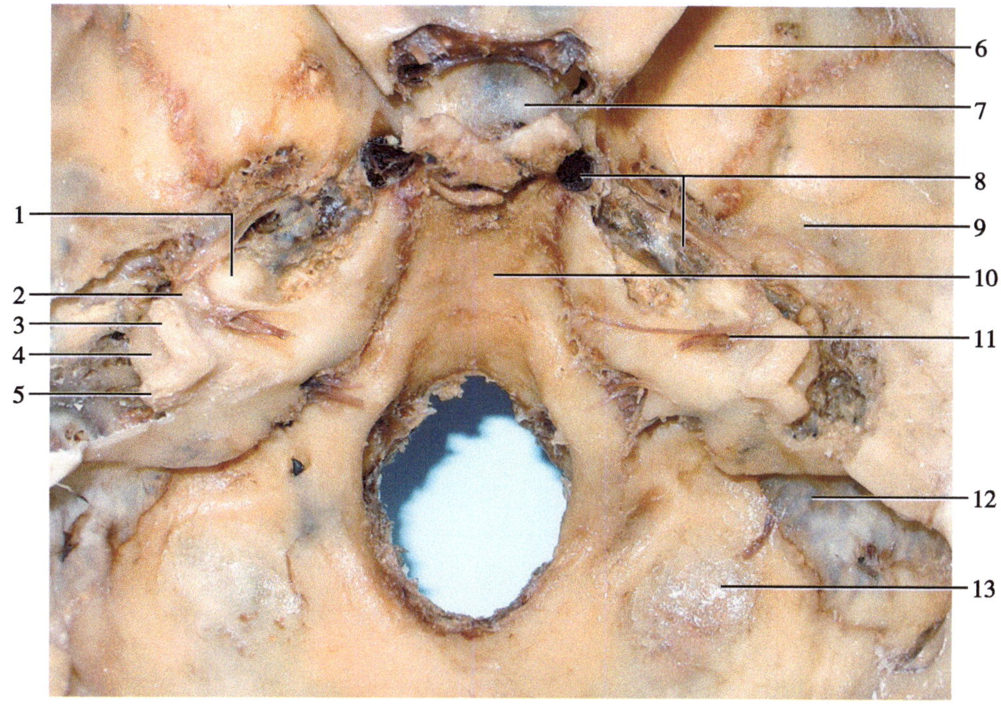

Fig. 1.34 Corresponding positions of inner ear at skull base. (1) Cochlea. (2) Vestibule. (3) Anterior semicircular canal. (4) Lateral semicircular canal. (5) Posterior semicircular canal. (6) Sphenoid bone. (7) Sella turcica. (8) Internal carotid artery. (9) Middle cranial fossa. (10) Slope. (11) Internal acoustic meatus. (12) Sigmoid sulcus. (13) Posterior cranial fossa

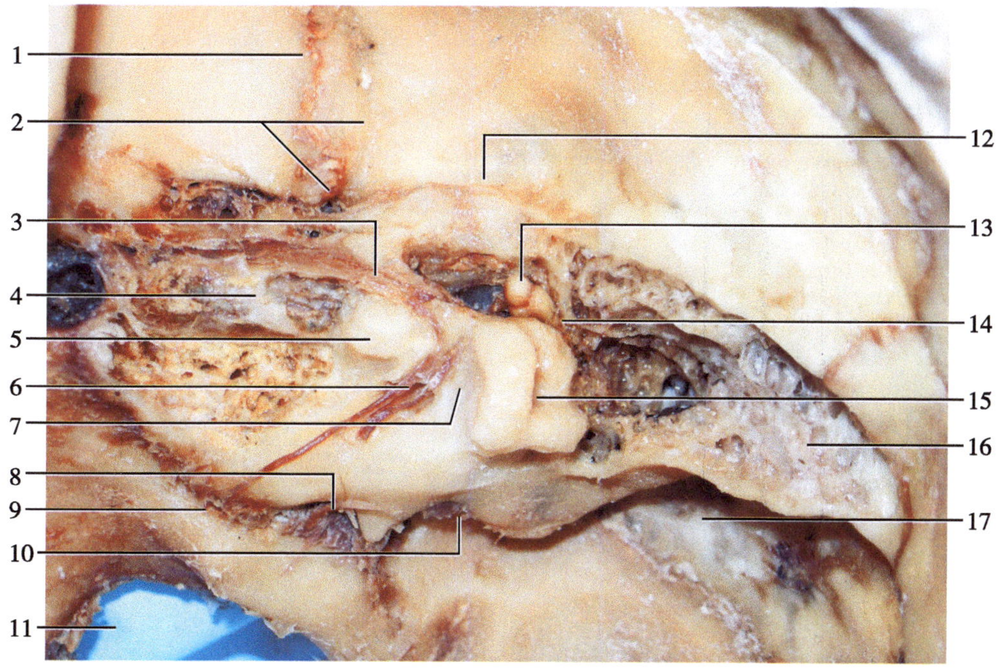

Fig. 1.35 Location of inner ear at petrous part of temporal bone (right). (1) Sphenoid squamous fissure. (2) Middle meningeal artery groove. (3) Superficial petrosal nerve. (4) Carotid artery canal. (5) Cochlea. (6) Auditory nerve at internal acoustic meatus. (7) Vestibule. (8) Nerve part of jugular vein foramen. (9) Petrooccipital fissure. (10) Vascular part of jugular vein foramen. (11) Large occipital foramen. (12) Petrosquamous fissure. (13) Auditory ossicles. (14) Aditus ad antrum. (15) Semicircular canal. (16) Mastoid air cells. (17) Sigmoid groove

cochlear window membrane, containing the perilymph. The spiral plate hook is formed at the top of the bony spiral plate, and the spiral plate is formed at the top of the modiolus; the spiral plate hook, the modiolus plate, and the top blind end of the membrane-cochlear canal form a cochlear hole (helicotrema). The perilymph of the scala tympani communicates with the perilymph of the scala vestibuli through the helicotrema. There is an inner opening of the cochlear canaliculus at the beginning of the scala tympani (hook region of cochlea) and the modiolus near the cochlear window.

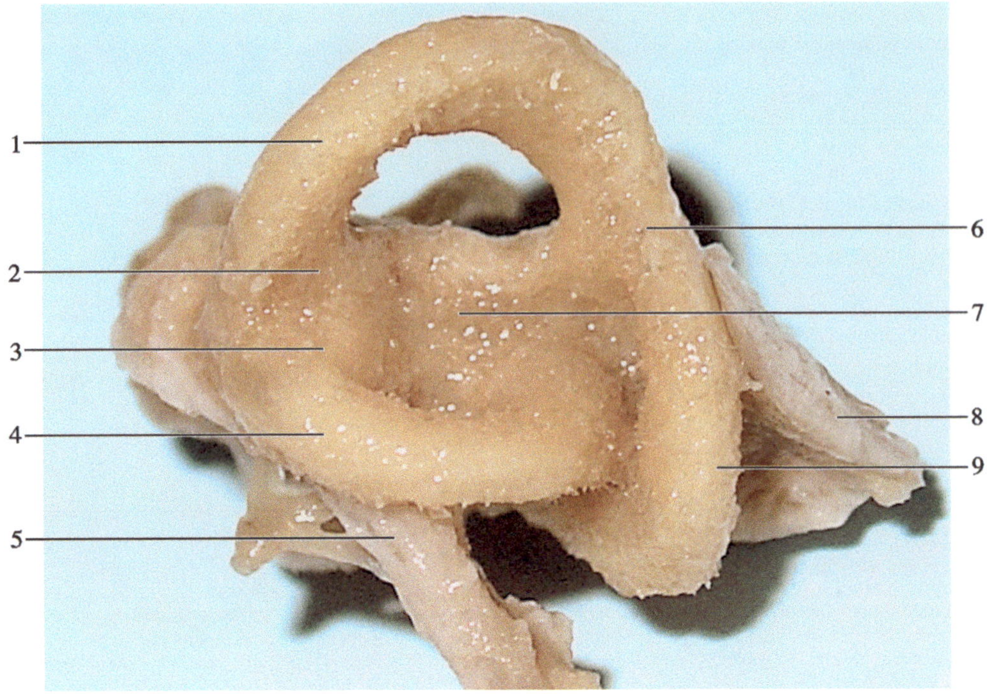

Fig. 1.36 Semicircular canal and vestibule, endolymphatic sac (left). (1) Anterior semicircular canal. (2) Ampulla of anterior semicircular canal. (3) Ampulla of lateral semicircular canal. (4) Lateral semicircular canal. (5) Facial nerve. (6) Common crus. (7) Vestibule. (8) Endolymphatic sac. (9) Posterior semicircular canal

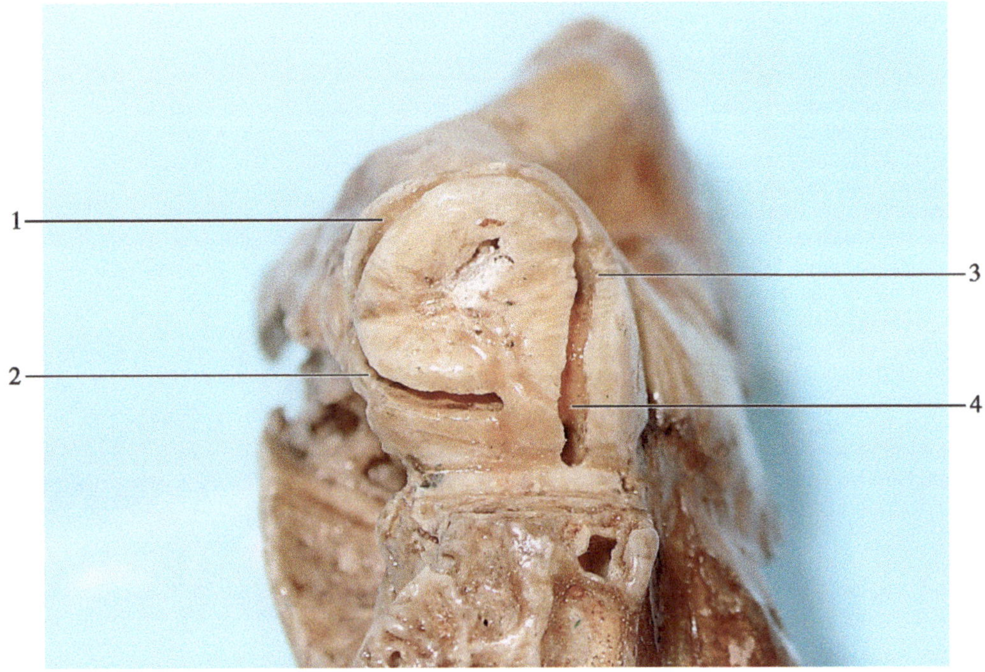

Fig. 1.37 Spatial position of semicircular canal (section, left). (1) Anterior semicircular canal. (2) Lateral semicircular canal. (3) Common crus. (4) Posterior semicircular canal. The planes of the three semicircular canals are approximately perpendicular to each other

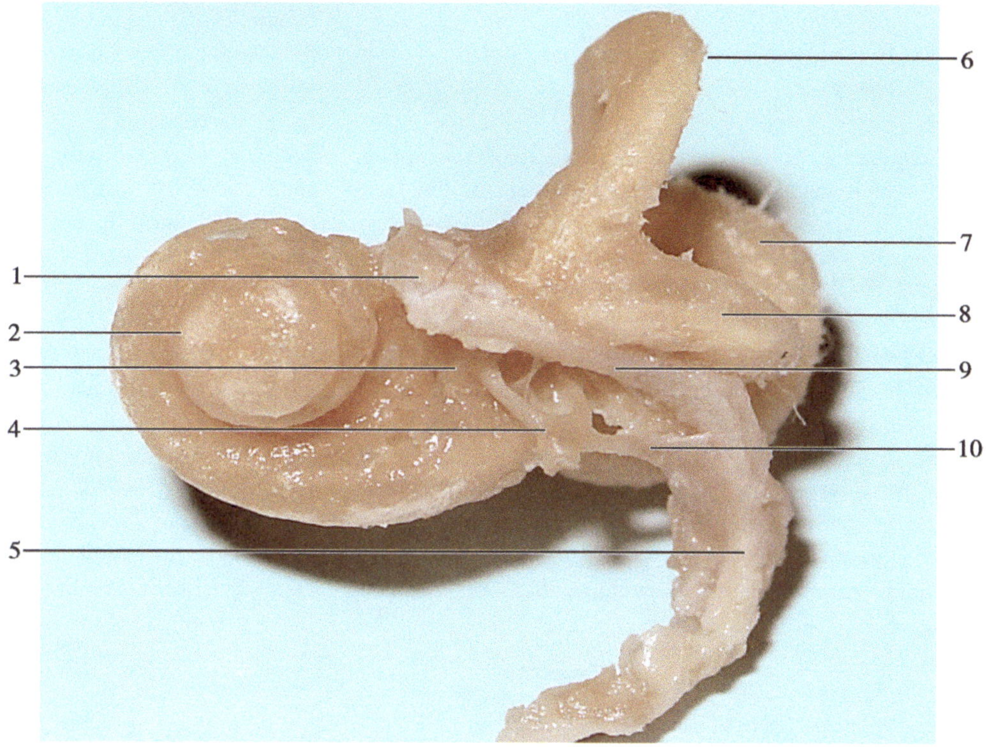

Fig. 1.38 Inner ear anatomy (left). (1) Geniculate ganglion. (2) Cochlea. (3) Vestibule. (4) Stapes. (5) Vertical segment of facial nerve. (6) Anterior semicircular canal. (7) Posterior semicircular canal. (8) Lateral semicircular canal. (9) Horizontal segment of facial nerve. (10) Stapedial muscle. The left cochlear duct runs clockwise, between the cochlea and semicircular canal is the vestibule, and its vestibular window is closed by the footplate of the stapes; The horizontal (tympanic) segment of the facial nerve is located below the lateral semicircular canal and above the vestibular window

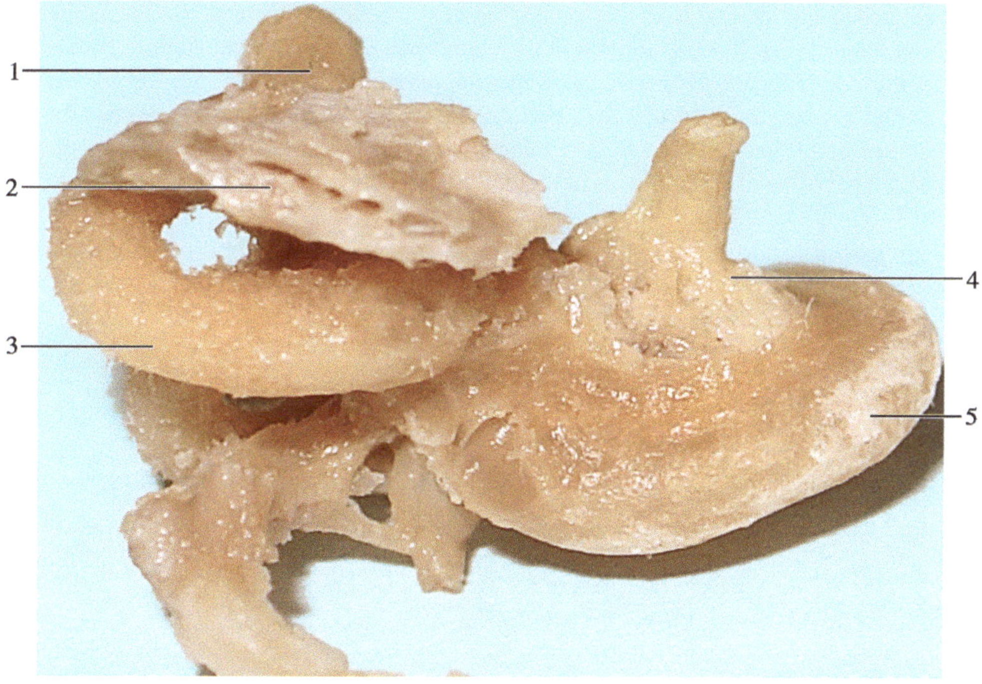

Fig. 1.39 Cochlear nerve and cochlea (left). (1) Anterior semicircular canal. (2) Endolymphatic sac. (3) Posterior semicircular canal. (4) Cochlear nerve. (5) Basal turn of cochlea

1.5 Intratemporal Anatomy of Facial Nerve

The facial nerve, or the seventh cranial nerve, is a compound nerve, which mainly controls the movement of the facial expression muscles (except the levator palpebrae superioris muscle), the secretion of the lacrimal gland and the taste of the anterior 2/3 of the tongue. The facial nerve traverses about 28.5 mm in the temporal bone. It is the longest cranial nerve traversing in the skull. The thickness of the facial nerve is only 30–50% of the volume of the bone canal, the rest is filled with blood vessels and connective tissue outside the nerve bundle. The ratio of the area of sectioned facial nerve to that facial nerve canal are significant larger in horizontal segment and vertical segment of facial nerve than in labyrinthine segment (Ogawa and Sando 1982). Facial nerve receives blood supply from peripheral blood vessels along the way.

1.5.1 Intratemporal Course of Facial Nerve

After leaving the pons, the facial nerve fibers juxtaposes with the vestibulocochlear nerve and enters the internal acoustic meatus (called the internal acoustic meatus segment, about 8 mm in length) (Fig. 1.40) is located at the anterosuperior part of the vestibulocochlear nerve and enters the labyrinth segment with bony canal through the fundus of the internal acoustic meatus (Fig. 1.41), about 3–5 mm in length. The bony facial nerve canal at the fundus of the internal acoustic meatus is the thinnest, with the smallest diameter of only 0.68–1 mm. There is almost no gap between the nerve and the bone canal, which is the most easily squeezed place when facial nerve edema; This segment is located between the cochlea and the anterior semicircular canal, and in the bone canal above the vestibule. It is inclined forward to reach the geniculate ganglion. The upper wall of the facial nerve bone canal can be absent, and the facial nerve directly contacts the dural mater of the middle cranial fossa (Lang 1992). Spontaneous cerebrospinal fluid otorrhea can occasionally occur here, which is difficult to diagnose (MRI hydrography is helpful for the diagnosis). After that, the geniculate ganglion turned sharply to the posterolateral (the intersection angle between the labyrinth segment and the tympanum segment is about 75°) (Jäger and Reiser 2001) and entered the medial wall of the tympanum, which is the tympanic segment or the horizontal segment (Fig. 1.42), with a length of about 7–12 mm. The lateral-inferior wall of this segment of facial nerve (fallopian) canal, especially the upper part of the vestibular window, often has dehiscence (in adults, accounting for 41–75% of the horizontal segment (Baxter 1971; Dimopoulos et al. 1996; Takahashi and Sando 1992; Yu et al. 2011). The latter part of this segment is located below the lateral semicircular canal and above the vestibular window, turns at the posterior crus of the lateral semicircular canal (known as the second genu of facial nerve) vertically downward and slightly backward outward (the intersection angle between the horizontal and vertical segments is about 95–125°), then enters the posterior wall of the tympanic cavity (mastoid segment or vertical segment) (Fig. 1.42), about 16 mm in length, and sends out the stapes muscle branch at

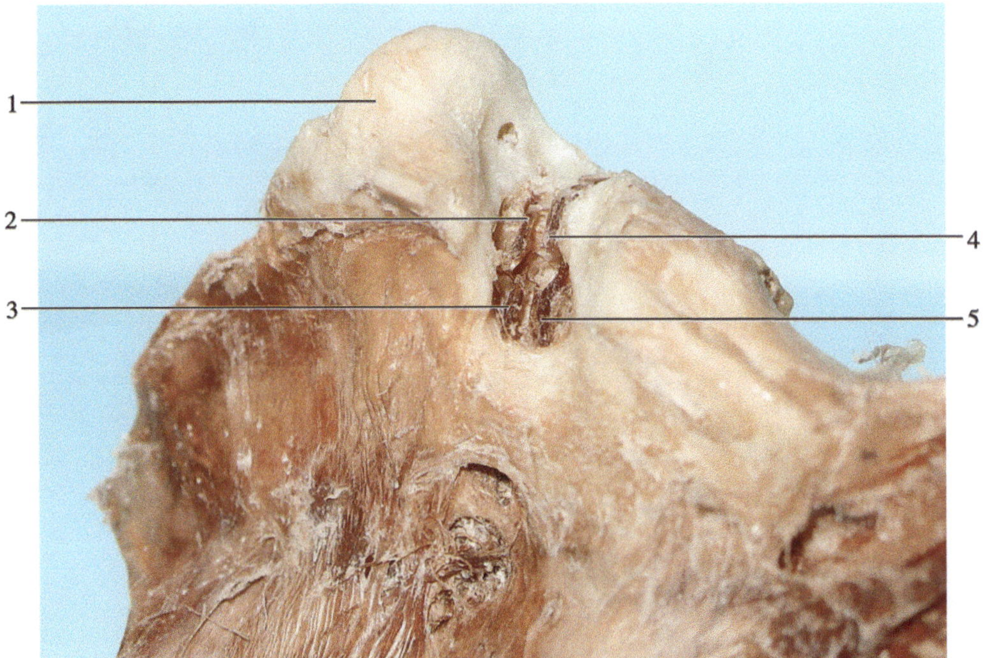

Fig. 1.40 Internal acoustic meatus segment of facial nerve (left). (1) Anterior semicircular canal. (2) Superior vestibular nerve. (3) Inferior vestibular nerve. (4) Facial nerve. (5) Cochlear nerve. The facial nerve is located in the anterosuperior area of the internal acoustic meatus

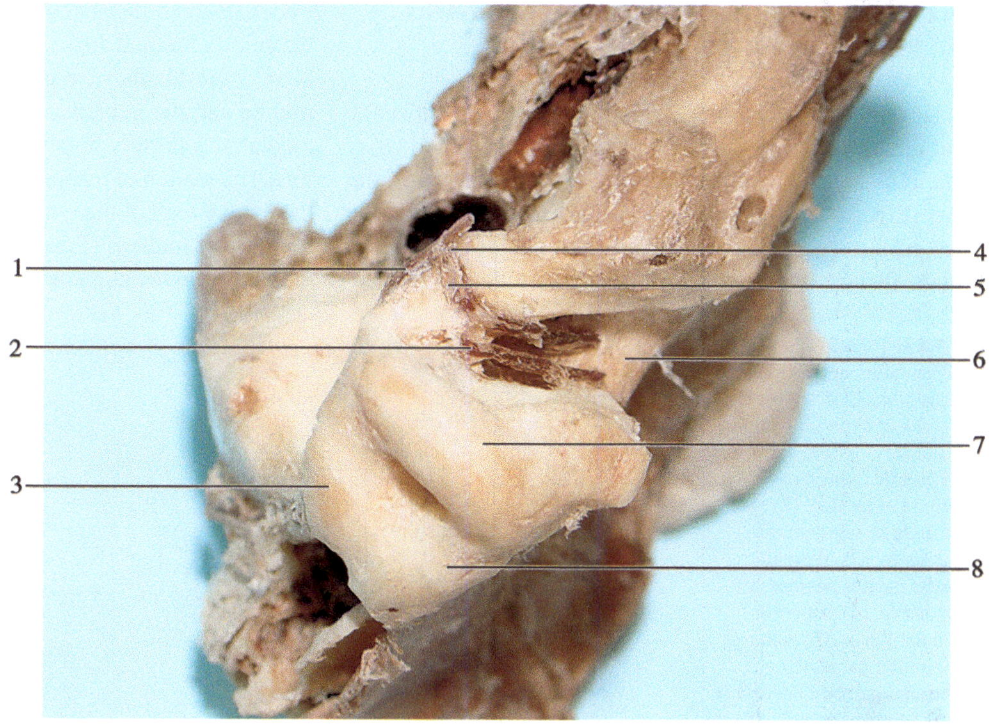

Fig. 1.41 Labyrinthine segment of facial nerve (left). (1) Horizontal segment of facial nerve. (2) Superior vestibular nerve. (3) Lateral semicircular canal. (4) Geniculate ganglion. (5) Labyrinthine segment of facial nerve. (6) Internal acoustic meatus. (7) Anterior semicircular canal. (8) Posterior semicircular canal

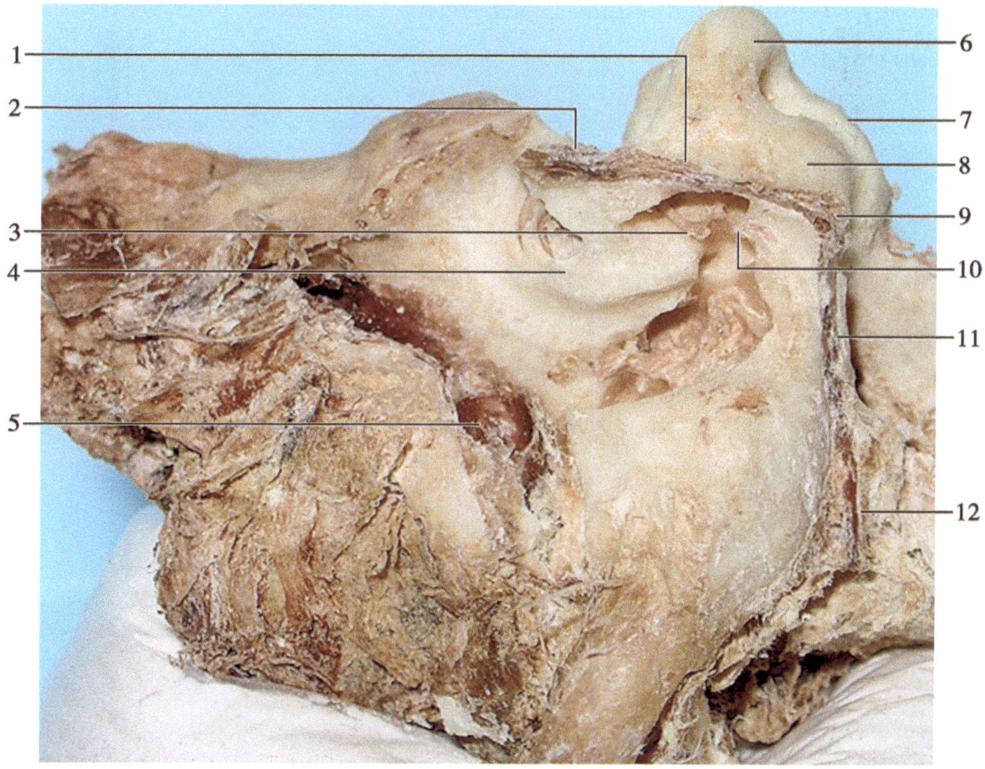

Fig. 1.42 Horizontal and second genu & vertical segments of facial nerve (left). (1) Horizontal (tympanic) segment of facial nerve. (2) Geniculate ganglion. (3) Stapes. (4) Cochlea. (5) Internal carotid artery. (6) Anterior semicircular canal. (7) Posterior semicircular canal. (8) Lateral semicircular canal. (9) Second genu of facial nerve. (10) Pyramidal eminence and stapes. (11) Vertical (mastoid) segment of facial nerve. (12) Stylomastoid foramen

the beginning of the vertical segment to innervate the stapes muscle. The facial nerve sends out the chorda tympani nerve before emerging from the skull through the stylomastoid foramen, to serve the taste of the anterior 2/3 of the tongue, the facial nerve of this segment is surrounded by dense bone, Congenital dehiscence of bone canal is rare, and HRCT scan is of great value in the diagnosis of pathological exposure of facial nerve in this segment (Yu et al. 2007).

1.5.2 Intratemporal Anatomical Landmarks of Facial Nerve

The labyrinthine segment of facial nerve is located above the vestibule, in the bone between the cochlea and the anterior semicircular canal, and in front of the superior vestibular nerve (Fig. 1.43). In this region facial nerve canal runs in close proximity to the upper first turn of cochlea which can explain facial nerve excitement during stimulation of electrodes in some instances (Erixon et al. 2009). Viewing from the middle cranial fossa, the geniculate ganglion is located behind the hiatus of facial nerve canal; viewing from the middle ear, the geniculate ganglion is located in the anteromedial and slightly upper part of the processus cochleariformis. The tendon of tensor tympani, which is perpendicular to the medial wall of the tympanum and outward attached to the neck of the malleus (Figs. 1.43 and 1.44). The facial nerve is emitted from the geniculate ganglion and moves almost hori-

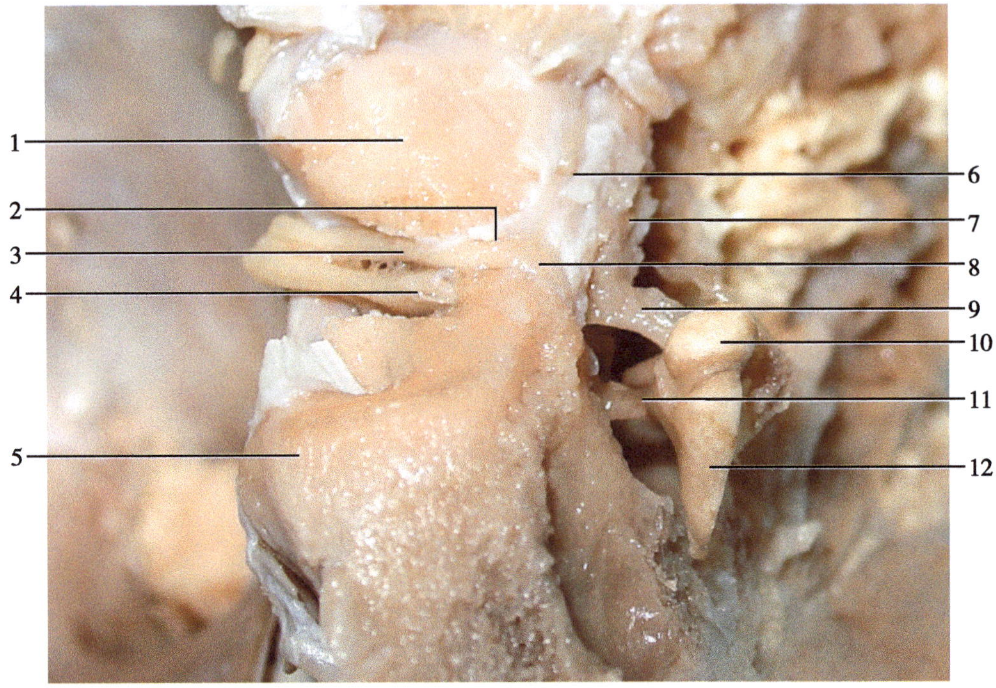

Fig. 1.43 Relationship between facial nerve in petrous portion of temporal bone and semicircular canal and auditory ossicle viewed from middle cranial fossa (right). (1) Cochlea. (2) Labyrinthine segment of facial nerve. (3) Internal acoustic meatus segment of facial nerve. (4) Superior vestibular nerve. (5) Anterior semicircular canal. (6) Superficial petrosal nerve. (7) Tensor tympani muscle. (8) Geniculate ganglion. (9) Tensor tympani tendon. (10) Head of malleus. (11) Lenticular process. (12) Incus

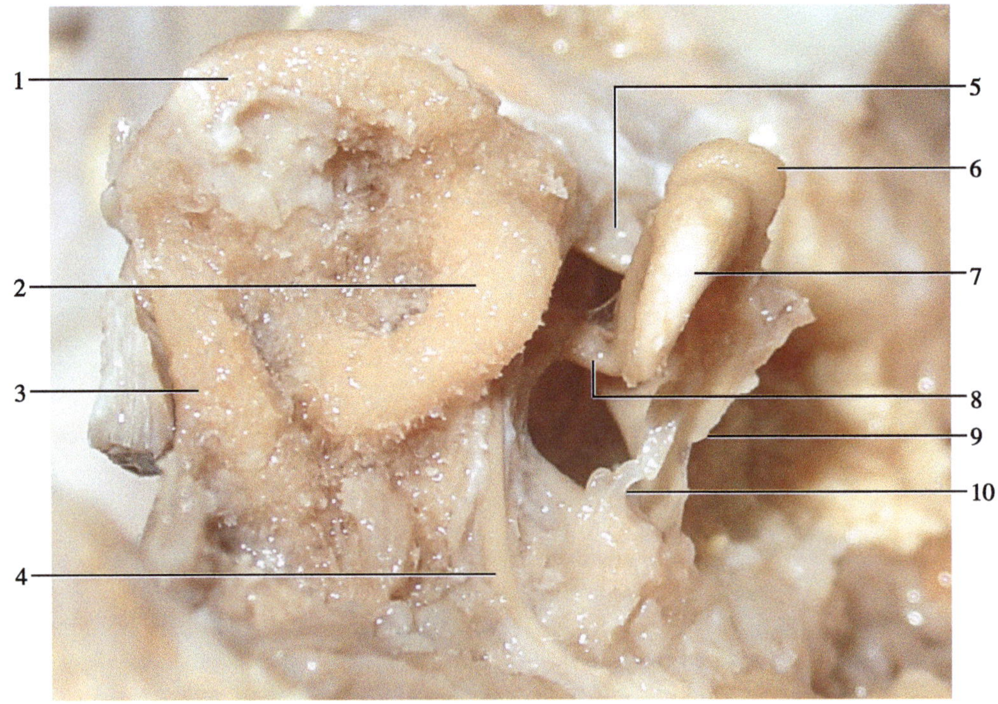

Fig. 1.44 Relationship between facial nerve and semicircular canal and ossicular viewed from tympanic antrum (right). (1) Anterior semicircular canal. (2) Lateral semicircular canal. (3) Posterior semicircular canal. (4) Second genu of facial nerve. (5) Tensor tympani tendon. (6) Head of malleus. (7) Body of incus. (8) Lenticular process. (9) Tympanic membrane. (10) Chorda tympani nerve

zontally backward and slightly outward, this part is called a horizontal segment or tympanic segment. This segment is located at the junction level of the meso- and epitympanum and the medial side of the slightly lower level of the incudomalleolar articulation (Fig. 1.45), the middle and posterior parts of the horizontal segment are located above the vestibular window and below the lateral semicircular canal (Fig. 1.42). The second genu of facial nerve is located in the deep side of the incudial fossa (the shortest distance from the rearmost end of the short crus of the incus to the facial nerve is 1.8–3.9 mm, with an average of 2.7 mm) (Luntz et al. 2000) (Fig. 1.46), and below the posterior crus of the lateral semicircular canal. The vertical segment is located between the posterior crus of the lateral semicircular canal and the convex part of the posterior semicircular canal (Figs. 1.42 and 1.45), and the posteromedial side of the tympanomastoid

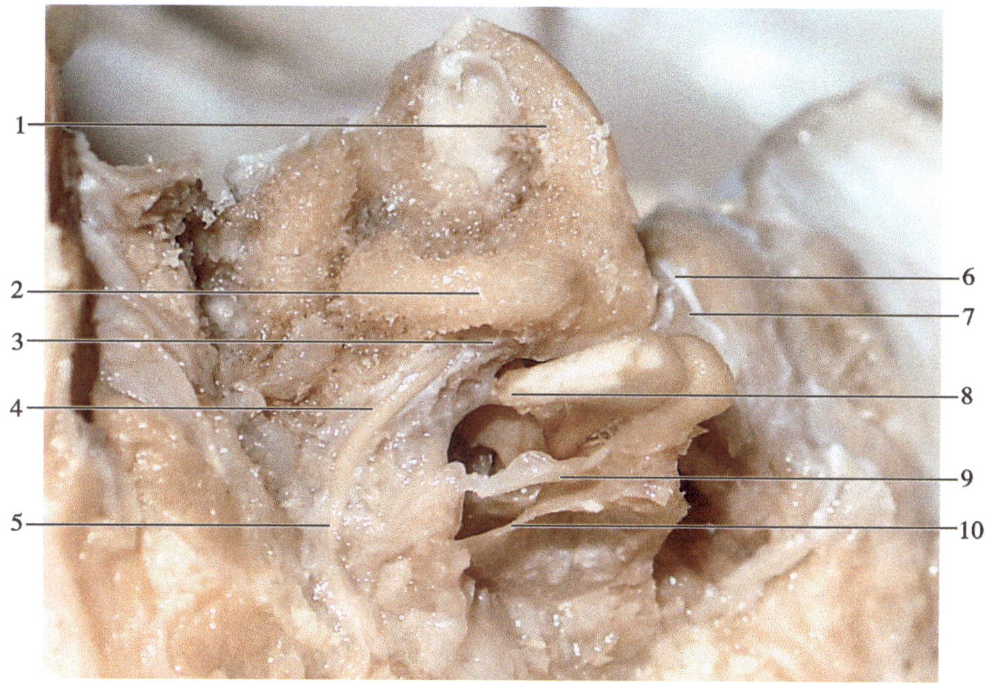

Fig. 1.45 Relationship between facial nerve and semicircular canal and ossicles viewed from mastoid cavity(right). (1) Anterior semicircular canal. (2) Lateral semicircular canal. (3) Horizontal segment of facial nerve. (4) Second genu of facial nerve. (5) Vertical segment of facial nerve. (6) Labyrinthine segment of facial nerve. (7) Geniculate ganglion. (8) Short crus of incus. (9) Chorda tympani nerve. (10) Tympanic membrane

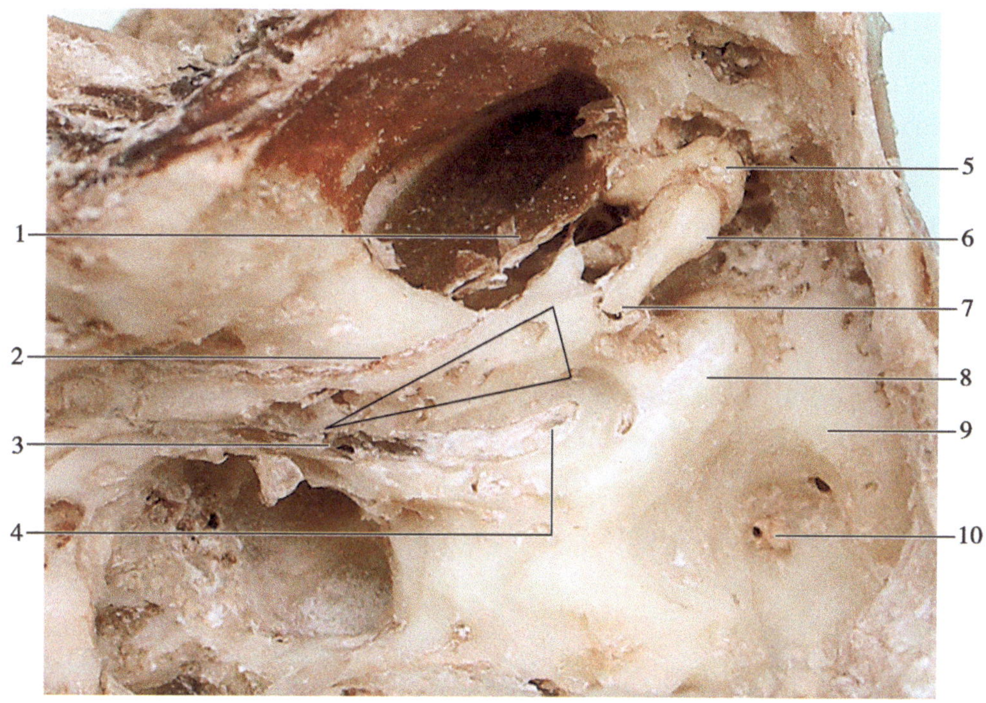

Fig. 1.46 Relationship between short crus of incus and second genu of facial nerve (left). (1) Pars tensa of the tympanic membrane. (2) Chordal tympanic nerve. (3) Vertical segment of facial nerve. (4) Second genu of facial nerve. (5) Head of malleus. (6) Body of incus. (7) Short crus of incus. (8) Convex of lateral semicircular canal. (9) Anterior semicircular canal. (10) Mastoid end of petromastoid canal. The chordal tympanic nerve (anterior boundary), the facial nerve (posterior boundary) and the short crus of the incus (superior boundary) form the boundary of the facial nerve recess (triangle in the figure)

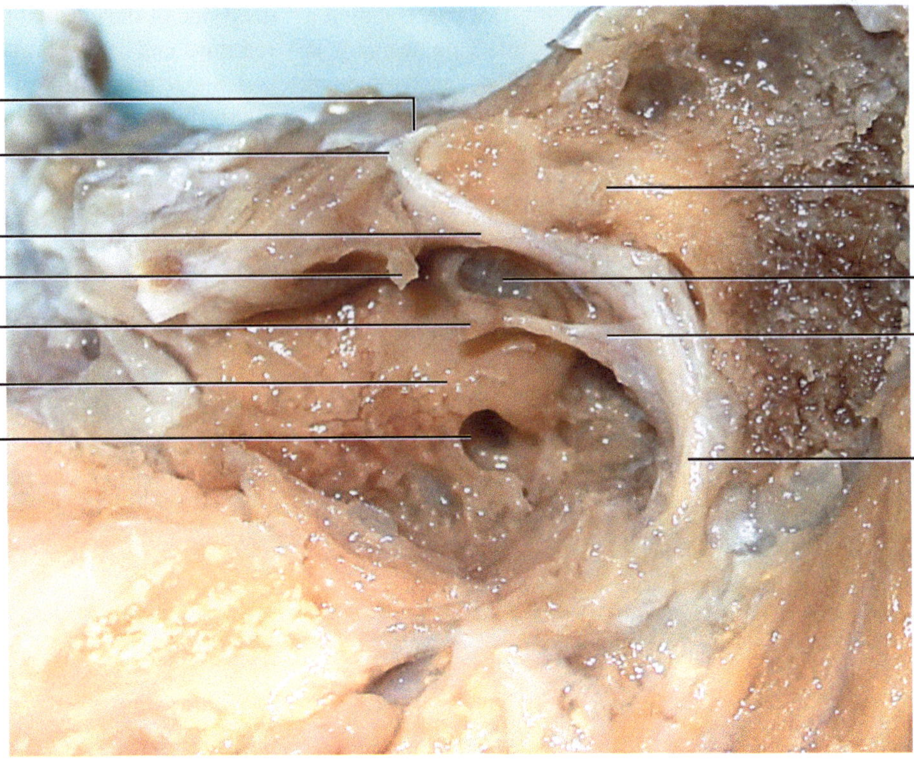

Fig. 1.47 Relationship between facial nerve, tensor tympani tendon, stapes and lateral semicircular canal (left). (1) Labyrinthine segment of facial nerve. (2) Geniculate ganglion. (3) Horizontal segment of facial nerve (tympanic segment). (4) Tensor tympani tendon. (5) Head of stapes. (6) Promontory. (7) Cochlear window niche. (8) Lateral semicircular canal. (9) Footplate of stapes. (10) Stapedial muscle. (11) Vertical segment of facial nerve (mastoid segment)

fissure. The vertical segment is also downward and slightly outward or downward and slightly forward to the stylomastoid foramen. The stapedius branch of facial nerve extends from the second genu forward and inward (Fig. 1.47). If the mastoid process is well pneumatized, the line between the intersection of the digastric crest and the posterior wall of the external auditory canal and the incudal fossa can be used as one of the landmarks for removing the lateral bone of the vertical segment of the facial nerve (facial nerve ridge) during mastoidectomy with canal wall down. The stylomastoid foramen is located between the styloid process and the digastric groove.

1.5.3 The Anatomical Relationship Between Vertical Segment of Facial Nerve and Posterior Wall of External Auditory Canal and Tympanic Membrane

The vertical segment (mastoid segment) of facial nerve started from the inferior edge of the second genu (pyramid eminence) to the stylomastoid foramen is not vertically downward, but slightly outward (50–70% of cases) and/or slightly forward (30–50% of cases). Therefore, this segment of facial nerve forms a certain intersection with the outward and anteroinferior inclined tympanic membrane plane at the coronal position. The upper segment of the vertical segment of facial nerve walks in the wall of the retro-tympanum, and the more the facial nerve runs inferiorly, the closer to the posteroinferior wall of the external auditory canal. The shortest distance from the facial nerve to the posterior point on the tympanic sulcus is range from 1.79 to 4.19 mm (Aslan et al. 2001; Yasumura et al. 1993). The measurement at the plane of the tympanic annulus, posteroinferior quadrant of external auditory canal in most specimens are closest to the vertical segment of the facial nerve (Figs. 1.48, 1.49, 1.50, and 1.51) and at this quadrant, the facial nerve is located at the outside of the extended line of the plane of the tympanic annulus (coronal view) (Adad et al. 1999) (Fig. 1.52). When the cholesteatoma of the external auditory canal invades the posteroinferior medial wall of the external auditory canal, this segment of the facial nerve may be

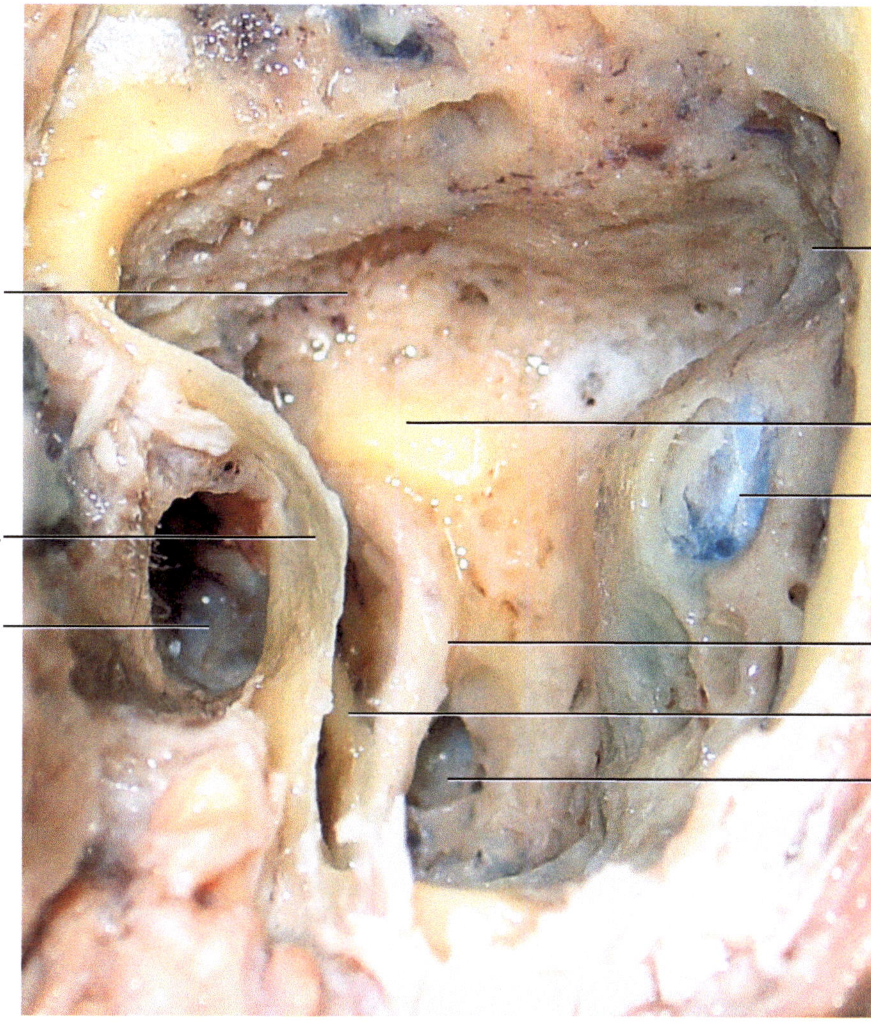

Fig. 1.48 Spatial relationship between posterior wall of external auditory canal and vertical segment of the facial nerve (external auditory canal view). (1) Aditus ad antrum. (2) Posterior wall of external auditory canal. (3) Tympanic membrane. (4) Sinus-meningeal angle. (5) Lateral semicircular canal. (6) Sigmoid sinus. (7) Vertical segment of facial nerve. (8) Chorda tympani nerve. (9) Glomus jugular

exposed. In addition, the external auditory canal approach is often used for external auditory canaloplasty, tumor resection of external auditory canal, tympanoplasty, resection of lesions in the hypotympanum, mastoidectomy with canal wall down, etc., the vertical segment of facial nerve in the posteroinferior quadrant of external auditory canal is most vulnerable to injury. Therefore, understanding the relationship between the plane of the tympanic annulus, the posterior wall of the external auditory canal and the vertical segment of facial nerve plays an important role in guiding the operation at the level of the external auditory canal, the ear surgeon must be kept in mind the close relationship of the facial nerve with external auditory canal (Aslan et al. 2001).

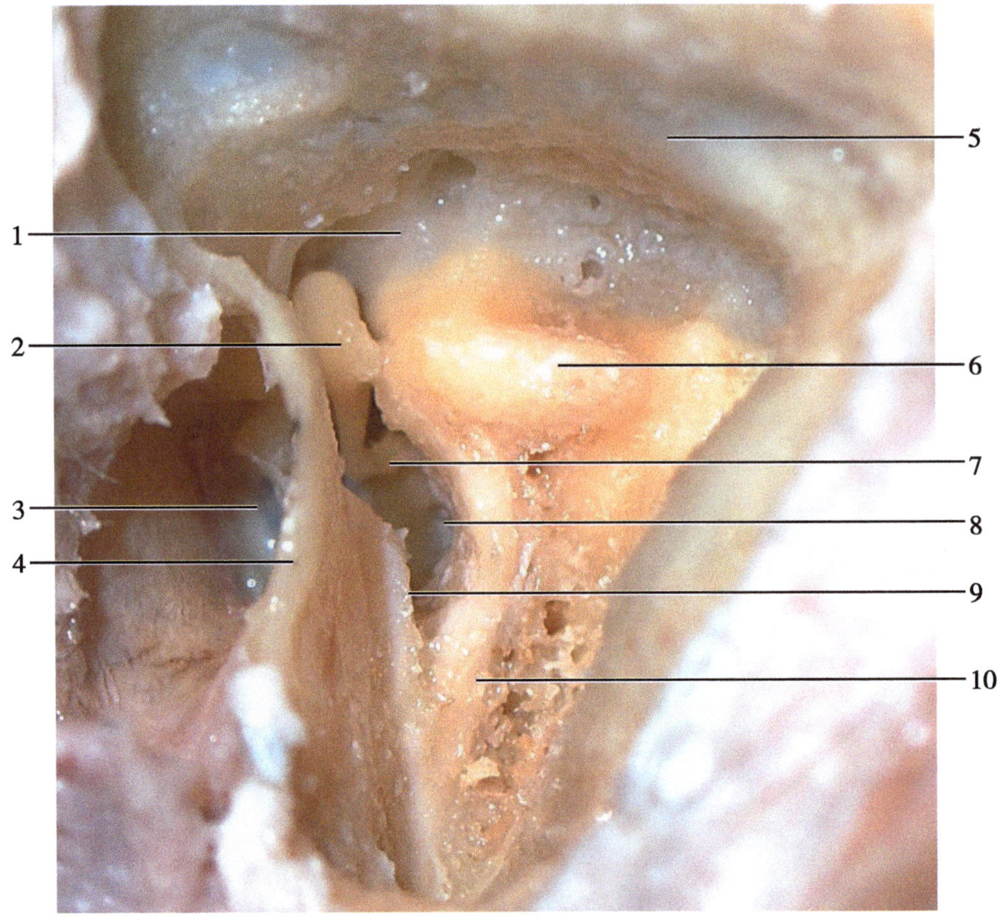

Fig. 1.49 Spatial relationship between posterior wall of external auditory canal and vertical segment of facial nerve (left, view of paralleling to the posterior wall of external auditory canal). (1) Incus. (2) Short crus of incus. (3) Posterior margin of tympanic membrane (overlapping of anterior and posterior margin of tympanic membrane). (4) Posterior wall of external auditory canal. (5) Sinus-meningeal angle. (6) Lateral semicircular canal. (7) Incudostapedial articulation. (8) Cochlear window niche (view from facial recess). (9) Chorda tympani nerve. (10) Vertical segment of facial nerve

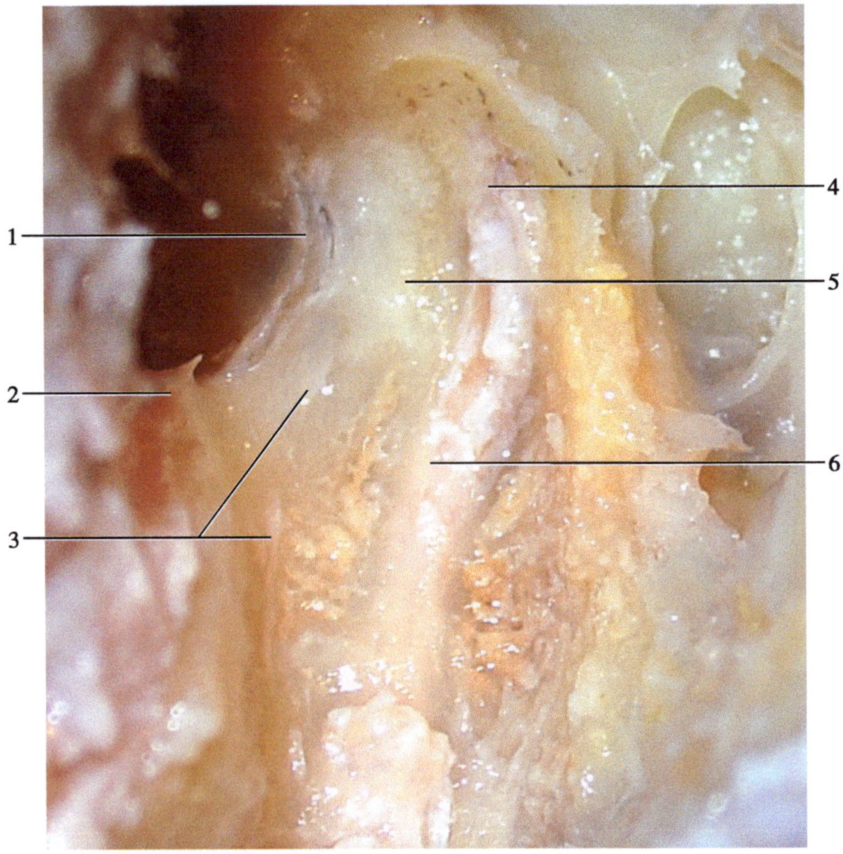

Fig. 1.50 Spatial relationship between tympanic annulus and inferior wall of external auditory canal and vertical segment of facial nerve (left). (1) Fibrous annulus of tympanic membrane. (2) Inferior wall of external auditory canal. (3) Chorda tympani nerve. (4) Second genu of facial nerve. (5) Lateral wall of retro-tympanum (facial recess). (6) Vertical segment of facial nerve. The posterior wall of the external auditory canal had been removed

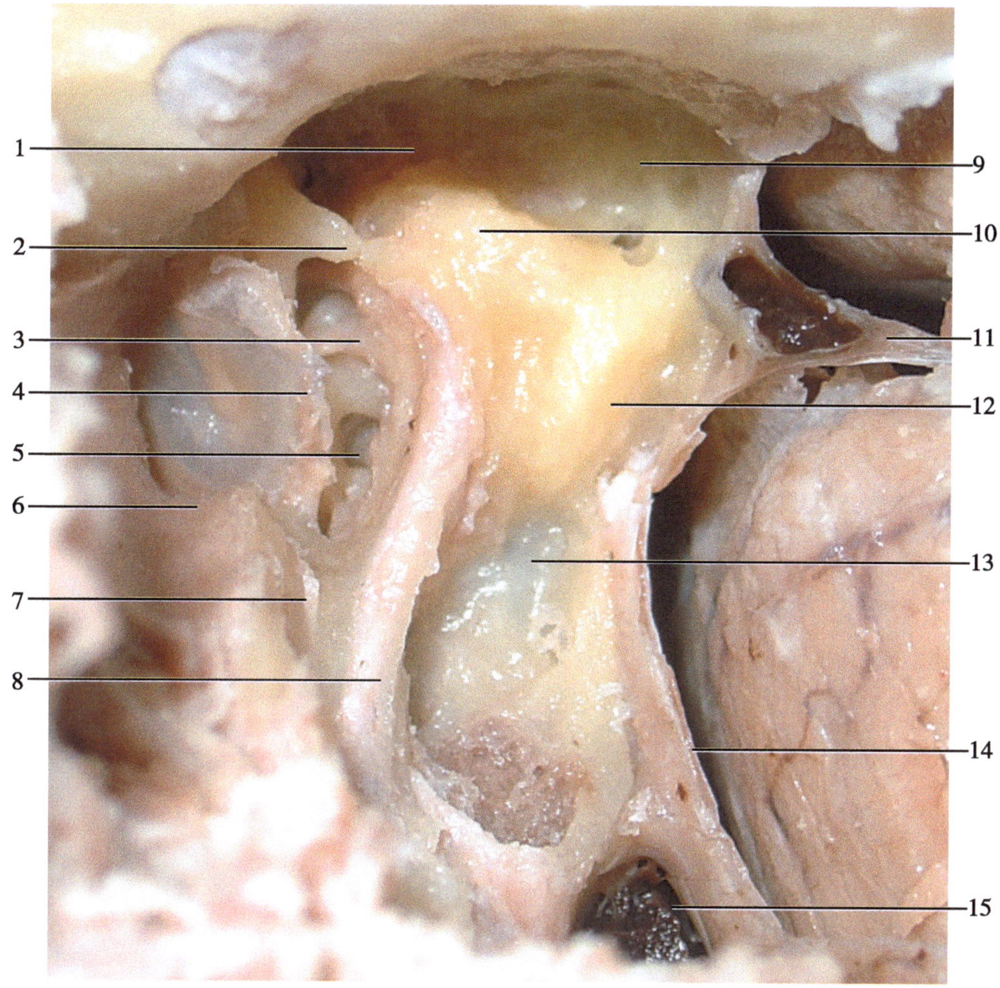

Fig. 1.51 Spatial relationship between tympanic annulus and inferior wall of external auditory canal & vertical segment of facial nerve (left). (1) Aditus ad antrum. (2) Short crus of incus. (3) Pyramidal eminence. (4) Fibrous annulus of tympanic membrane. (5) Cochlear window niche. (6) Inferior wall of external auditory canal. (7) Broken end of chorda tympani nerve. (8) Vertical segment of facial nerve. (9) Tympanic antrum. (10) Lateral semicircular canal. (11) Superior petrosal sinus. (12) Posterior semicircular canal. (13) Glomus jugular. (14) Dura mater of posterior cranial fossa. (15) Sigmoid sinus. The posterior wall of the external auditory canal had been removed and the facial recess was open

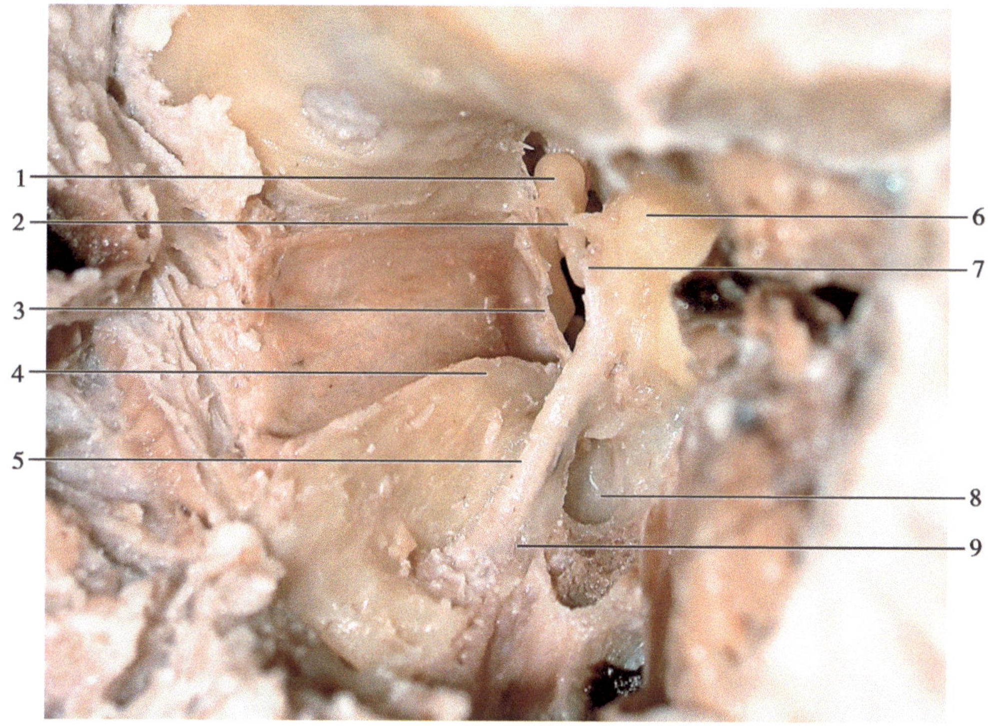

Fig. 1.52 Spatial relationship between plane of tympanic annulus(sulcus) and inferior wall of external auditory canal & vertical segment of facial nerve (left). (1) Incus. (2) Short crus of incus. (3) Posterior edge of tympanic membrane. (4) Inferior wall of external auditory canal. (5) Vertical segment of facial nerve. (6) Lateral semicircular canal. (7) Second genu of facial nerve. (8) Posterior cells of facial nerve. (9) stylomastoid foramen. View on overlapping plane of anterior and posterior edges of tympanic membrane

1.6 Anatomy of Cerebellopontine Angle and Petrous Apex

1.6.1 Anatomy of Cerebellopontine Angle

The medial boundary of the cerebellopontine angle is the outside of the pons, the posterolateral boundary is the front of the cerebellum, and the anterolateral boundary is the back of the petrous part of the temporal bone, which is an approximate triangular subarachnoid space composed by the three adjacent structures (Fig. 1.53).

The cerebellopontine angle is one of the most intensive areas where the cranial nerve roots enter and exit the brain. The vestibulocochlear nerve and facial nerve roots are located in this angle (Fig. 1.54). The facial nerve is located inside the vestibulocochlear nerve. There is a small nervus intermedius between it and the vestibulocochlear nerve. The nervus intermedius contains sensory (taste) fibers and parasympathetic fibers. The facial nerve exits the brain from the midcrus margin of the cerebellum, runs in the cerebellopontine angle cistern, and enters the internal acoustic meatus, which is called the cistern segment of facial nerve. The vestibulocochlear nerve consists of the cochlear nerve and the vestibular nerve, which enters the brain from the pons and medullary groove. Below this angle are glossopharynx, vagus and accessory nerve roots, which are located in the posterior olive groove. The lateral foramen of the fourth ventricle and the choroid plexus of the fourth ventricle are also located in the cerebellopontine angle, just below the facial nerve and vestibulocochlear nerve. The trigeminal nerve root is located at the junction of the pontine base and the cerebellar midcrus, above this angle; The abducent nerve is located in the pontine groove of the medulla oblongata, between the pontine and the medulla oblongata cone, and in the medial side of this angle. The anteroinferior cerebellar artery starts from the lower segment of the basilar artery and runs diagonally to the dorsolateral side. It runs on the ventral side of the abducent nerve, facial nerve and vestibulocochlear nerve. Before supplying the cerebellum, it branches to the upper and middle third of the medulla oblongata and the base of the pons near the medulla oblongata. When the anterior inferior cerebellar artery passes through the cerebellopontine angle, it often forms a wide loop curve of the artery, which can pass through the upper, lower or between the facial nerve and the vestibulocochlear nerve. Labyrinthine artery, also known as the internal auditory artery, is a slender artery, most of which originate from the anteroinferior cerebellar artery, and enter the internal acoustic meatus with the facial nerve and vestibulocochlear nerve. It is divided into cochlear branches and vestibular branches distributed in the inner ear, including semicircular canal, saccule, utricle and cochlea. The tumors of cerebellopontine angle mainly include acoustic neuromas, accounting for about 70–80% of these tumors. It is generally believed that they originate from the outside of the Obersteiner Redlich area of the vestibular nerve, that is, the place where the vestibular nerve penetrates the arachnoid membrane of the cerebellopontine angle cistern, where the nerve interstitium changes from glial fine cells to Schwann cells. Other tumors include meningioma, epithelioid cyst, glioma and metastatic tumor. In addition to the symptoms of

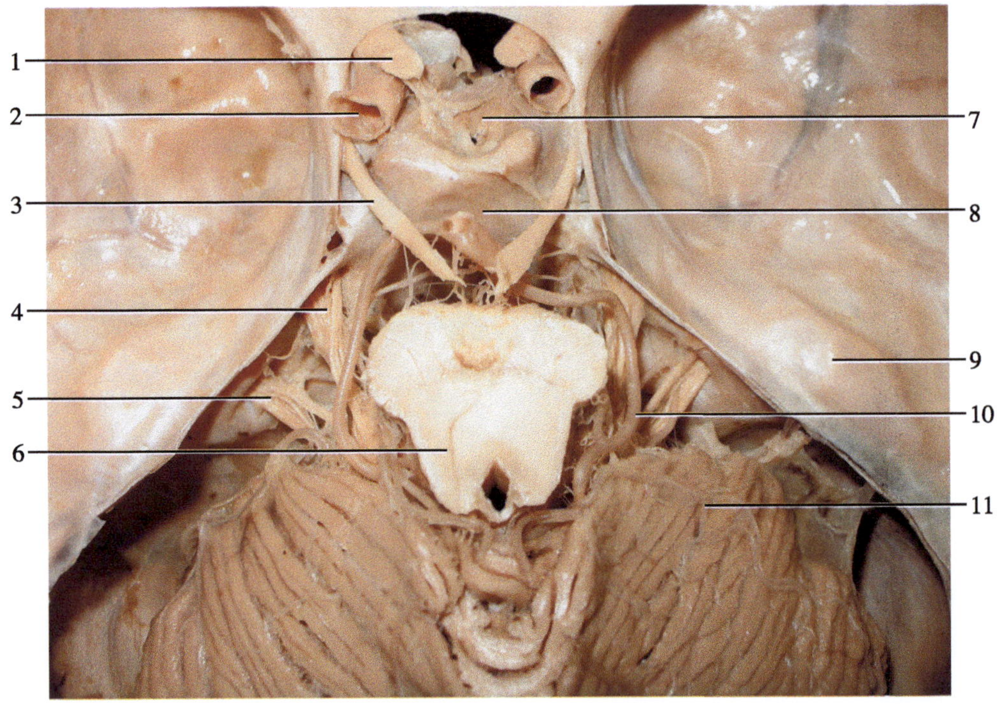

Fig. 1.53 Anatomy of cerebellopontine angle (view above). (1) Optic nerve. (2) Internal carotid artery. (3) Ocular nerve. (4) Trigeminal nerve. (5) Facial nerve and vestibulocochlear nerve bundle. (6) Pontine. (7) Pituitary fossa. (8) Clivus. (9) Petrous portion of temporal bone. (10) Superior cerebellar artery. (11) Cerebellum

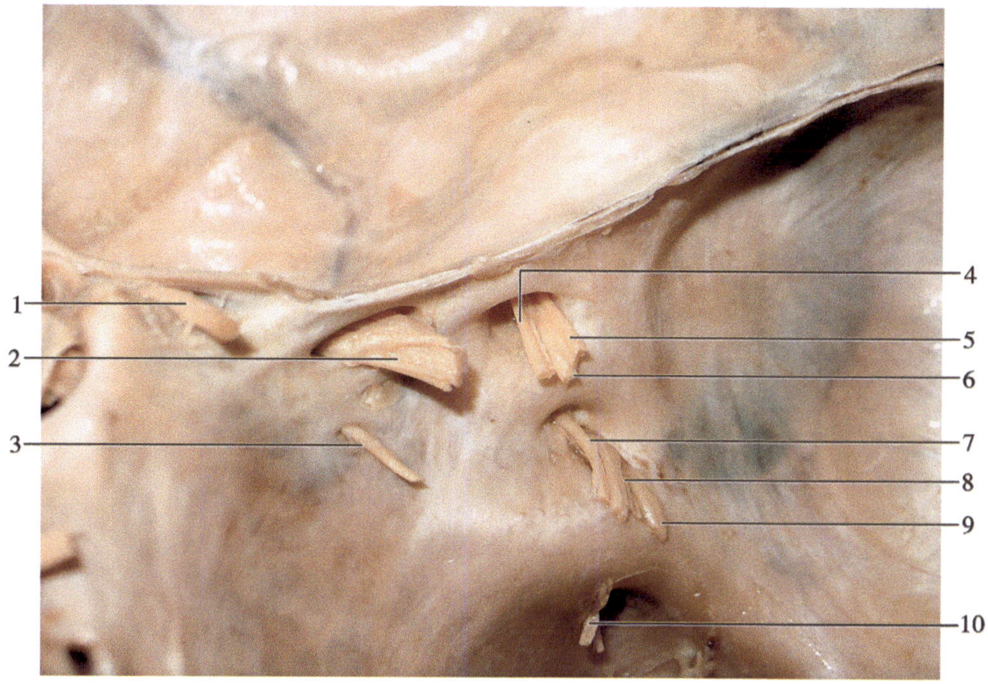

Fig. 1.54 Anatomy of posterior aspect of petrous portion of temporal bone (view of posterior cranial fossa, left). (1) Oculomotor nerve. (2) Trigeminal nerve. (3) Abducent nerve. (4) Facial nerve. (5) Vestibular nerve. (6) Cochlear nerve. (7) Glossopharyngeal nerve. (8) Vagus nerve. (9) Accessory nerve. (10) Hypoglossal nerve

hearing impairment and cerebellar damage, cerebellopontine angle tumors can also compress the facial nerve, glossopharyngeal nerve and vagus nerve nearby, resulting in corresponding clinical symptoms.

1.6.2 Anatomy of Petrous Apex

The tip part of petrous portion of temporal bone is called petrous apex (Figs. 1.3 and 1.7), which is located in the anteromedial sides of the cochlea and the internal acoustic meatus. Its medial side is connected with the occipital bone at the clivus, its anterolateral side is connected with the greater wing of the sphenoid bone, and its anterior side is the carotid artery canal (Fig. 1.34, 1.35 and 1.53) and foramen lacerum, which communicates the nasopharynx with the intracranial. Its anterosuperior part of petrous apex forms part of the middle cranial fossa base, and its posteroinferior surface extends outward along the clivus, forming the anterolateral part of the posterior cranial fossa. The irregular inferior surface is the attachment point of the infratemporal muscle (Fig. 1.2). A large number of nerves and blood vessels surround the petrous apex, which is a challenge for surgical treatment to some extent. The carotid artery canal crosses the petrous apex along the petrous long axis. The cavernous sinus and trigeminal nerve are located at the front and upper part. The abducent nerve, cavernous sinus and superior petrosal sinus intersect through their anteromedial sides. The posterolateral side of the petrous apex is the internal acoustic meatus and labyrinth. The petrous apex can interact with the surrounding diseases, and it is difficult to determine the primary location of the extensive or advanced tumor.

2 Comparison of Sectional Anatomy and CT of Temporal Bone

Zilong Yu

One of the difficulties in understanding the temporal bone CT image is the lack of temporal bone anatomy knowledge. Through the study of Ear Clinical Anatomy, we have understood the anatomy of temporal bone to some extent. In this chapter, the temporal bones were divided into several continuous parallel sectionals (axial, coronal, and sagittal), respectively, and compared with their own high-resolution CT images. The surgical landmarks in sectional samples and their corresponding CT images were marked in detail, their clinical significances were also illustrated in the meantime. This self-contrasting and mutually validating method will help beginners quickly grasp the relevant knowledge.

2.1 CT Scan of Temporal Bone and Preparation of Temporal Bone Sectional Specimen

2.1.1 Ear CT Scan

HRCT can clearly display the meticulous structures of the middle ear, inner ear, and temporal bone. This examination technology has been widely used in clinical practice. In this section, routine HRCT images were acquired in the axial, coronal, and sagittal planes using a Philips Brilliance 64 CT scanner (Philips, the Netherlands) before preparation of ear sectional specimen. The imaging parameters were as follows: voltage 120 Kv, current 200 mA, matrix 512x 512, reconstructing sectional thickness 0.65 mm. The images were reconstructed using a high resolution bone algorithm. A window width of 4000 Hounsfield Units (HU) and a window center of 700 HU were preferred for reading these high resolution images. Before scanning, the cadaver heads were dried until the fixed fluid in the middle ear mastoid process were disappeared and then scanned to avoid the false image of "middle ear effusion" which affected the structural observation of the temporal bone itself.

The two-dimensional image of ear (temporal bone) was usually reconstructed with axial (horizontal), coronal, and sagittal views. Each position had their own advantages and shortcomings when displaying a certain structure. However, one common characteristic is: the structure parallel to the scanning plane could only be partially displayed or could not be displayed at all (Valvassori et al. 1985). For example, the horizontal position could clearly display the front, back, and inside structures of the scanned structure; The coronal position could clearly show the upper and lower, the inner and outer structures of the scanning objective; Sagittal position had its advantages in displaying anterior, posterior, upper and lower structures, but they were not good at displaying some structures which parallel to them.

The protocol was approved by the Institutional Committee of the Beijing Institute of Otolaryngology.

2.1.2 Preparation of Ear Sectional Specimen

After the cadaver head had dried, the temporal bone was taken out, a small hole was drilled at the tegmen tympani, an appropriate amount of epoxy resin was injected into the tympanic cavity, then the temporal bone was turned up and down several times, Epoxy resin was evenly distributed around the ossicular chain, then polymerized at 60 °C for 48 hours, the corresponding structures of temporal bone were ground out layer by layer and compared with their temporal bone CT images. A digital camera was used to record the structure layer by layer, the post-processing was done by notebook computer.

Z. Yu (✉)
Department of Otolaryngology Head and Neck Surgery, Beijing Tongren Hospital, Capital Medical University, Beijing, China

Z. Yu (ed.), *Ear Diseases and CT*, https://doi.org/10.1007/978-981-99-7220-3_2

2.2 Comparison of Sectional Anatomy and CT of Temporal Bone: Axial View

Axial (horizontal) position view of temporal bone CT can clearly display: anterior and posterior wall of external auditory canal, auditory ossicles, bony eustachian tube, internal and external wall of facial nerve horizontal segment, geniculate ganglion, labyrinth segment of facial nerve, facial recess, labyrinth, vestibular window, cochlear window, pyramidal eminence, anterior and posterior wall and fundus of internal acoustic meatus, internal carotid tube, glomus jugular, sigmoid groove, and other structures. However, the upper and lower walls of some structures (such as tympanic cover, external auditory canal and internal acoustic meatus) are not well displayed. All the images shown here are from the right temporal bone, which are taken from the anterior semicircular arch to the stylomastoid foramen (Figs. 2.1, 2.2, 2.3, 2.4, 2.5, 2.6, 2.7, 2.8, 2.9, 2.10, 2.11, 2.12, 2.13, 2.14, 2.15, 2.16, 2.17, 2.18, and 2.19).

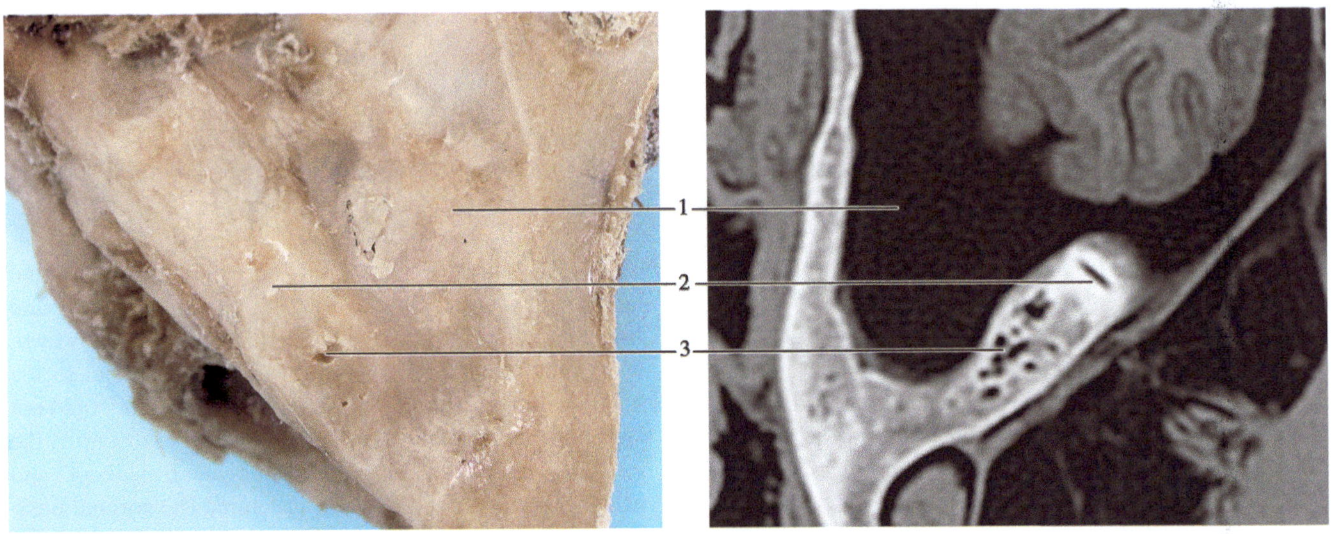

Fig. 2.1 Anterior semicircular canal arch plane (right) (1) Middle cranial fossa. (2) Anterior semicircular canal. (3) Petrous Cells.

Note: Anterior semicircular canal arch is the highest part of the inner ear, located under the arcuate eminence, and is one of the surgical landmarks of the middle cranial fossa. The axial position can diagnose the lower position of the middle cranial fossa, but it is not easy to make accurate diagnosis for its integrity, and it is also of little value for the diagnosis of anterior semicircular fissure (Fig. 2.1)

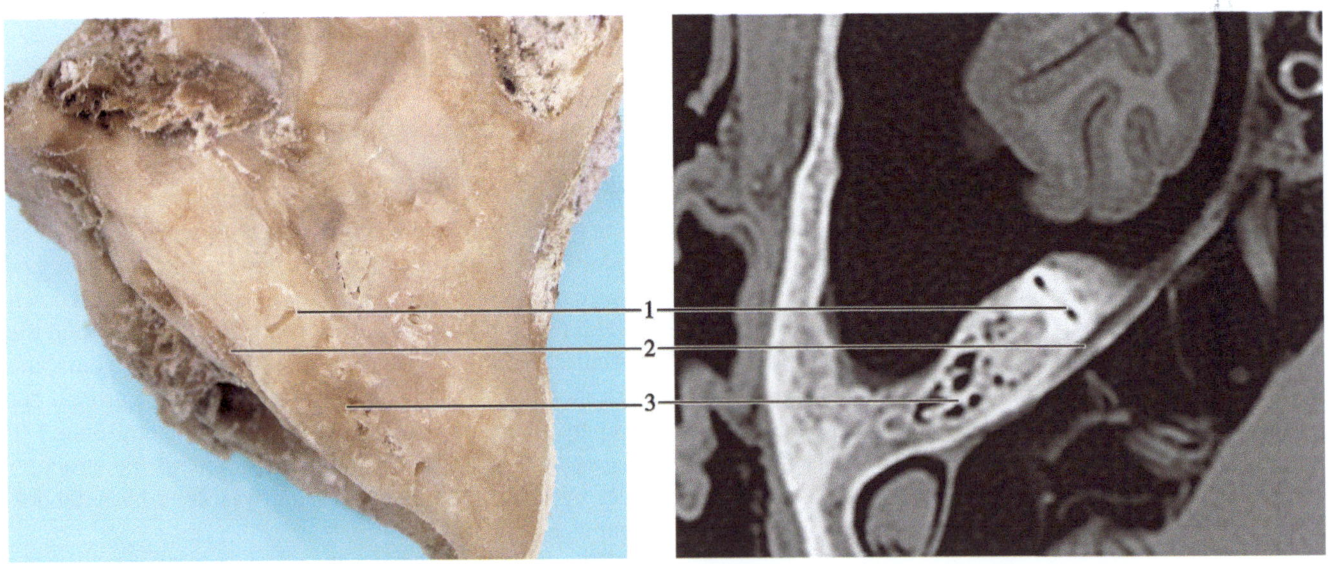

Fig. 2.2 Anterior semicircular canal arch plane (right) (1) Anterior semicircular canal arch. (2) Superior petrosal sulcus. (3) Cells around the anterior semicircular canal.

Note: The anterior semicircular canal arch is perpendicular to the long axis of the petrous portion (or perpendicular to the superior petrosal sulcus) (Fig. 2.2)

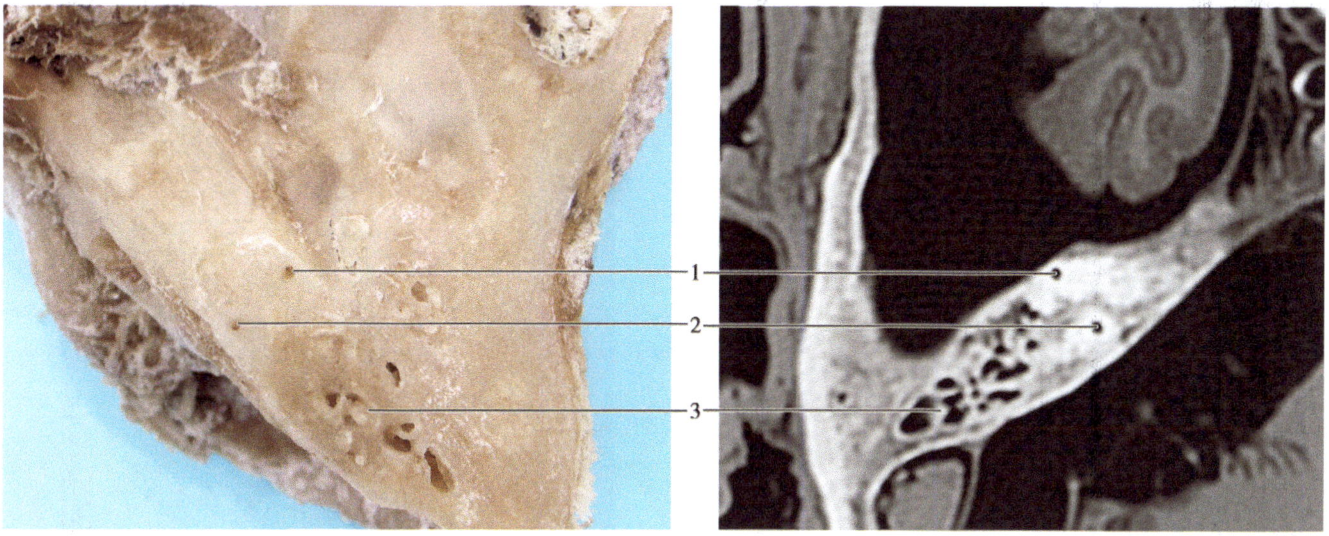

Fig. 2.3 Anterior semicircular canal crus plane (right). (1) Anterior semicircular canal crus. (2) Posterior semicircular canal crus. (3) Petrous Cells

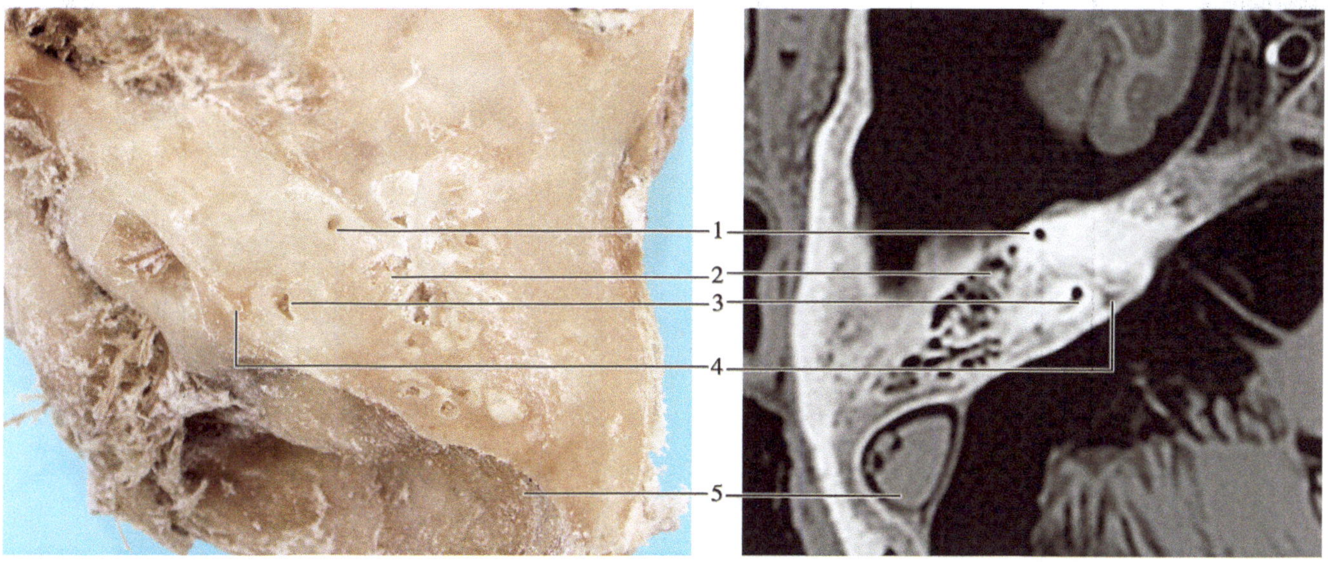

Fig. 2.4 Common crus level plane (right). (1) Anterior crus of anterior semicircular canal. (2) Petrous Cells. (3) Common crus. (4) Petromastoid canal. (5) Sigmoid sulcus.

Note: Petromastoid canal is a potential channel to communicate the tympanic sinus and intracranial, with subarchic artery and vein inside, located under the arch of anterior semicircular canal and above the lateral semicircular canal. Inflammation of the mastoid process of the middle ear can cause intracranial complications through this canal (Fig. 2.4)

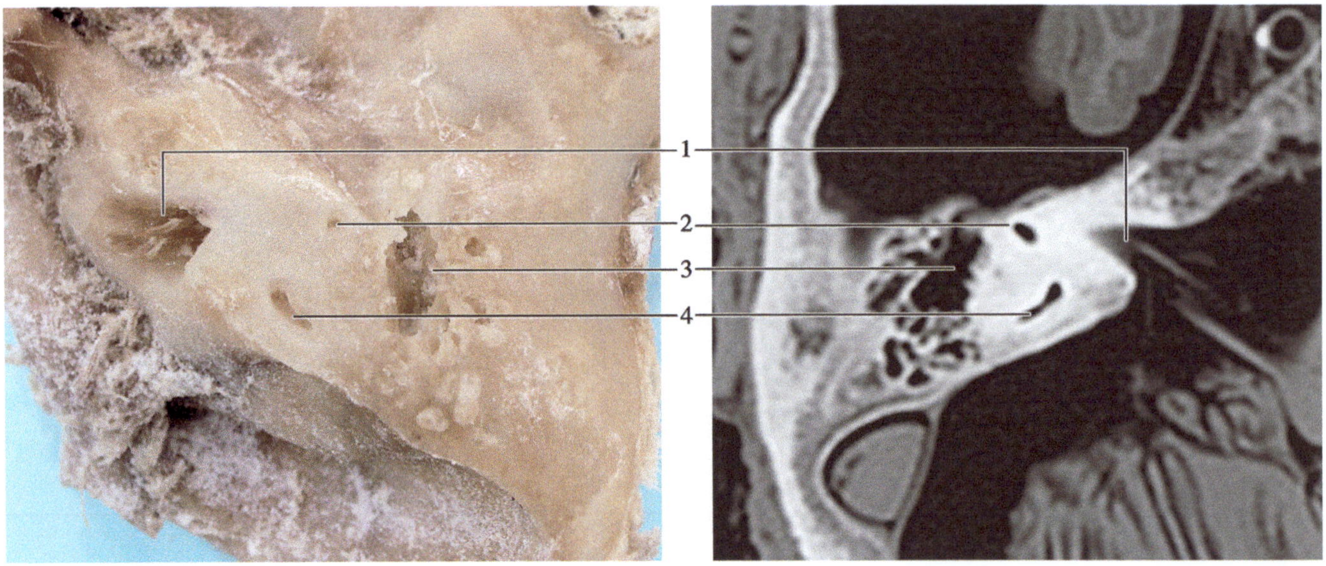

Fig. 2.5 Posterior semicircular canal arch plane (right). (1) Internal acoustic meatus. (2) Anterior crus of the anterior semicircular canal. (3) Tympanic antrum. (4) Posterior semicircular canal arch.

Note: The posterior semicircular canal arch is parallel to the long axis of the petrous part; All cells of mastoid open to the tympanic sinus and mastoid cavity (Fig. 2.5)

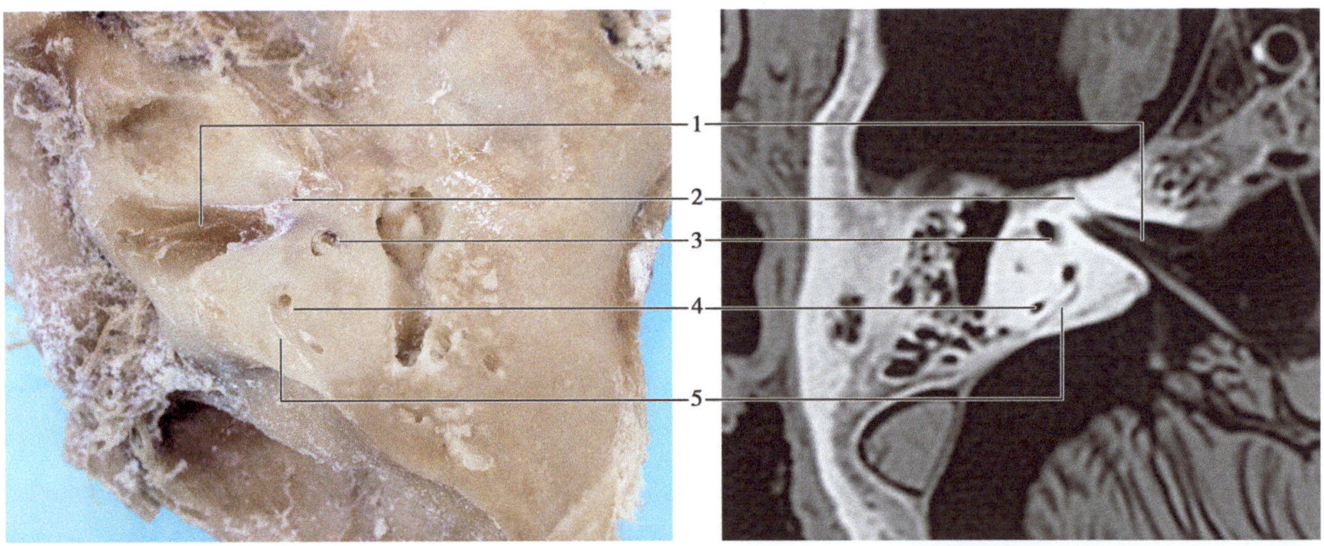

Fig. 2.6 Labyrinth segment of facial nerve (canal) and vestibular aqueduct plane (right). (1) Internal acoustic meatus. (2) Labyrinth segment of the facial nerve (canal). (3) Ampulla of the anterior semicircular canal. (4) Posterior semicircular canal. (5) Vestibular aqueduct.

Note: The internal acoustic meatus can be present as tubular and ampullary, about 10 mm in length, and slightly wider at the fundus of the internal acoustic meatus. The compression of the posterior wall of the internal acoustic porus can make the internal acoustic meatus expand like a cone, which is one of the typical manifestations of acoustic neuroma. Stenosis of the internal acoustic meatus can result in the sensorineural hearing loss. At the same time, the internal acoustic meatus is one of the weaker parts of the temporal bone. Transverse fracture of the temporal bone can lead to rupture of the inner ear and facial nerve injury. This segment of facial nerve enters the temporal bone through the fundus of the internal acoustic meatus, which is called labyrinthine segment of facial nerve, about 3–5 mm in length (Fig. 2.6)

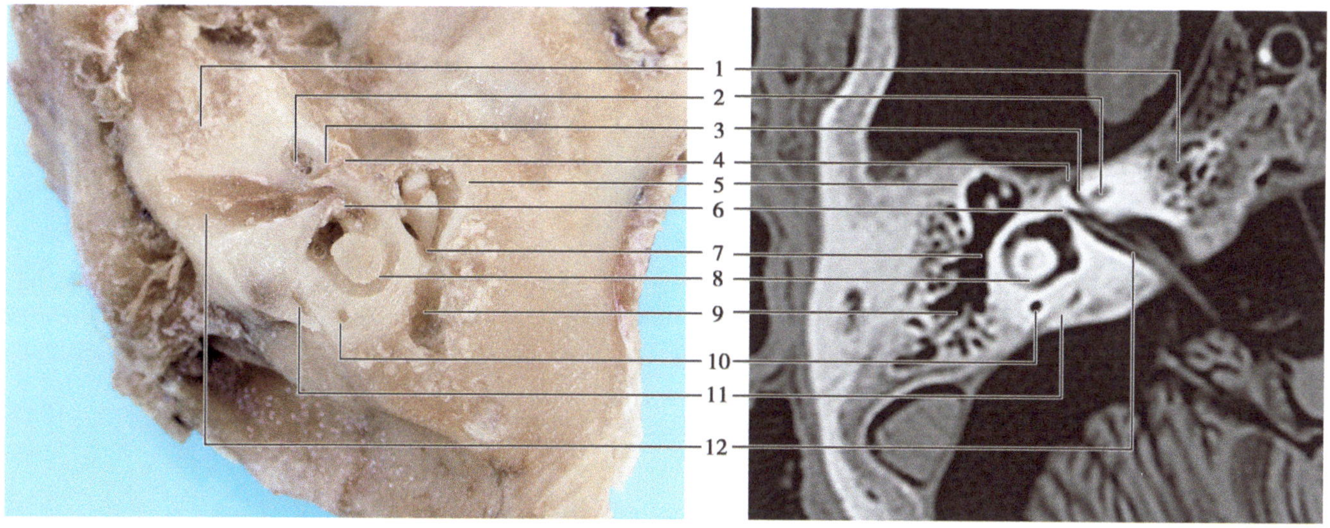

Fig. 2.7 Lateral semicircular canal plane (right). (1) Petrous apex cells. (2) Cochlea. (3) Labyrinth segment of facial nerve (canal). (4) Geniculate ganglion. (5) Tympanic scutum. (6) Superior vestibular nerve. (7) Aditus ad antrum. (8) Lateral semicircular canal. (9) Tympanic antrum. (10) Posterior semicircular canal arch. (11) Vestibular aqueduct (endolymphatic canal). (12) Internal acoustic meatus.

Note: The vestibular aqueduct can be clearly displayed at the level of lateral semicircular canal plane. Enlargement of vestibular aqueduct is one of the most common malformations of the inner ear, which often occurs simultaneously in both ears. The inner diameter of the middle segment of the vestibular aqueduct in enlargement of vestibular aqueduct syndromes is usually more than 1.5 mm.

The lateral semicircular canal protrudes to the aditus ad antrum, it is also one of the important landmarks of the tympanic segment of the facial nerve. Aditus ad antrum is a narrow channel from the epitympanic cavity to the tympanic antrum and mastoid process, when the attic cholesteatoma extends to the mastoid process, it can destroy the lateral semicircular canal arch, leading to the formation of labyrinthine fistula (Fig. 2.7)

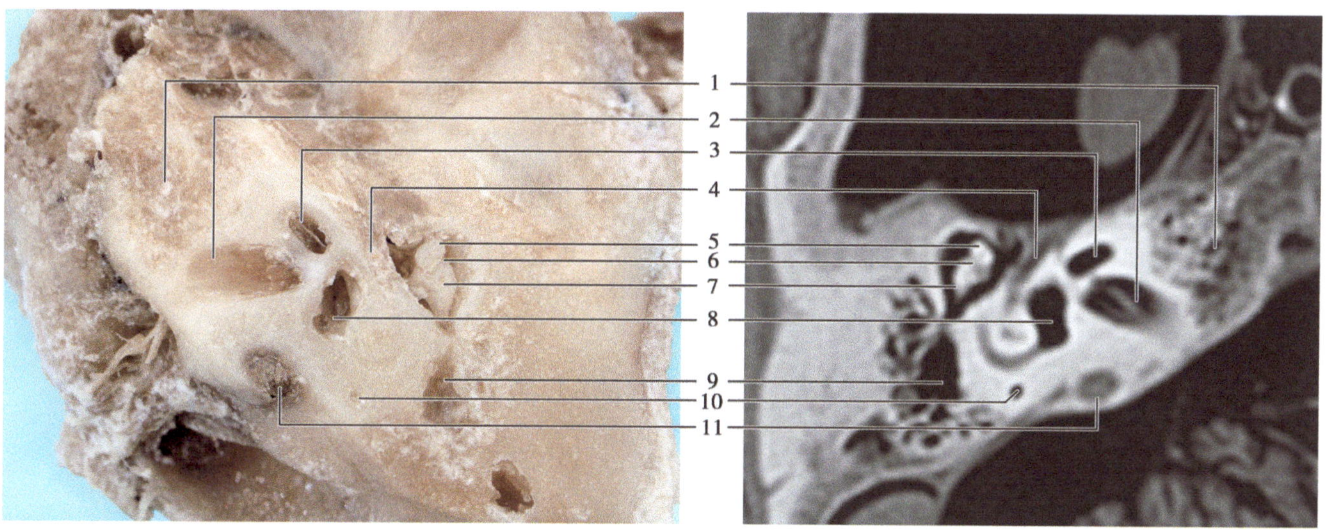

Fig. 2.8 Horizontal segment of facial nerve and incudomalleolar articulation plane (right). (1) Petrous apex cells. (2) Internal acoustic meatus. (3) Cochlea. (4) Horizontal segment of facial nerve canal (tympanic segment). (5) Head of malleus. (6) Incudomalleolar articulation. (7) Body of incus. (8) Vestibule. (9) Tympanic antrum. (10) Posterior semicircular canal arch. (11) Glomus jugular (higher position).

Note: The petrous apex is located in the anteromedial part of the petrous portion of the temporal bone, which is one of the most common sites of cholesterol granuloma and congenital cholesteatoma occurred in temporal bone. The head of the malleus and the body of the incus are located in the epitympanic cavity, arranged anteromedially and posterolaterally, and the medial side of the incudomalleolar articulation is the tympanic segment of the facial nerve. This segment of facial nerve is about 11 mm long, and its lateroinferior canal wall is very thin, and dehiscence of facial nerve canal often occurs here. In the meantime, iatrogenic injure of facial nerve usually take place here during middle ear mastoid surgery (Fig. 2.8)

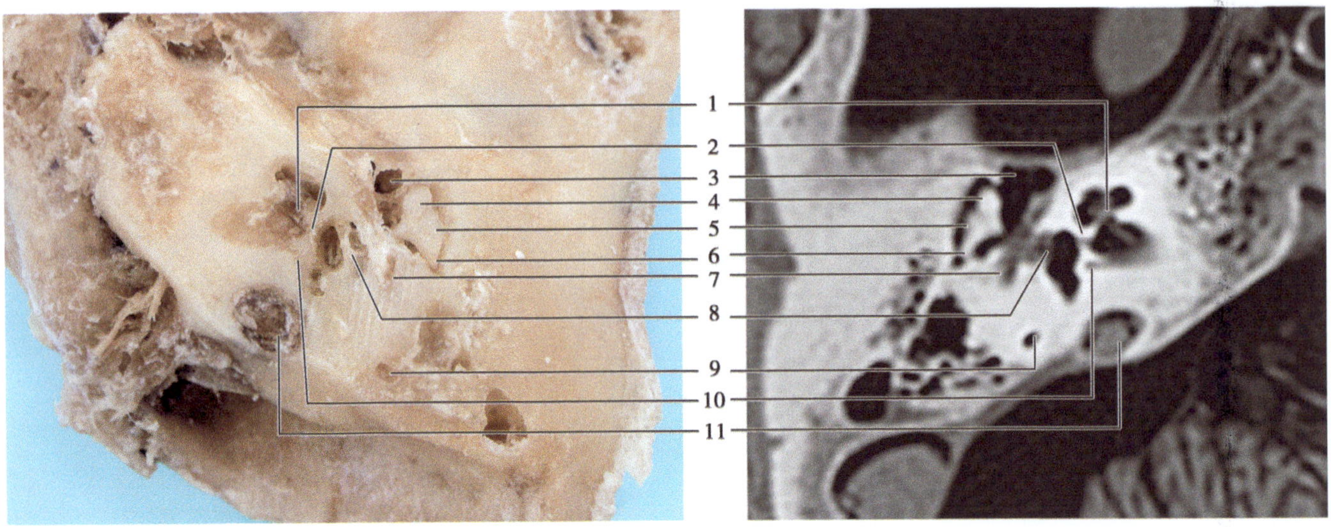

Fig. 2.9 Vestibular window plane (right). (1) Cochlear nerve (foramen). (2) Inferior vestibular nerve (foramen). (3) Anterior recess of epitympanum. (4) Malleus head. (5) Incus body. (6) Short crus of incus and incudal fossa (7) Posterior end of horizontal segment of facial nerve. (8) Footplate of stapes (vestibular window). (9) Posterior semicircular canal arch. (10) Single foramen (posterior ampullary nerve). (11) Glomus jugular.

Note: This plane can clearly show cochlear nerve foramen, inferior vestibular nerve foramen and single foramen. Cochlear foramen stenosis often leads to sensorineural hearing loss, which is mostly unilateral. The anterior recess of the epitympanum, located in the anteromedial part of the malleus head, is often hidden by the Cog's ridge (Fig. 2.9)

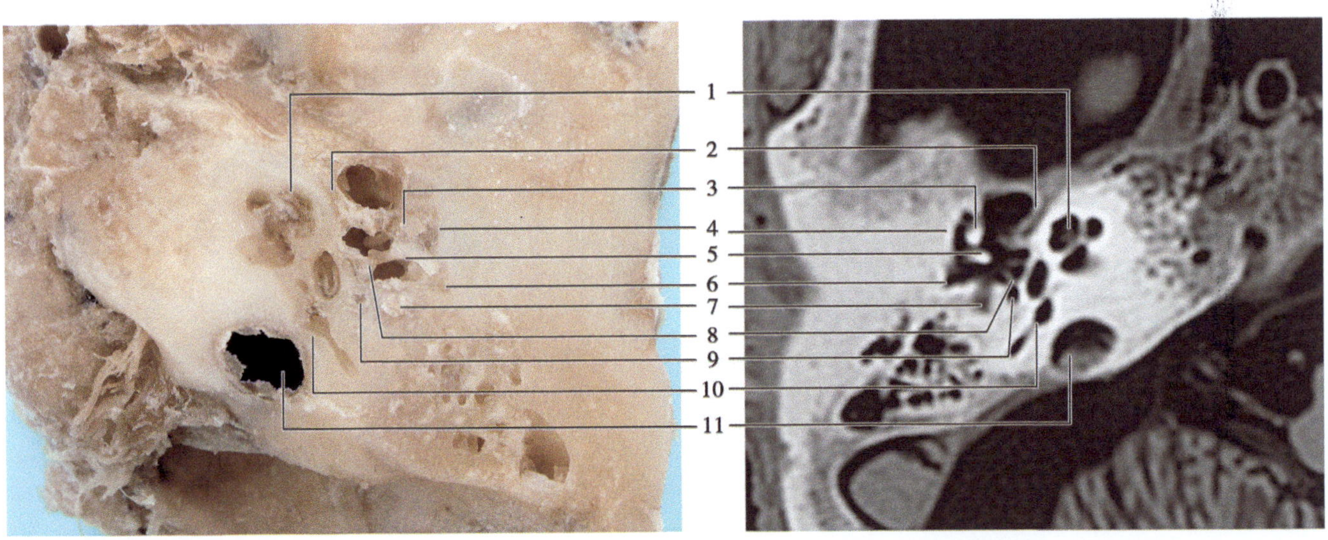

Fig. 2.10 Second genu of facial nerve and stapes & tensor tympani muscle plane (right). (1) Cochlea. (2) Tensor tympani muscle (semicanal). (3) Neck of malleus. (4) Tympanic scutum. (5) Long crus of incus. (6) Facial recess. (7) Second genu of facial nerve. (8) Stapes. (9) Tympanic sinus. (10) Posterior semicircular canal and its ampulla. (11) Glomus jugular.

Note: This plane can display the three turns of cochlea, through which can judge the development of cochlea; Facial recess is one of the approaches for cochlear implantation and exploration of retrotympanum. The anterior and posterior crus of stapes are faintly visible (Fig. 2.10)

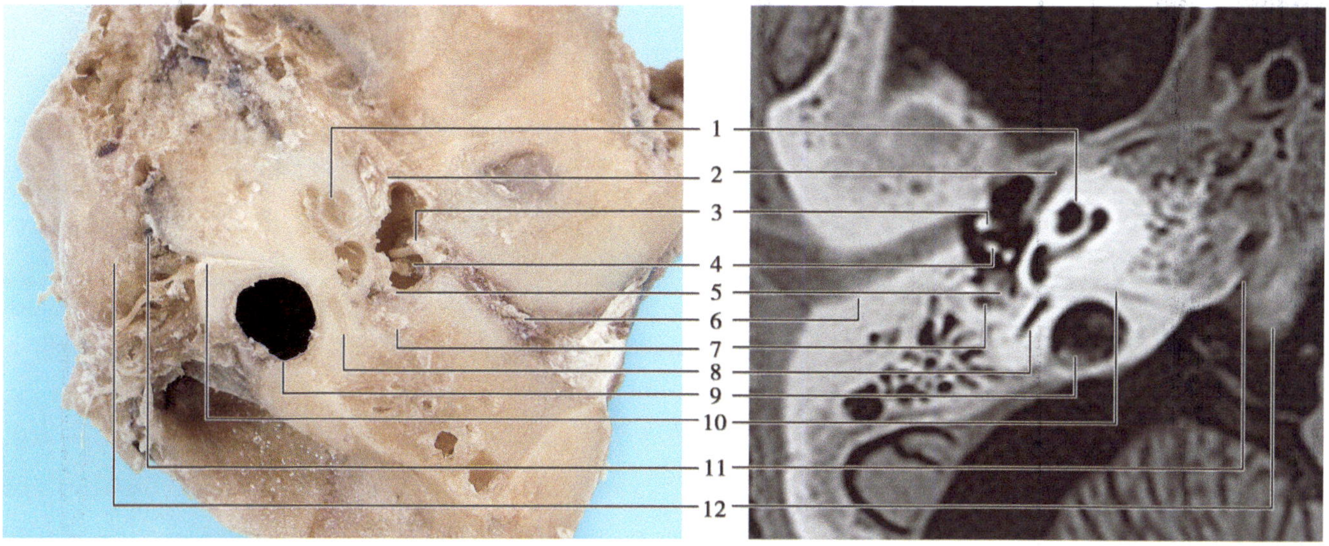

Fig. 2.11 Incudostapedial articulation and pyramidal eminence & cochlear canaliculus plane (right). (1) Cochlea. (2) Tensor tympani muscle (semicanal tube). (3) Manubrium. (4) Incudostapedial articulation (lenticular process, stapes head). (5) Pyramidal eminence. (6) Superior wall of the external auditory canal. (7) Second genu of facial nerve. (8) Posterior semicircular canal. (9) Glomus jugular. (10) Cochlear canaliculus. (11) Petrooccipital fissure. (12) Occipital bone.

Note: Pyramid eminence (stapes tendon) is located at the anteromedial side of the facial nerve trunk; Cochlear canaliculus is also one of the common sites of temporal bone transverse fracture (Fig. 2.11)

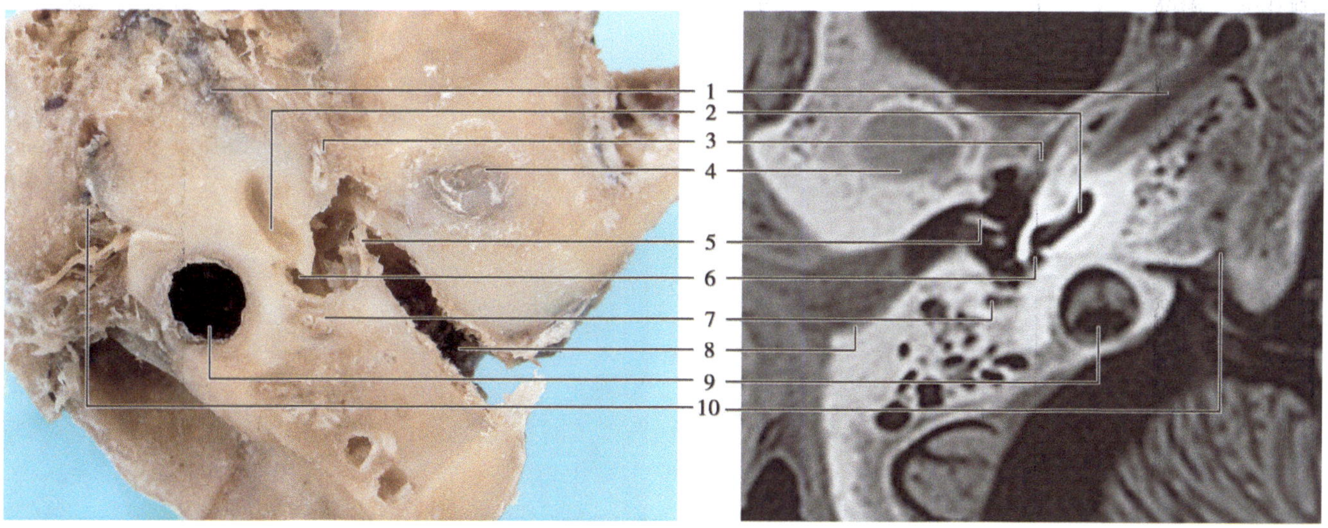

Fig. 2.12 Cochlear window niche plane (right). (1) Horizontal portion of carotid canal. (2) Cochlea. (3) Tensor tympani muscle (semicanal). (4) Top wall of temporomandibular joint. (5) Manubrium. (6) cochlear window niche. (7) Vertical segment of facial nerve (mastoid segment). (8) External auditory canal. (9) Glomus jugular. (10) Petrooccipital fissure.

Note: Cochlear window niche is located in the posteroinferior part of the promontory, which is an important landmark of cochlear implant and Vibrant Soundbridge middle ear implant (Fig. 2.12)

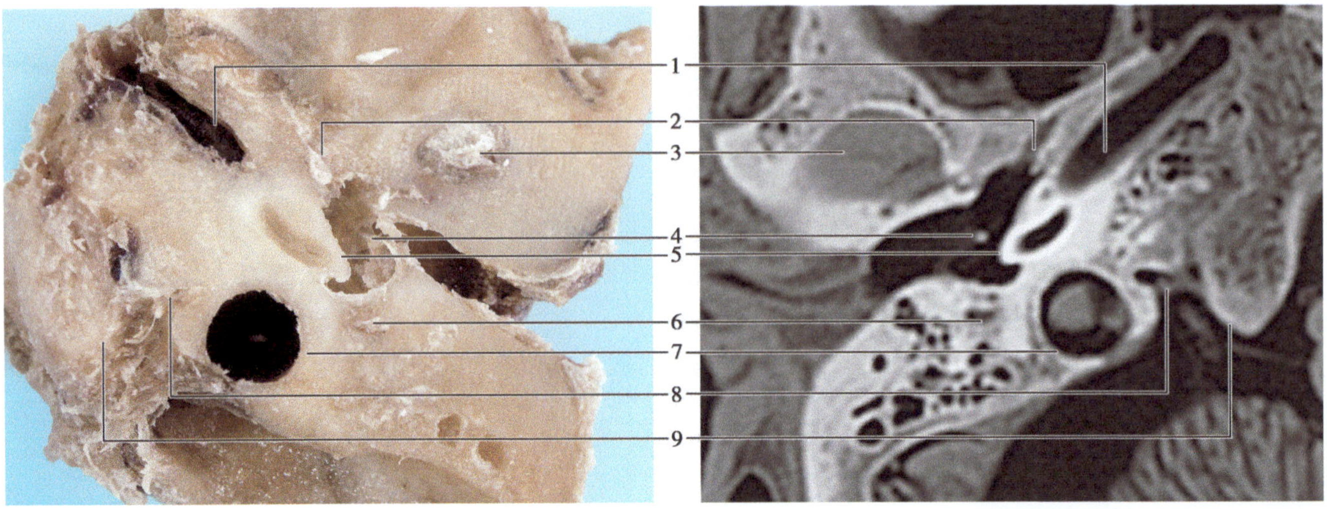

Fig. 2.13 Carotid canal and umbo of manubrium plane(right). (1) Carotid canal. (2) Tensor tympani muscle (semicanal). (3) Temporomandibular joint capsule. (4) Manubrium. (5) Promontory. (6) Vertical segment of facial nerve. (7) Vascular part of jugular foramen. (8) Nerve part of jugular foramen. (9) Occipital bone.

Note: Eustachian tube is located at the middle and upper part of the anterior wall of tympanic cavity, carotid canal is located at the medial-anterior side of the anterior wall of tympanic cavity, and the bone between the eustachian tube and the carotid canal is thin, even cracked. The carotid canal is located at the anteroinferior part of the cochlea, and the jugular fossa is located at the posteromedial-inferior part of the cochlea. The mastoid segment of the facial nerve is about 16 mm long. In the sclerotic mastoid, the facial nerve is surrounded by the surrounding dense bone, and the chances of natural dehiscence of the bone canal are less (Yu et al. 2007); When the mastoid process is well pneumatized, it is difficult to recognize the facial nerve in axial view, especially when there is obstructive inflammation or bone destruction in the surrounding cells (Fig. 2.13)

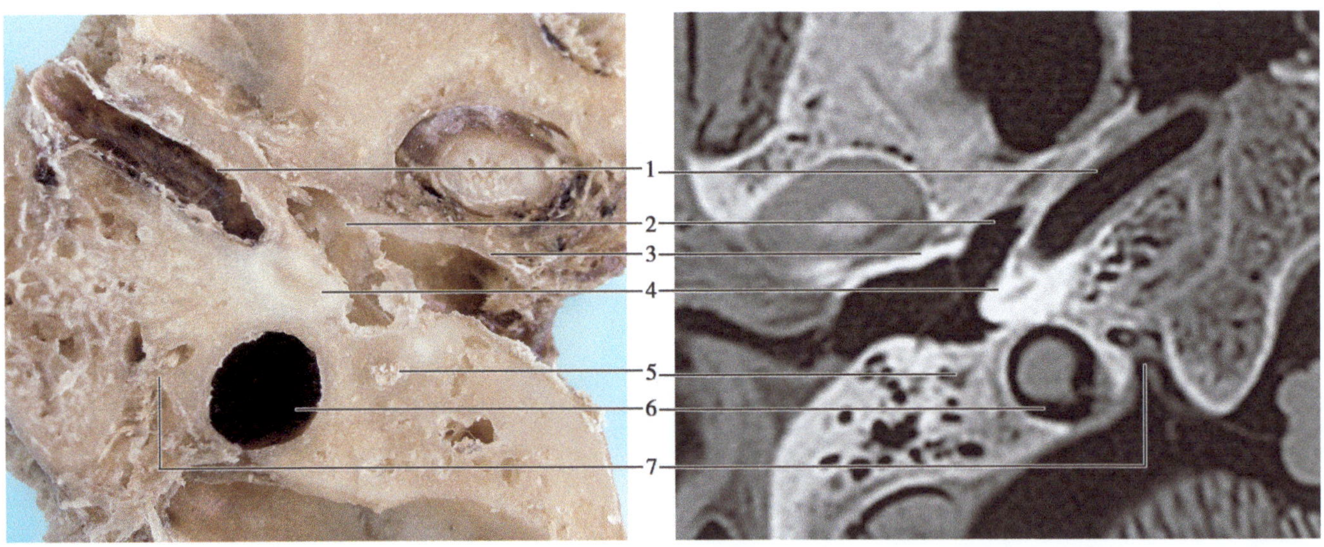

Fig. 2.14 Basal turn of cochlea plane (right). (1) Horizontal portion of internal carotid. (2) Tympanic orifice of eustachian tube. (3) Anterior wall of external auditory canal. (4) Basal turn of cochlea. (5) Facial nerve. (6) Vascular part of jugular foramen. (7) Nerve part of jugular foramen.

Note: Tympanic portion of temporal bone forms the posterior wall of temporomandibular joint, namely the anterior wall of external auditory canal (Fig. 2.14)

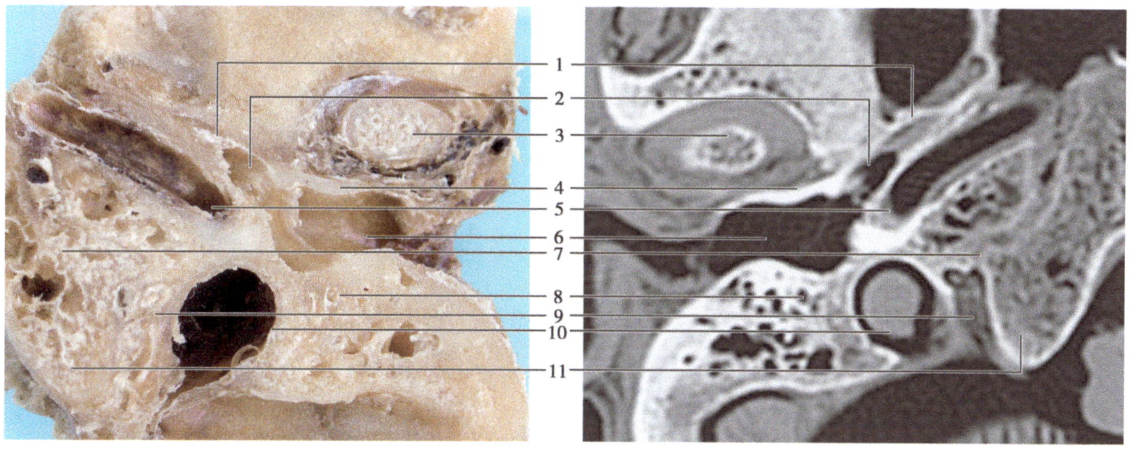

Fig. 2.15 Eustachian tube and carotid canal plane (right). (1)Tube of tensor tympani muscle. (2) Eustachian tube. (3) Process of temporomandibular joint. (4) Anterior wall of external auditory canal. (5) Horizontal portion of carotid canal. (6) External auditory canal. (7) Petroccipital fissure. (8) Facial nerve. (9) Nerve part of jugular foramen. (10) Vascular part of jugular foramen. (11) Occipital bone.

Note: The outer wall of the carotid tube at this layer is very thin, so when dealing with the lesions of the eustachian tube, we should avoid squeezing the inner wall in order to avoid fatal hemorrhage caused by internal carotid injury (Fig. 2.15)

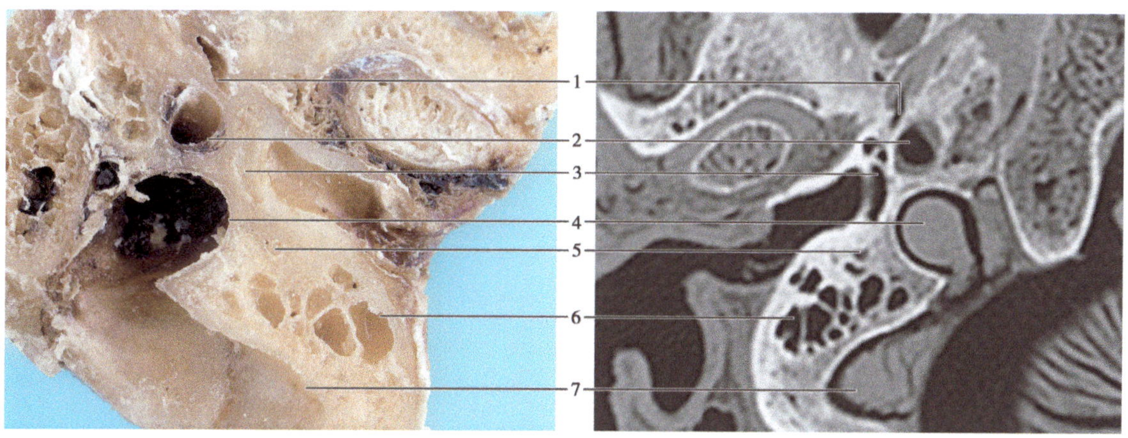

Fig. 2.16 Hypotympanum plane (right). (1) Eustachian tube. (2) Vertical portion of carotid canal. (3) Hypotympanum. (4) Glomus jugular. (5) Facial nerve. (6) Mastoid air cell. (7) Sigmoid sulcus.

Note: This plane of eustachian tube is at the junction of bone and cartilage, with a smaller diameter; the semicanal of the tensor tympani muscle is approximately parallel to the eustachian tube and moves forward, inward and downward. In addition, the facial nerve at this level is located on the longitudinal extension line of the tympanic membrane (tympanic annulus plane). When cholesteatoma of the external auditory canal erodes the bone of the external auditory canal, the facial nerve may be exposed. Osteoporosis, loss or destruction of the anterior wall of the sigmoid sulcus is one of the important signs of intracranial complications caused by otitis media and mastoiditis (Fig. 2.16)

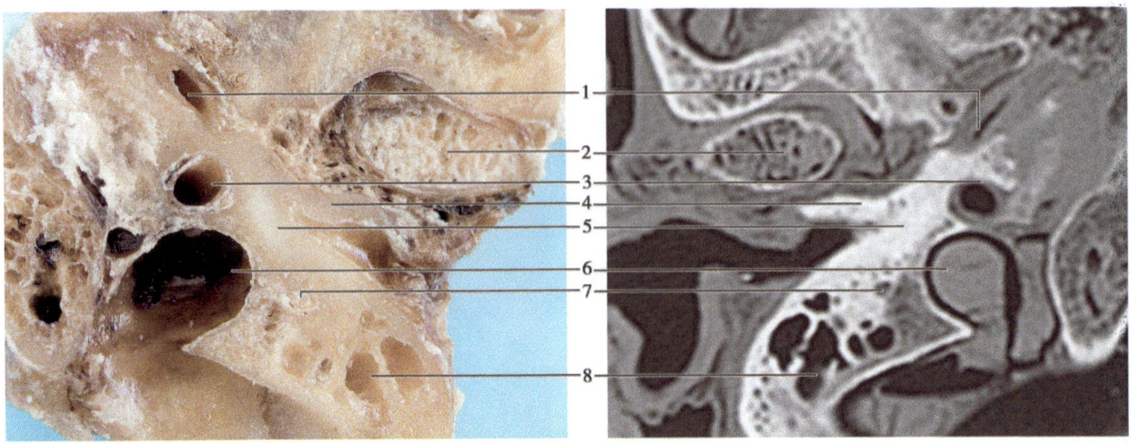

Fig. 2.17 Inferior wall of tympanic cavity plane(right). (1) Eustachian tube cartilage. (2) Mandibular ascending branch. (3) Carotid canal. (4) Anterior wall of external auditory canal. (5) Inferior wall of tympanic cavity. (6) Glomus jugular. (7) Vertical portion of facial nerve. (8) Cells of mastoid tip

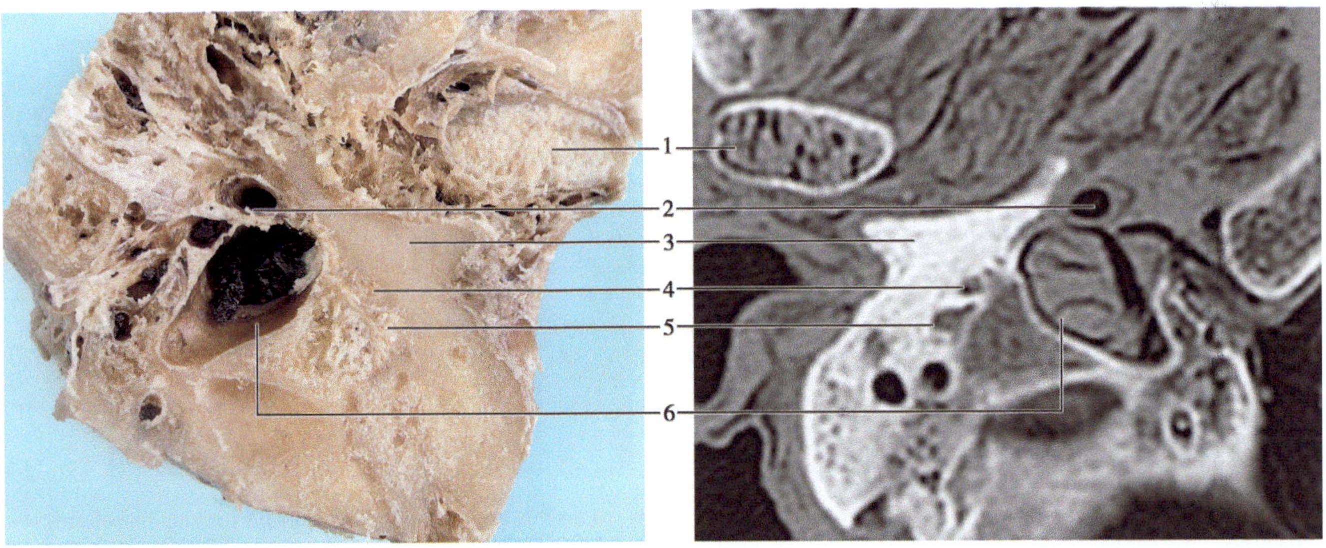

Fig. 2.18 Inferior wall of external auditory canal plane(right). (1) Ascending branch of the mandible. (2) Internal carotid. (3) Inferior wall of external auditory canal. (4) Bone marrow of styloid process. (5) Stylomastoid foramen. (6) Internal jugular vein.

Note: The inferior wall of the external auditory canal is composed of tympanic portion of temporal bone. The stylomastoid foramen is the place where the facial nerve comes out of the skull and is located between the styloid process and the mastoid tip. The styloid bone marrow is easily confused with the facial nerve canal (Fig. 2.18)

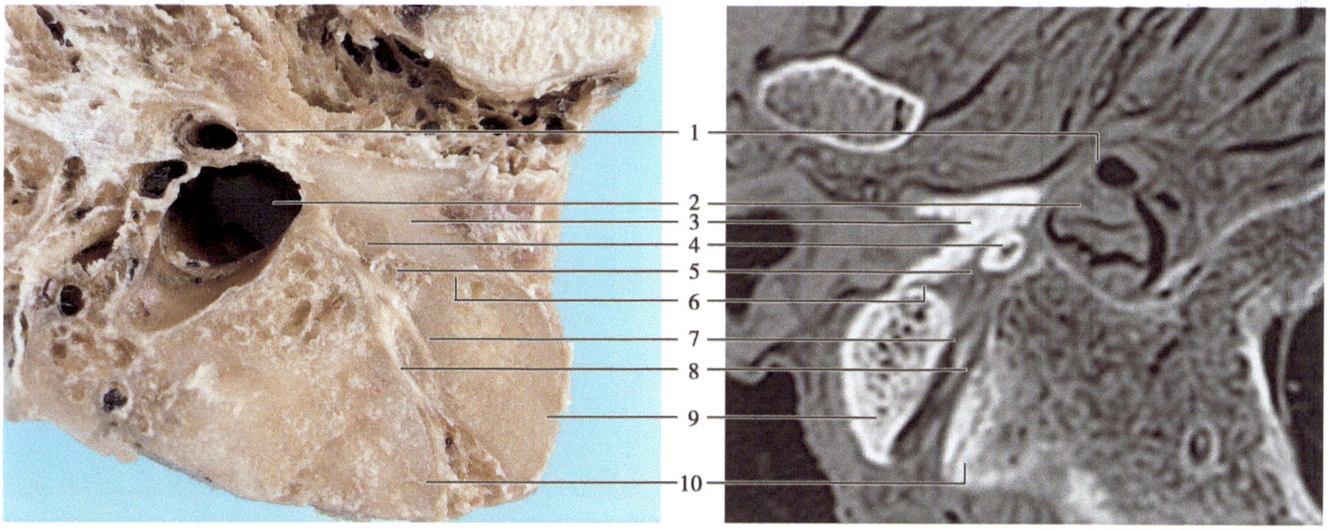

Fig. 2.19 Digastric muscle groove plane (right). (1) Internal carotid. (2) Internal jugular vein. (3) Inferior wall of external auditory canal. (4) Styloid process. (5) Facial nerve. (6) Tympanomastoid fissure. (7) Digastric muscle groove. (8) Occipital artery groove. (9) Mastoid tip. (10) Occipital bone.

Note: Tympanomastoid fissure can be used as one of the mastoid segment landmarks of facial nerve. Pus in mastoid can spread along the sternocleidomastoid muscle to the neck via the destroyed medial bone cortex of the mastoid process, forming Bezold abscess, deep neck abscess, etc.

2.3 Comparison of Sectional Anatomy and CT of Temporal Bone: Coronal View

Coronal CT scan of temporal bone can clearly display the structures of superior and inferior(basal)walls of external auditory canal, tympanic scutum, auditory ossicles (including malleolus and incus joints), tegmen tympani, bony labyrinth, vestibular window and cochlear window niche, medial and lateral walls of vertical segment of facial nerve canal, superior and inferior walls & fundus of internal acoustic meatus, etc., but it is poor in the display of anterior and posterior crus of stapes, inferior wall of tympanic segment of facial nerve, bony canal of second genu of facial nerve, facial recess, vestibular aqueduct, cochlear canaliculus, and anterior wall of sigmoid sulcus. This chapter will show the coronal sectional anatomy of the left temporal bone and its corresponding two-dimensional CT images, from the cartilaginous part of the eustachian tube to the endolymphatic sac (Figs. 2.20, 2.21, 2.22, 2.23, 2.24, 2.25, 2.26, 2.27, 2.28, 2.29, 2.30, 2.31, 2.32, 2.33, 2.34, 2.35, 2.36, 2.37, and 2.38).

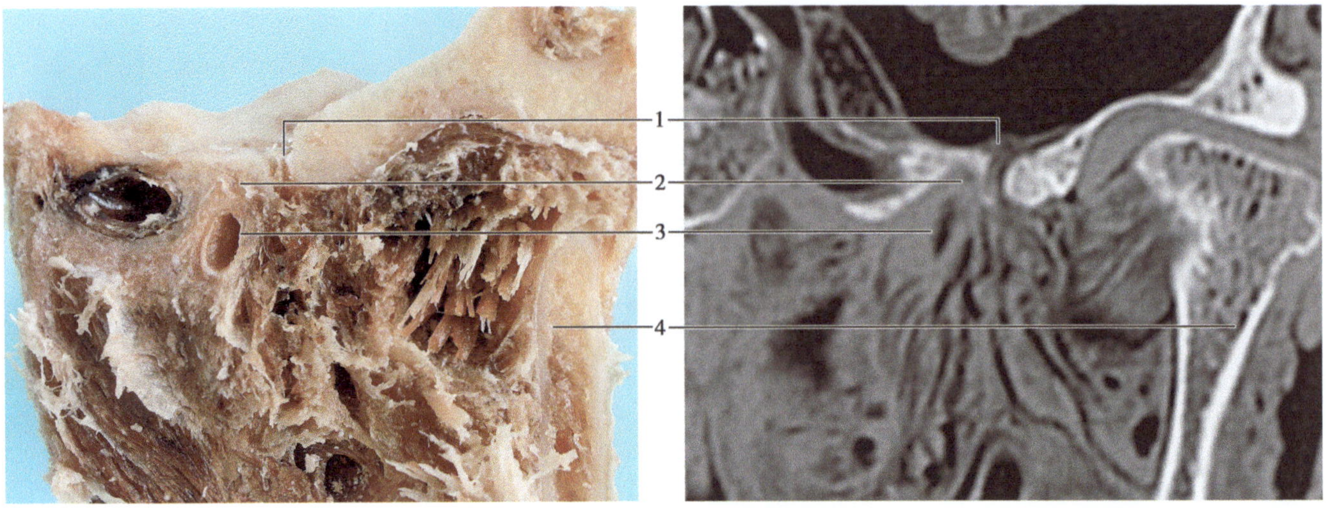

Fig. 2.20 Cartilage portion of eustachian tube and spinous foramen plane (left). (1) Spinous foramen. (2) Semicanal of tensor tympani. (3) Eustachian tube. (4) Mandible

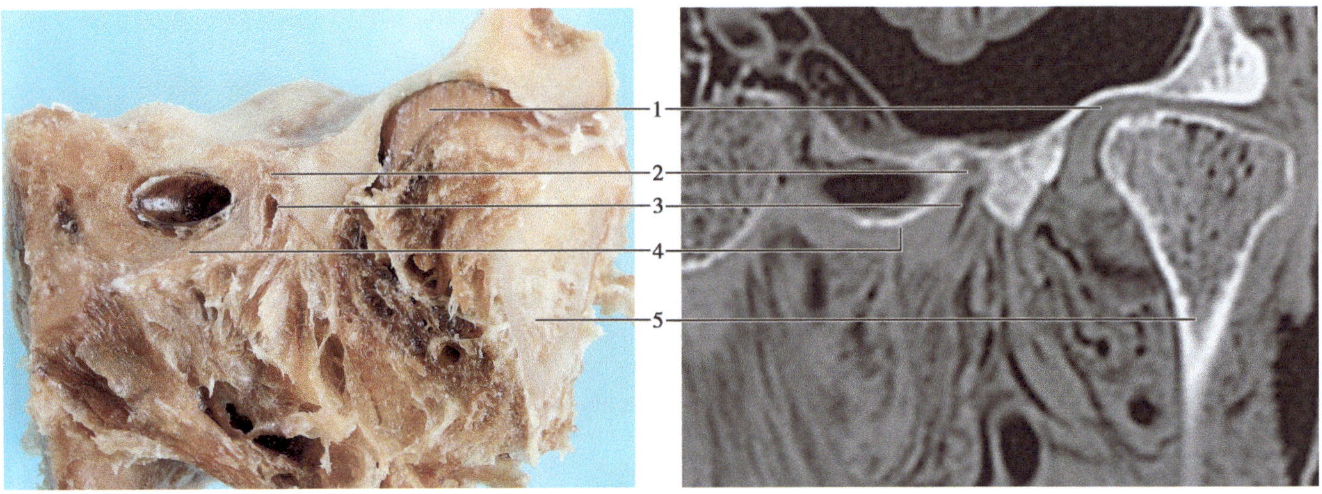

Fig. 2.21 Junction plane of bone and cartilage portion of eustachian tube (left). (1) The temporomandibular joint fossa and joint disc. (2) Semicanal of tensor tympani muscle. (3) Eustachian tube. (4) Horizontal portion of carotid canal. (5) Ascending branch of the mandible

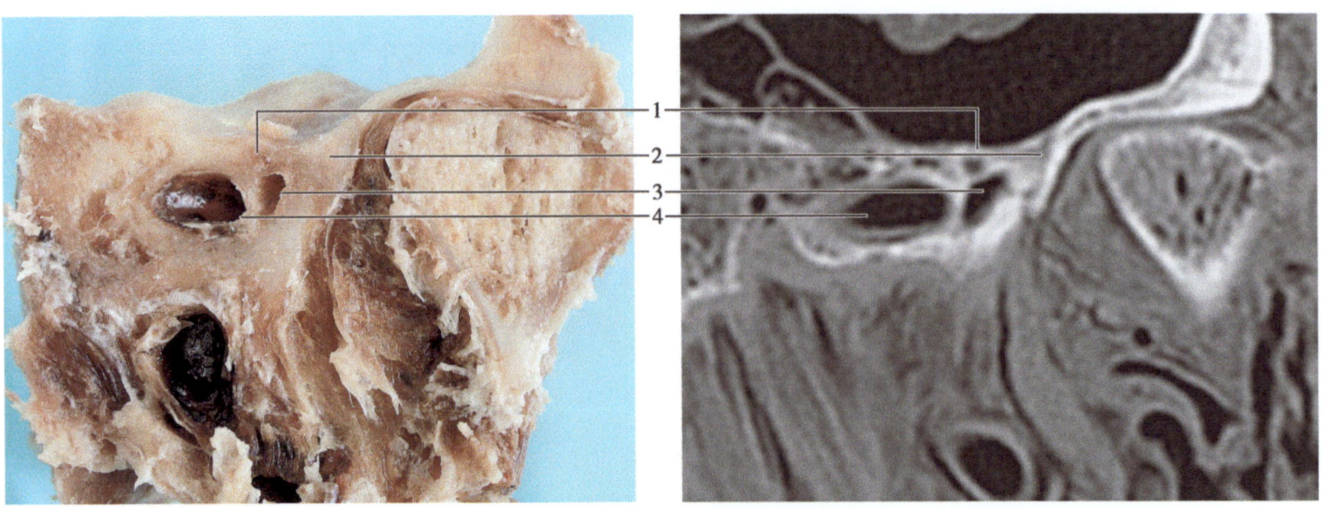

Fig. 2.22 Bony portion of eustachian tube plane (left). (1) Semicanal of tensor tympanic muscle. (2) Petrosquamous fissure. (3) Eustachian tube. (4) Horizontal portion of carotid canal.

Note: The semicanal of tensor tympanic muscle and eustachian tube arrange up and down; The horizontal portion of the carotid canal is located medial side the eustachian tube (Fig. 2.22)

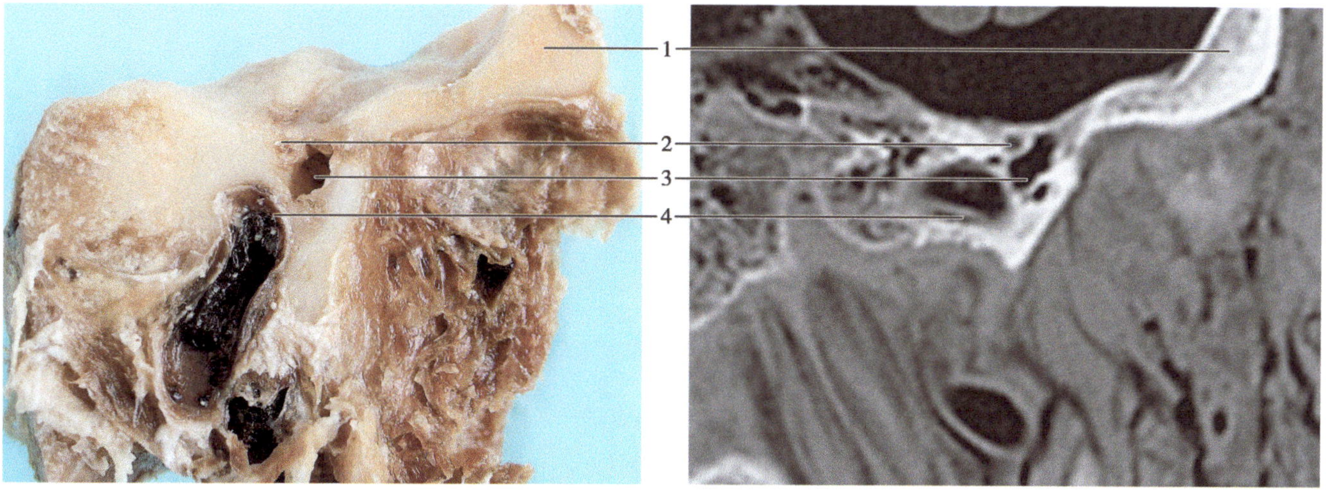

Fig. 2.23 Tympanic orifice of eustachian tube plane (left). (1) Squamous portion of temporal bone. (2) Semicanal of tensor tympanic muscle. (3) Eustachian tube. (4) Carotid canal.

Note: This plane is only separated by very thin bone plane between internal carotid canal and eustachian tube

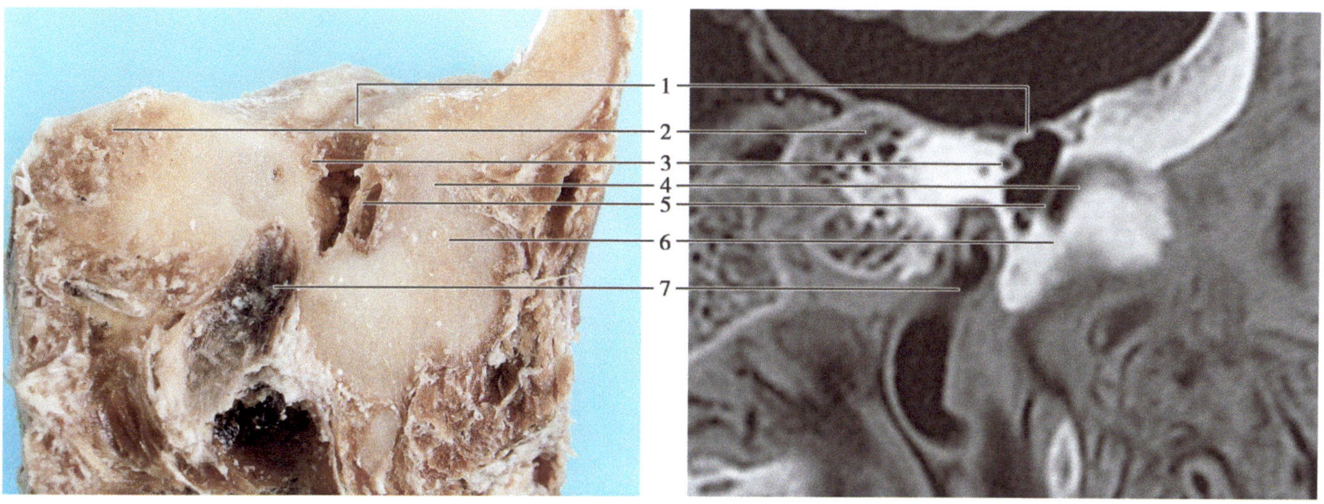

Fig. 2.24 Anterior inferior corner of external auditory canal plane (left). (1) Tegmen tympani. (2) Cells of petrous apex. (3) Semicanal of tensor tympanic muscle. (4) Anterior wall of external auditory canal. (5) Tympanic membrane. (6) Inferior wall of external auditory canal. (7) Vertical portion of the carotid canal.

Note: The anterior wall of the external auditory canal is mainly composed of the tympanic portion of the temporal bone (Fig. 2.24)

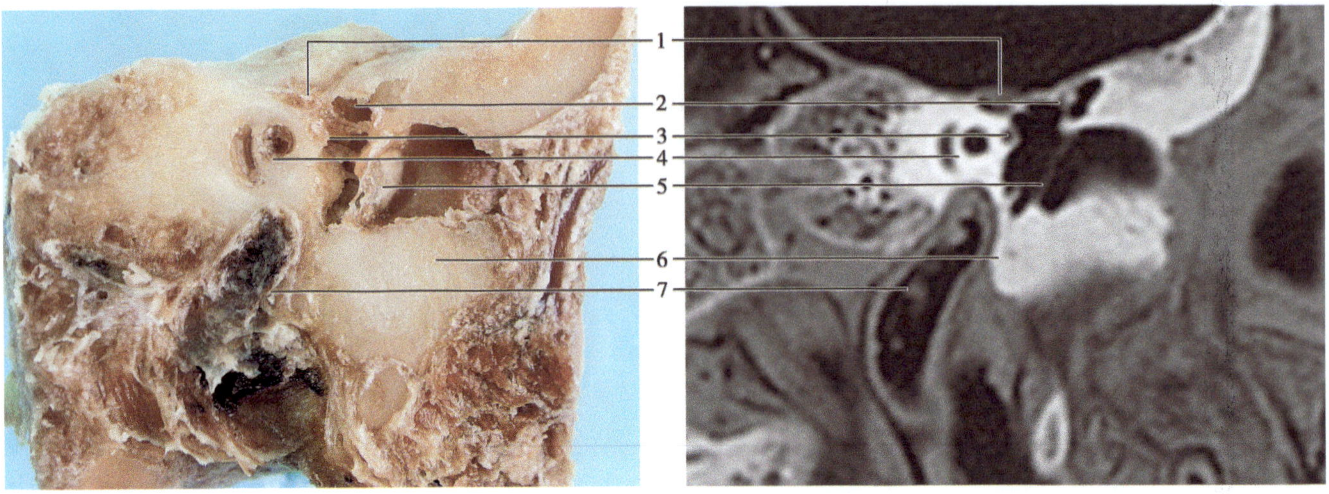

Fig. 2.25 Geniculate ganglion of facial nerve plane (left). (1) Geniculate ganglion of facial nerve. (2) Epitympanum(attic). (3) Semicanal of tensor tympani muscle. (4) Cochlea. (5) Tympanic membrane. (6) Inferior wall of external auditory canal. (7) Carotid canal.

Note: The geniculate ganglion of facial nerve is located in the medial-superior part of the semicanal of tensor tympani muscle, the distance between them is very short (Fig. 2.25)

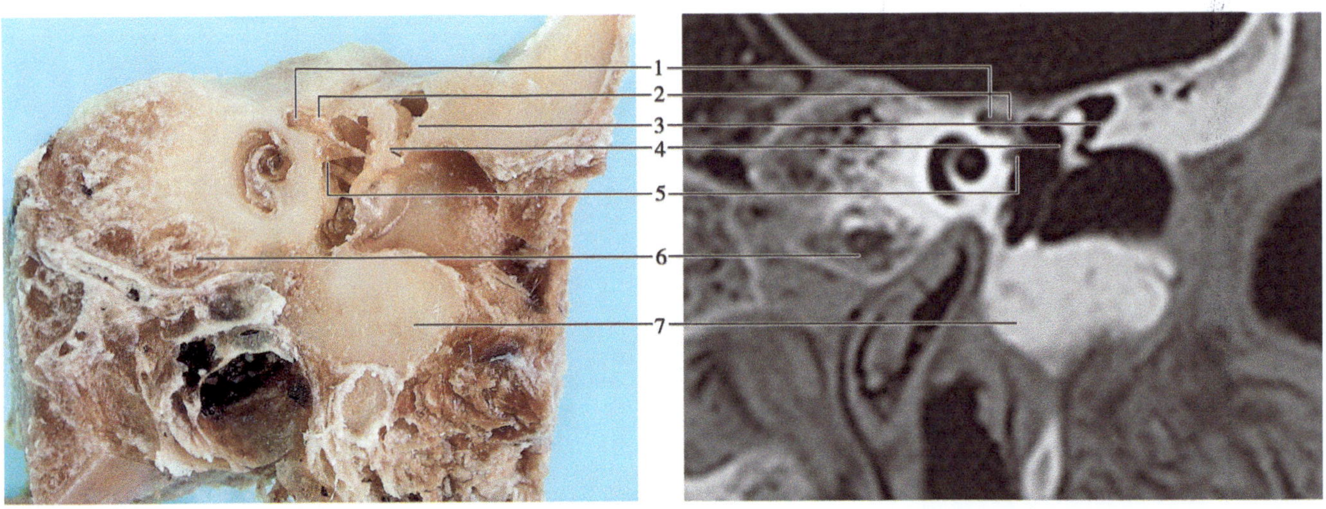

Fig. 2.26 Horizontal segment of facial nerve and malleus head (left). (1) Labyrinth segment of facial nerve. (2) Horizontal segment of facial nerve (tympanic segment). (3) Tympanic scutum. (4) Malleus. (5) Processus cochleariformis. (6) Cells of petrous apex. (7) Tympanic portion of the temporal bone (inferior wall of external auditory canal).

Note: At the level of the malleus head, the facial nerve is divided into the labyrinth segment (located in the bone above the cochlea) and the tympanic segment of facial nerve, both of which are arranged in a hawk-eye shape in coronal CT view. The head of malleus is located in the epitympanum, and its outer side is the tympanic scutum. The gap between the pars flaccida of the tympanic membrane, the tympanic scutum and the neck of the malleus is called the Prussak space, which is a favored location for a secondary acquired cholesteatoma (Barath et al. 2011). On CT, erosion of the scutum and ossicles by a focal rounded opacity in Prussak space is highly suggestive of an acquired attic cholesteatoma (Juliano, 2018) (Fig. 2.26)

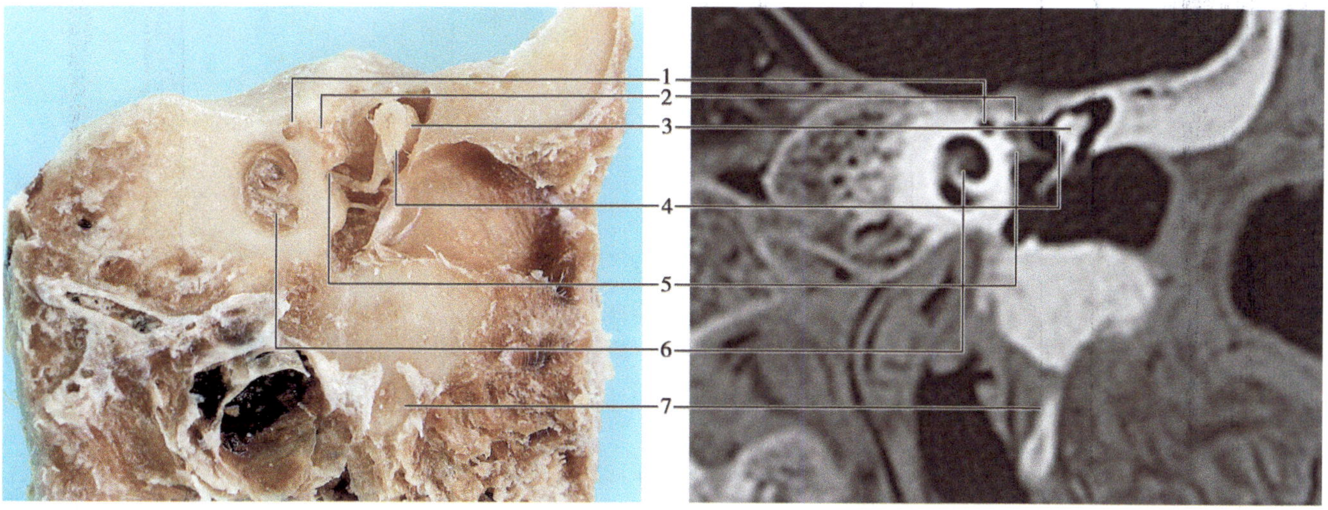

Fig. 2.27 Incudomalleolar articulation and processus cochleariformis plane (left). (1) Labyrinth segment of facial nerve. (2) Horizontal segment of facial nerve. (3) Body of incus. (4) Head of malleus. (5) Processus cochleariformis. (6) Cochlea. (7) Styloid process.

Note: The horizontal segment of facial nerve at this plane is located above the processus cochleariformis. Tensor tympani tendon extends outward to and attaches to the medial side of the neck of the malleus (Fig. 2.27)

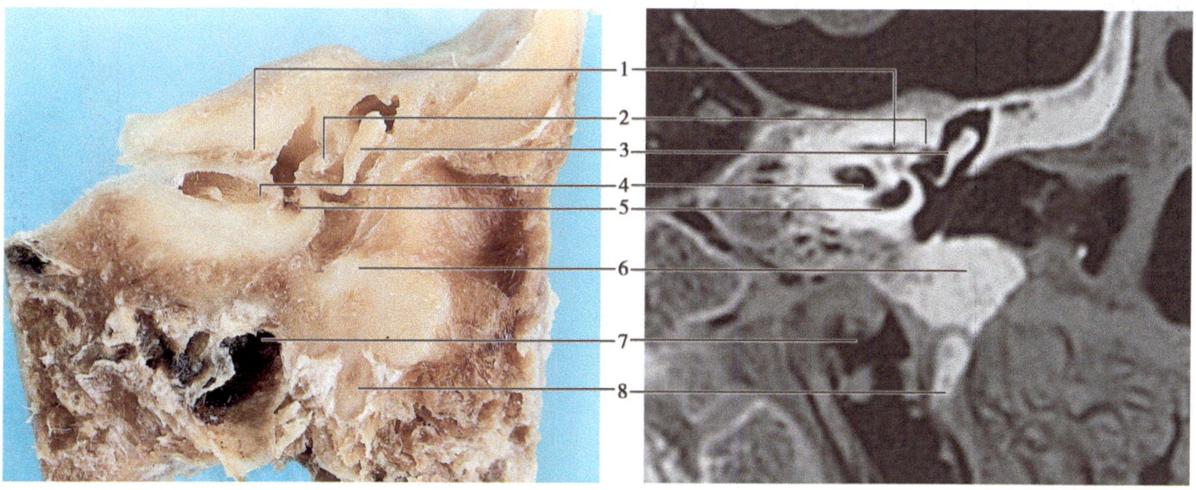

Fig. 2.28 Long crus and body of incus plane (left). (1) Internal acoustic meatus segment of facial nerve. (2) Horizontal segment of facial nerve. (3) Body and long crus of incus. (4) Cochlear nerve. (5) Cochlea. (6) Inferior wall of external auditory canal. (7) Internal jugular vein. (8) Styloid process

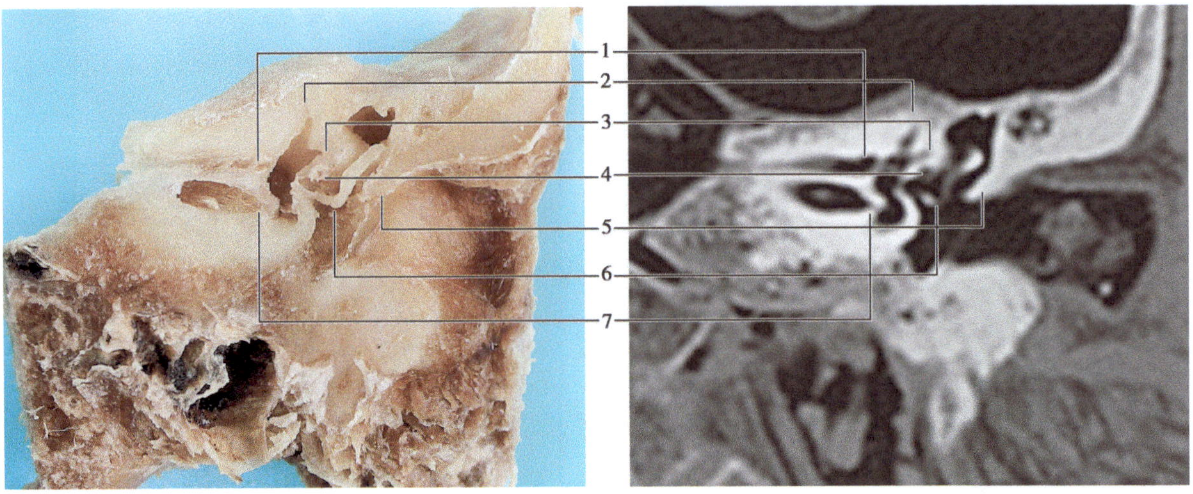

Fig. 2.29 Incudostapedial articulation plane (left). (1) Internal acoustic meatus segment of facial nerve. (2) Arcuate eminence and anterior semicircular canal. (3) Lateral semicircular canal. (4) Horizontal portion of facial nerve. (5) Tympanic scutum. (6) Incudostapedial articulation. (7) Cochlear nerve foramen.

Note: Facial nerve at this plane is located below the lateral semicircular canal (Fig. 2.29)

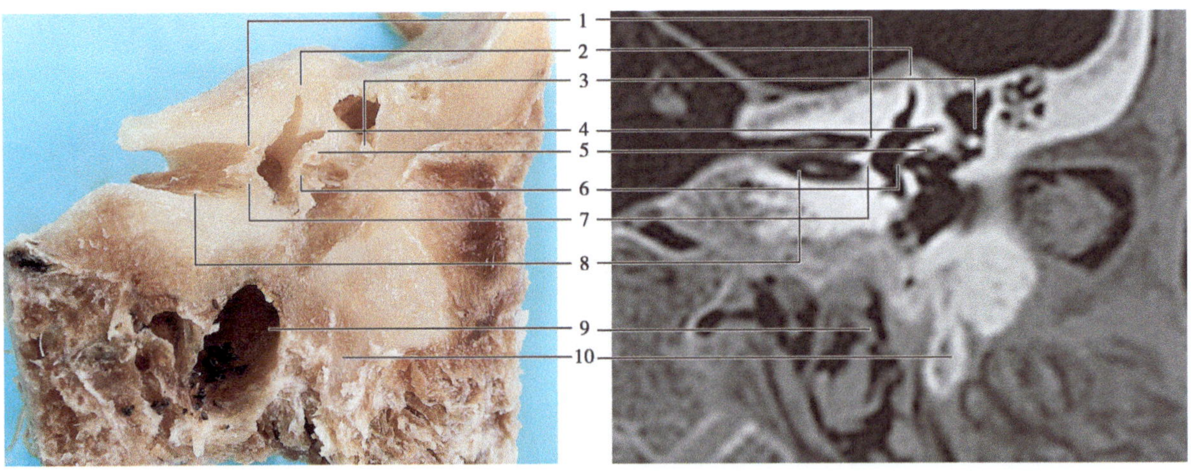

Fig. 2.30 Vestibular window plane (left). (1) Superior vestibular nerve. (2) Anterior crus of anterior semicircular canal. (3) Short crus of the incus and aditus ad antrum. (4) Anterior crus of lateral semicircular canal. (5) Facial nerve. (6) Vestibular window. (7) Inferior vestibular nerve. (8) Internal acoustic meatus. (9) Jugular fossa. (10) Styloid process.

Note: This segment of the facial nerve is located between the vestibular window and the lateral semicircular canal, and the dehiscence of the facial nerve canal often occurs above the vestibular window. The vestibular window is approximately oval, slightly inclined outward, and occasionally the stenosis or atresia of this window can occur. The short crus of the incus is located at the inferior wall of the aditus ad antrum and is an important sign of the second genu of the facial nerve (Fig. 2.30)

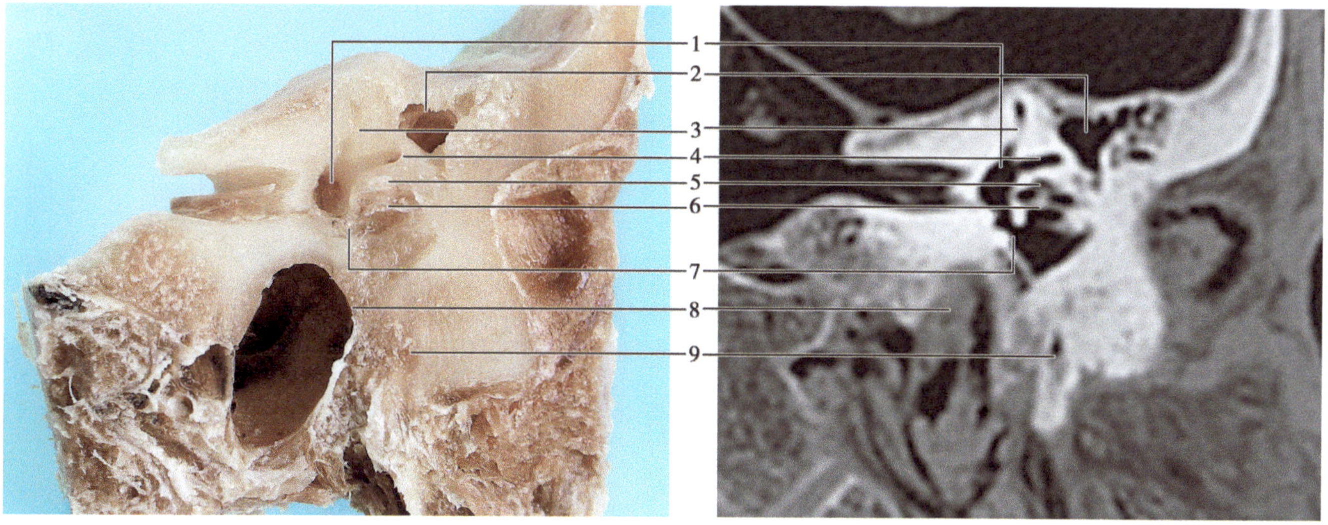

Fig. 2.31 Cochlear window plane (left). (1) Vestibule. (2) Aditus ad antrum. (3) Anterior crus of anterior semicircular canal. (4) Anterior crus of lateral semicircular canal. (5) Facial nerve. (6) Pyramidal eminence. (7) Cochlear window niche. (8) Jugular fossa. (9) Bone marrow of styloid process.

Note: The cochlear window niche opens in posterior inferior tympanum (Fig. 2.31)

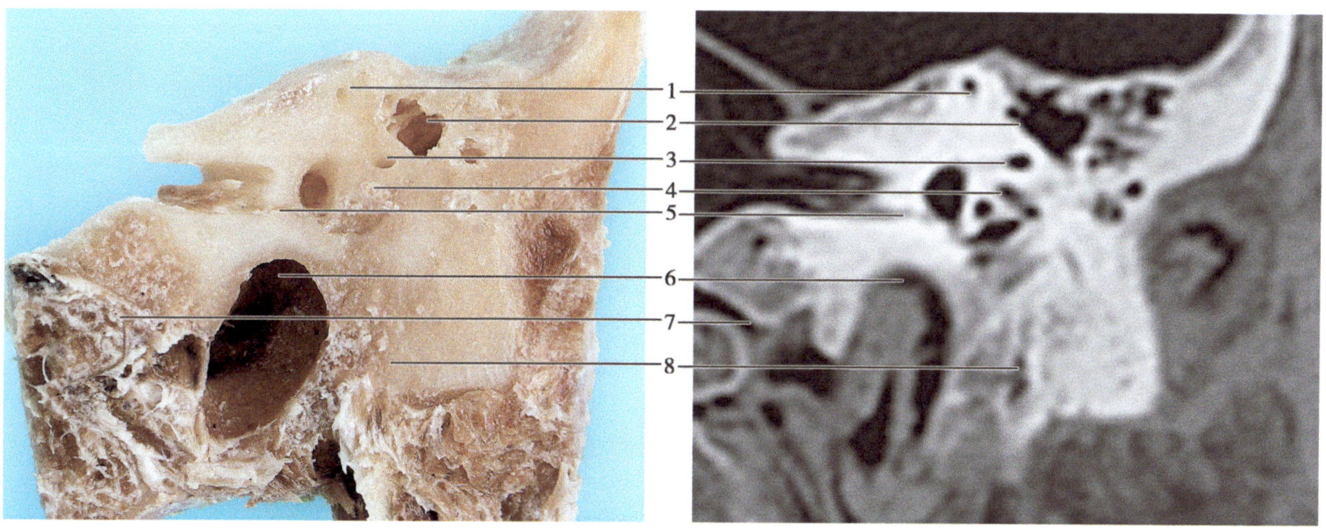

Fig. 2.32 Singular foramen nerve plane (left). (1) Anterior semicircular canal. (2) Tympanic antrum. (3) Lateral semicircular canal. (4) Facial nerve. (5) Singular foramen nerve. (6) Jugular fossa. (7) Petroccipital fissure. (8) Bone marrow of styloid process

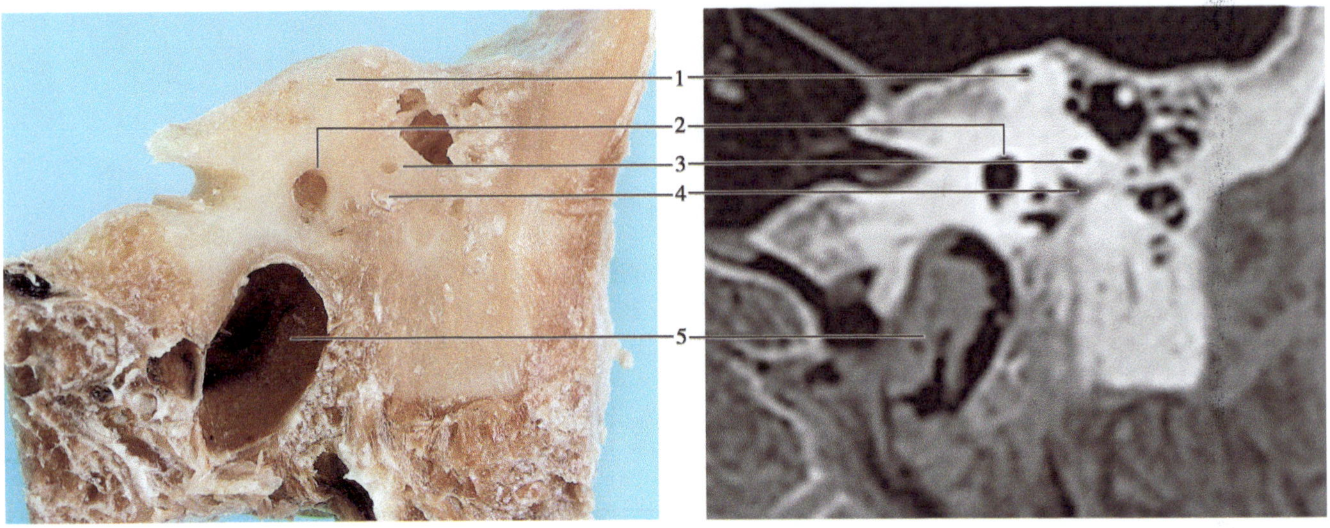

Fig. 2.33 Second genu of facial nerve plane(left). (1) Anterior semicircular canal. (2) Vestibule. (3) Lateral semicircular canal. (4) Second genus of facial nerve. (5) Jugular fossa.

Note: The second genu of facial nerve is not easy to recognize in coronal view, but it is under the lateral semicircular canal, so the lateral semicircular canal can be one of its landmarks. The natural dehiscence of the anterior semicircular canal is easier to find on the coronal view, but the size and position of the dehiscence are easier to observe on the oblique sagittal view (Fig. 2.33)

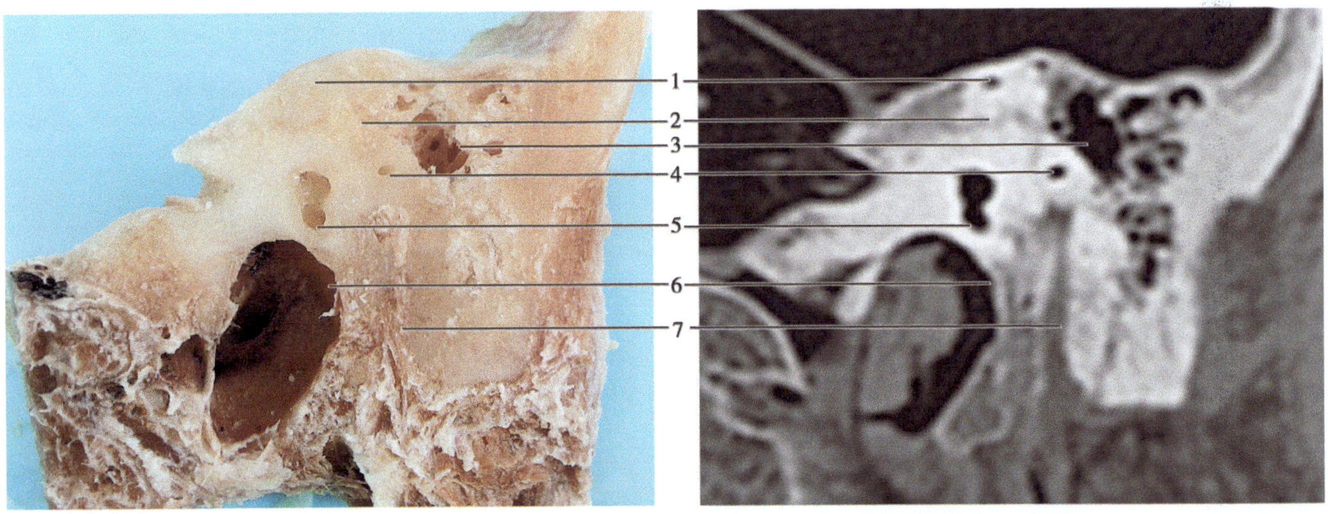

Fig. 2.34 Petromastoid canal plane (left). (1) Anterior semicircular canal. (2) Petromastoid canal. (3) Tympanic antrum. (4) Lateral semicircular canal. (5) Posterior semicircular canal ampulla. (6) Jugular fossa. (7) Vertical (mastoid) segment of facial nerve.

Note: The petromastoid canal is located under the anterior semicircular canal arch and above the lateral semicircular canal in the relatively loose bone, communicating the tympanic antrum and posterior cranial fossa (Fig. 2.34)

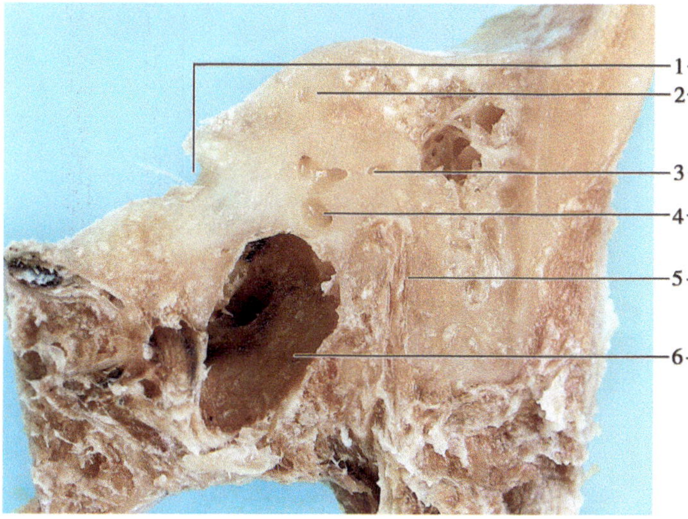

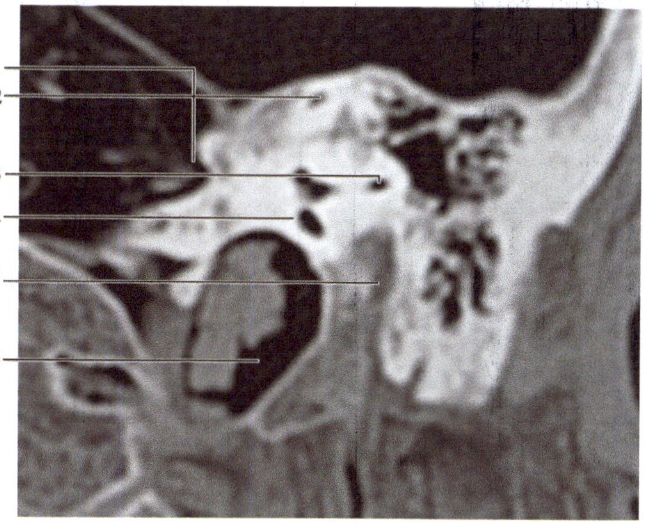

Fig. 2.35 Vertical segment of facial nerve plane (left). (1) Internal acoustic porus. (2) Anterior semicircular canal. (3) Posterior crus of lateral semicircular canal. (4) Ampulla of posterior semicircular canal. (5) Vertical segment of facial nerve. (6) Glomus jugular.

Note: The vertical (mastoid) segment of facial nerve is located between the posterior crus of lateral semicircular canal and the arch of posterior semicircular canal, and courses slightly outward downward (Fig. 2.35)

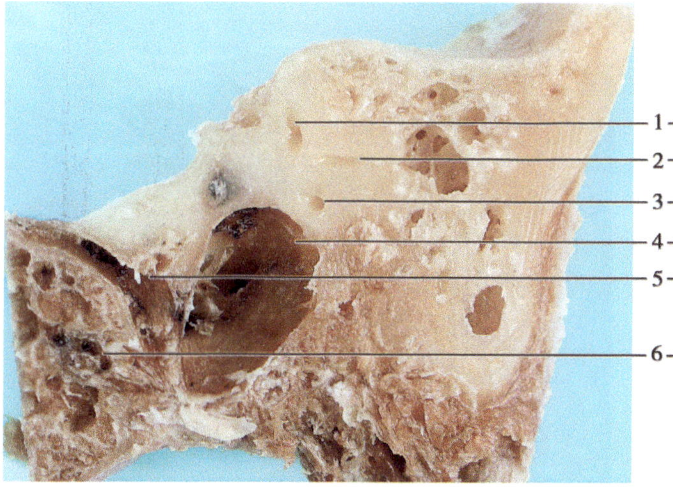

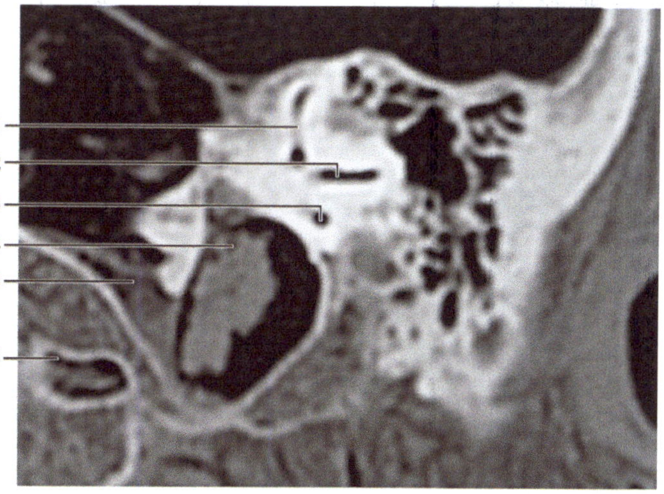

Fig. 2.36 Posterior crus of lateral semicircular canal (left). (1) Posterior crus of anterior semicircular canal. (2) Posterior crus of lateral semicircular canal. (3) Inferior crus of posterior semicircular canal. (4) Vascular part of jugular foramen. (5) Nerve part of jugular foramen. (6) Hypoglossal canal

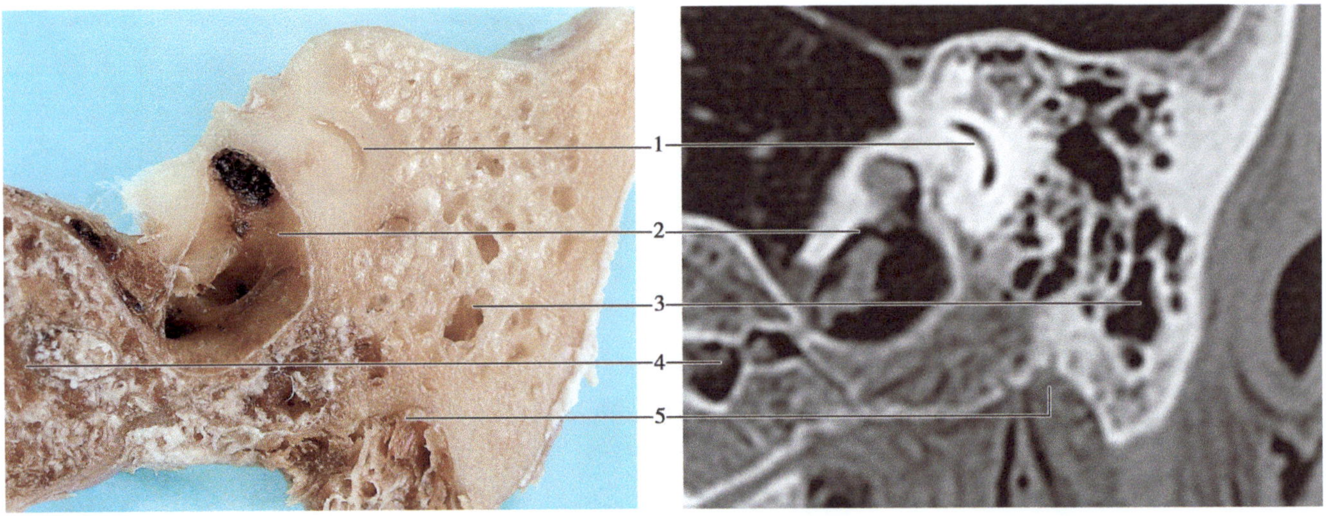

Fig. 2.37 Posterior semicircular canal arch plane (left). (1) Posterior semicircular canal arch. (2) Glomus jugular. (3) Cells of mastoid tip. (4) Hypoglossal nerve canal (in occipital bone). (5) Digastric muscle groove.

Note: The posterior semicircular canal is in an outward semicircular shape with dense surrounding bone; The inflammation of the pneumatized mastoid process can penetrate the lateral bone cortex to form a subperiosteal abscess behind the ear, and the inflammation can penetrate the medial bone cortex of the mastoid process tip to form Bezold abscess

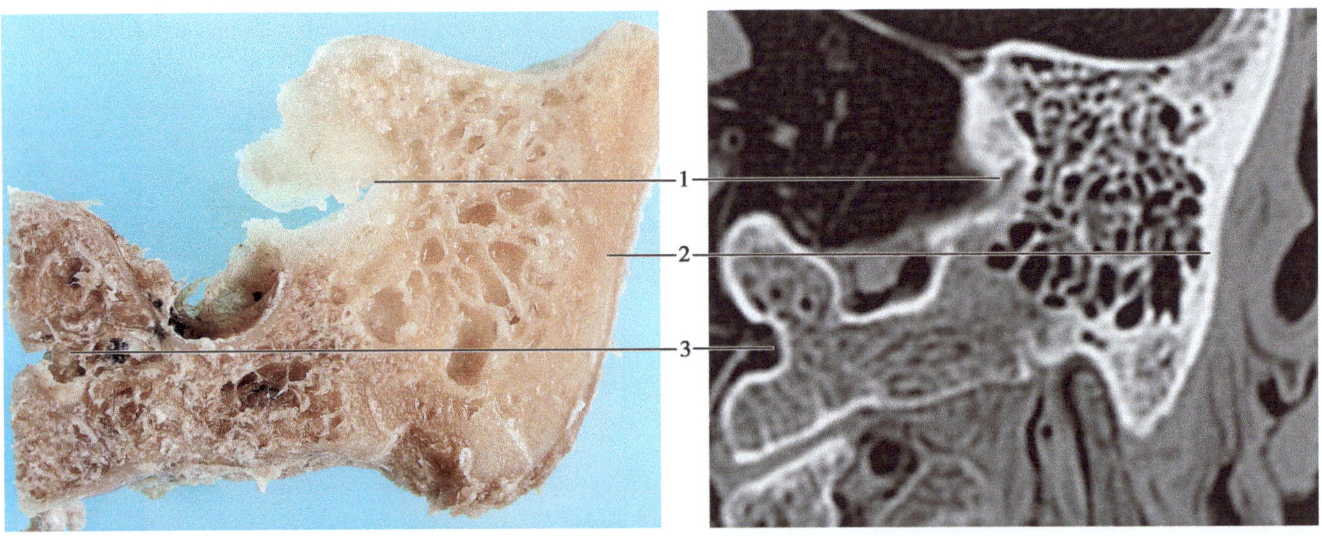

Fig. 2.38 Endolymphatic sac fissure plane (left). (1) Endolymphatic sac fissure. (2) Bone cortex of mastoid process. (3) Internal opening of sublingual nerve canal

2.4 Comparison of Sectional Anatomy and CT of Temporal Bone: Sagittal View

As an important supplement, sagittal CT view is found to be extremely useful for evaluating the diseases which involved the external auditory canal, tegmen tympani, incudomalleolar articulation, infra- and supra-labyrinthine air cell, sigmoid sinus plate, sinodural angle, horizontal and mastoid segment of facial nerve, and internal acoustic meatus (Mafee et al. 1988), but the display of tympanic scutum, vestibular window, footplate of stapes, etc. is not good. This section shows the sagittal view of the left temporal bone and its corresponding two-dimensional CT images, from the bony external auditory canal to the internal acoustic porus (Figs. 2.39, 2.40, 2.41, 2.42, 2.43, 2.44, 2.45, 2.46, 2.47, 2.48, 2.49, and 2.50).

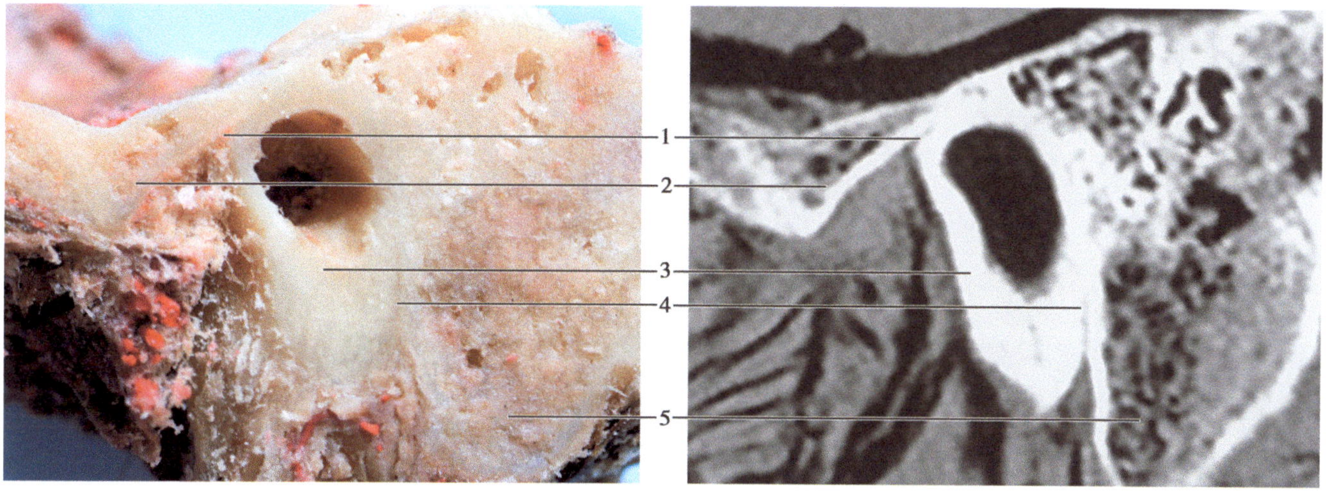

Fig. 2.39 Middle segment of external auditory canal plane (left). (1) Tympanosquamous fissure. (2) Zygomatic process root of temporal bone. (3) Tympanic portion of temporal bone. (4) Tympanomastoid fissure. (5) Mastoid process (Fig. 2.39).

Note: Sagittal CT can clearly show the size, shape, and changes of the bone in the four walls of the bony external auditory canal

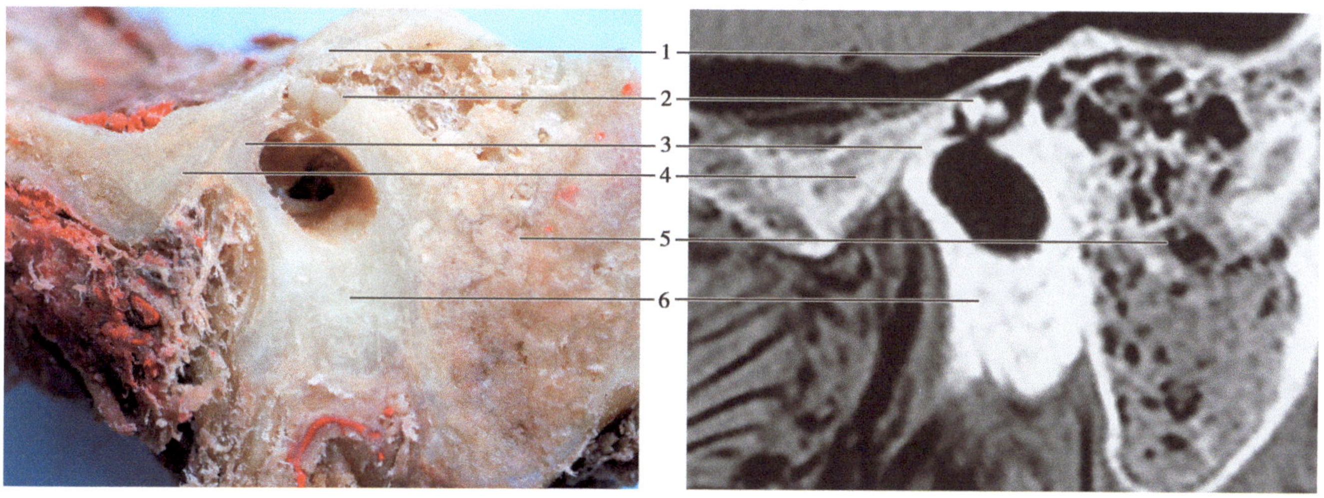

Fig. 2.40 Medial segment of external auditory canal plane (left). (1) Tegmen tympani. (2) Auditory ossicles. (3) Tympanosquamous fissure. (4) Zygomatic process root of temporal bone. (5) Mastoid process. (6) Tympanic portion of temporal bone

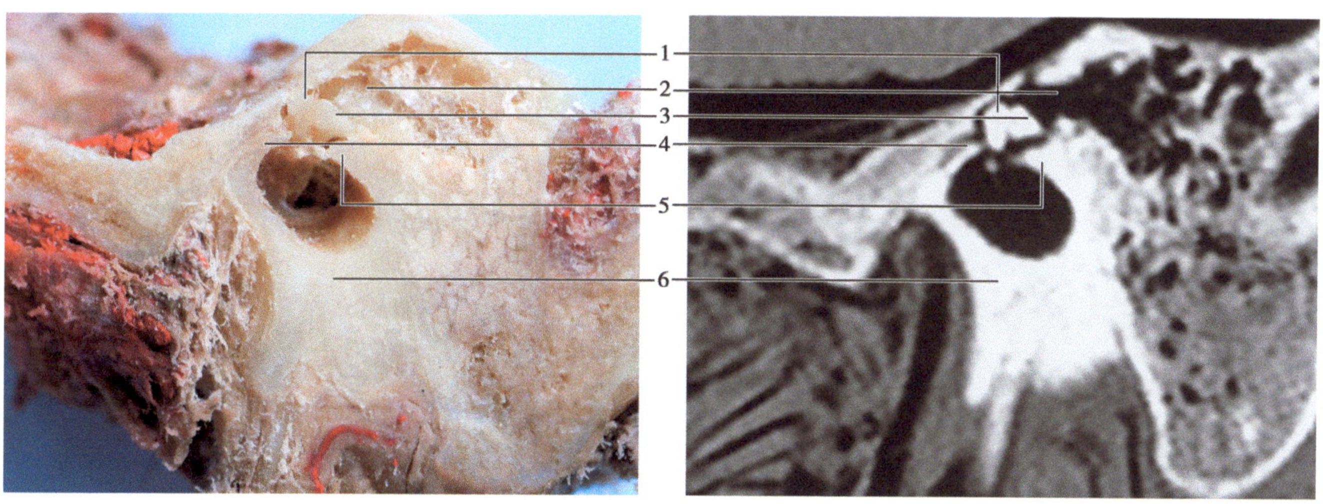

Fig. 2.41 Epitympanum and aditus ad antrum plane (left). (1) Head of malleus. (2) Aditus ad antrum. (3) Body of incus. (4) Anterior edge of tympanic scutum. (5) Posterior edge of tympanic scutum. (6) Tympanic portion of temporal bone

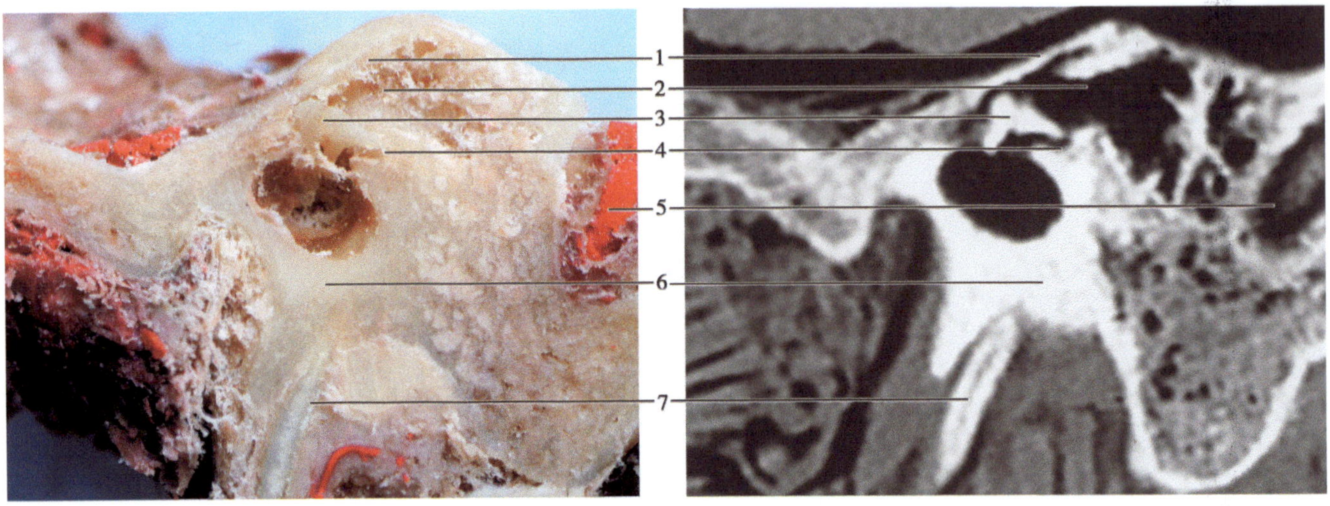

Fig. 2.42 Incudomalleolar articulation plane (left). (1) Tegmen tympani. (2) Aditus ad antrum. (3) Incudomalleolar articulation. (4) Incudal fossa (5) Sigmoid sinus. (6) Tympanic portion of temporal bone. (7) Styloid process.

Note: The sagittal view can continuously display the bony condition of tegmen tympani and tegmen of tympanic antrum; Aditus ad antrum is a narrow passage connecting the epitympanum and the tympanic antrum; The tympanic portion of temporal bone is U-shaped and the opening is backward and upward; This plane is of great value in the diagnosis of the status of the incudomalleolar articulation (Fig. 2.42)

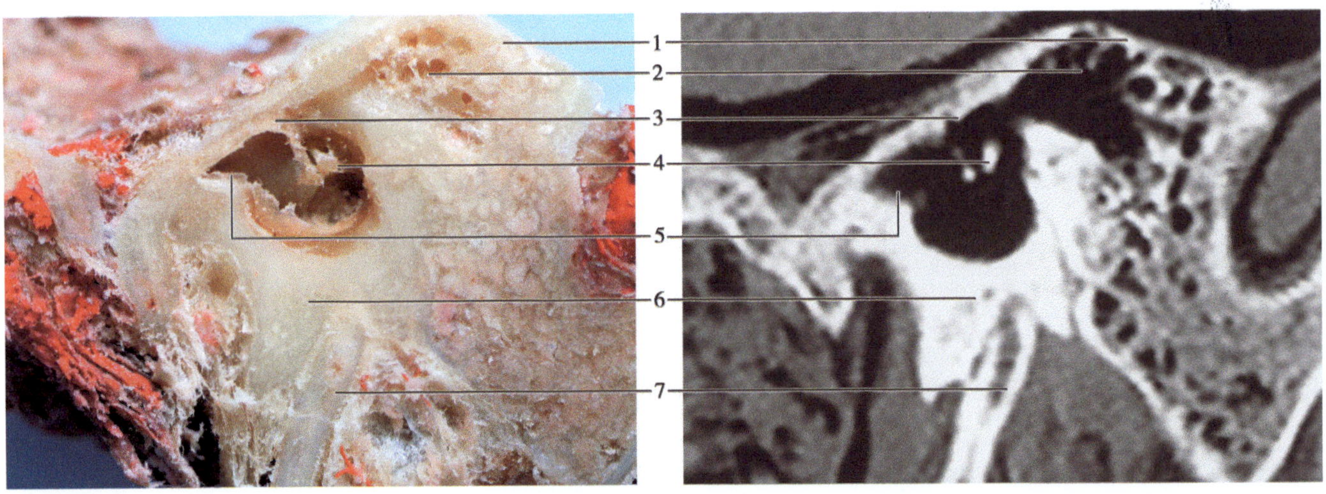

Fig. 2.43 Head of stapes and tympanic orifice of eustachian tube plane (left). (1) Tegmen of tympanic antrum. (2) Tympanic antrum. (3) Tegmen tympani. (4) Head of stapes. (5) Tympanic orifice of eustachian tube. (6) Tympanic portion of temporal bone. (7) Styloid process

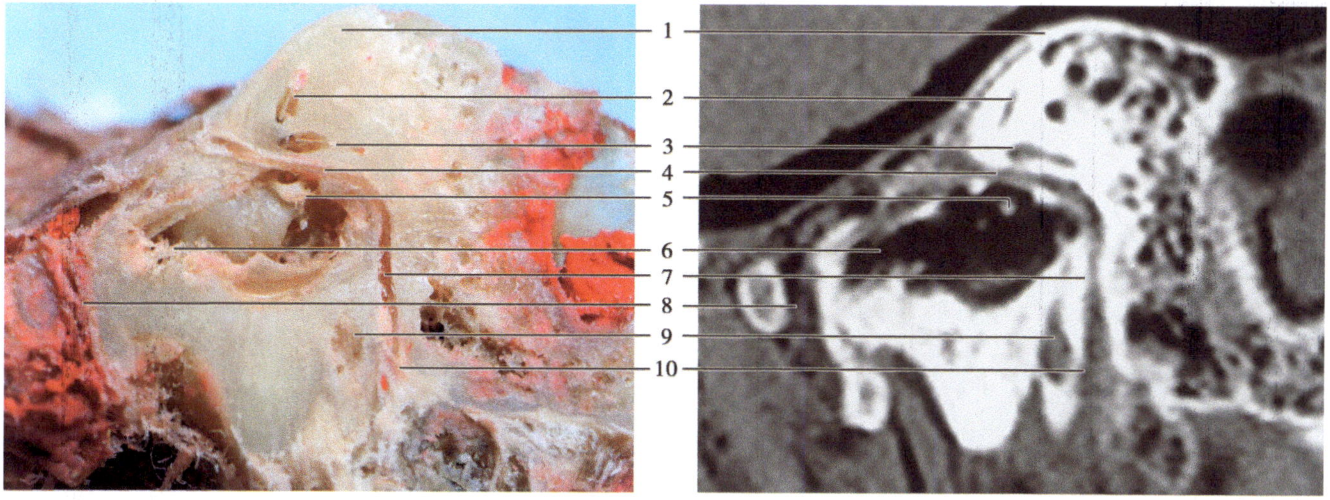

Fig. 2.44 Tympanic and mastoid segment of facial nerve plane (left). (1) Arcuate eminence. (2) Anterior crus of anterior semicircular canal. (3) Lateral semicircular canal. (4) Tympanic (horizontal) segment of facial nerve. (5) Head of stapes. (6) Eustachian tube. (7) Mastoid (vertical) segment of facial nerve. (8) Spinous foramen. (9) Bone marrow of styloid process. (10) Stylomastoid foramen.

Note: The posterosuperior cells of labyrinth can be connected with the cells of petrous apex, which is one of the important reasons for without dry ears after mastectomy with canal wall down. This plane can display the superior and inferior walls of tympanic segment, and the anterior and posterior walls of mastoid segment of facial nerve in one plane (Fig. 2.44)

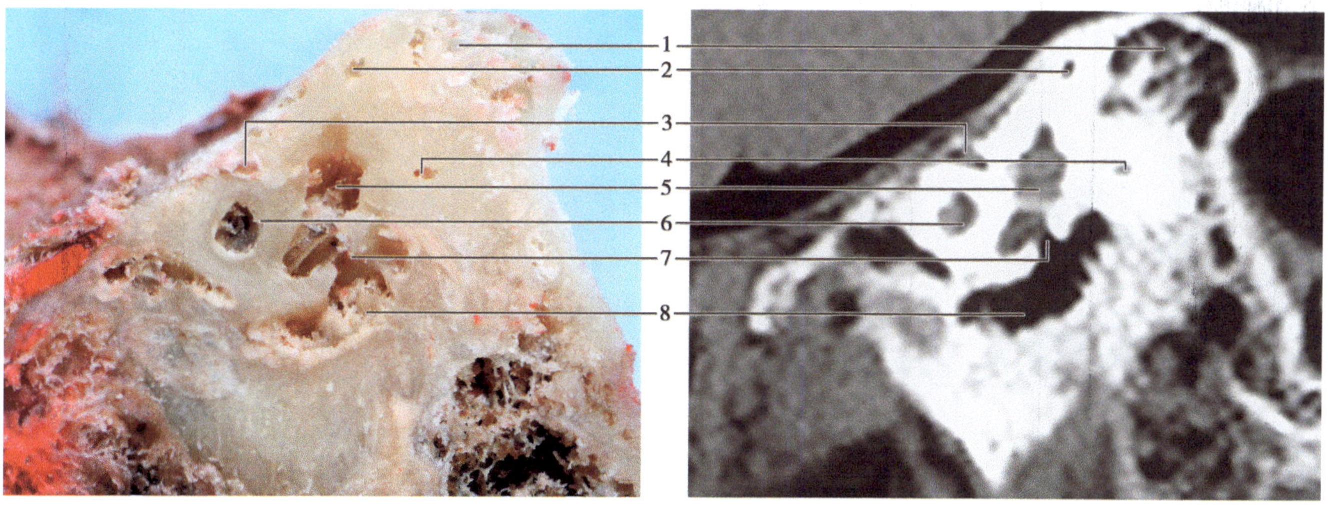

Fig. 2.45 Cochlear window niche and vestibule and geniculate ganglion plane (left).(1)Posterosuperior cells of labyrinth. (2) Arch of anterior semicircular canal. (3) Geniculate ganglion. (4) Arch of lateral semicircular canal. (5) Vestibule. (6) Cochlea. (7) Cochlear window niche. (8) Posteroinferior tympanum.

Note: The geniculate ganglion is located in the bone above the cochlea; The opening of the cochlear window niche is backward to the hypotympanum. When the temporal bone is well pneumatized, the mastoid cells are connected with the cells of petrous portion of the temporal bone through the cell tract around the labyrinth (Fig. 2.45)

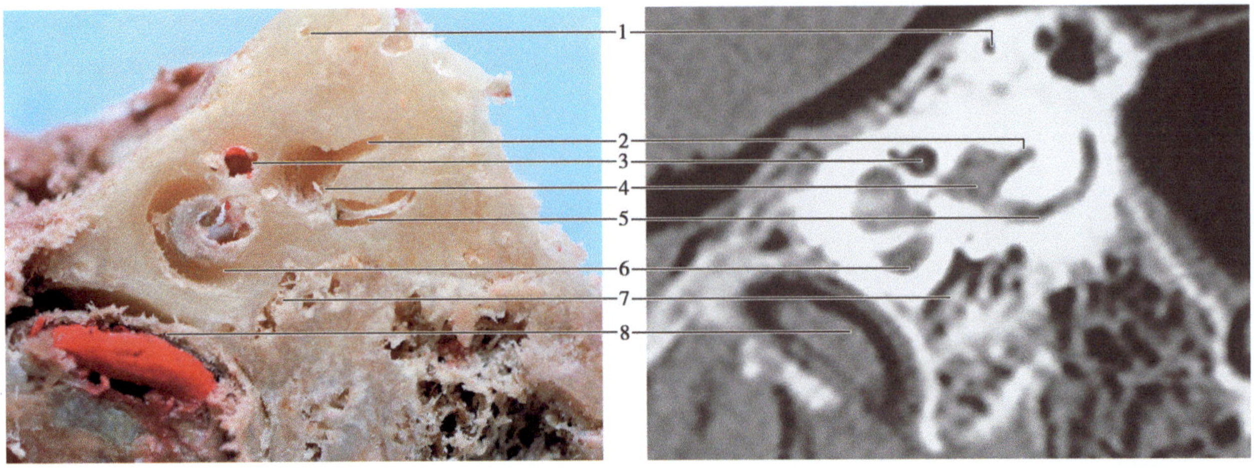

Fig. 2.46 Inferior crus of posterior semicircular canal and vestibule plane (left). (1) Arch of anterior semicircular canal. (2) Posterior crus of lateral semicircular canal. (3) Superior vestibular nerve foramen and facial nerve foramen. (4) Vestibular aqueduct. (5) Inferior crus of posterior semicircular canal. (6) Cochlear canaliculus. (7) Inferior cells of labyrinth. (8) Carotid canal

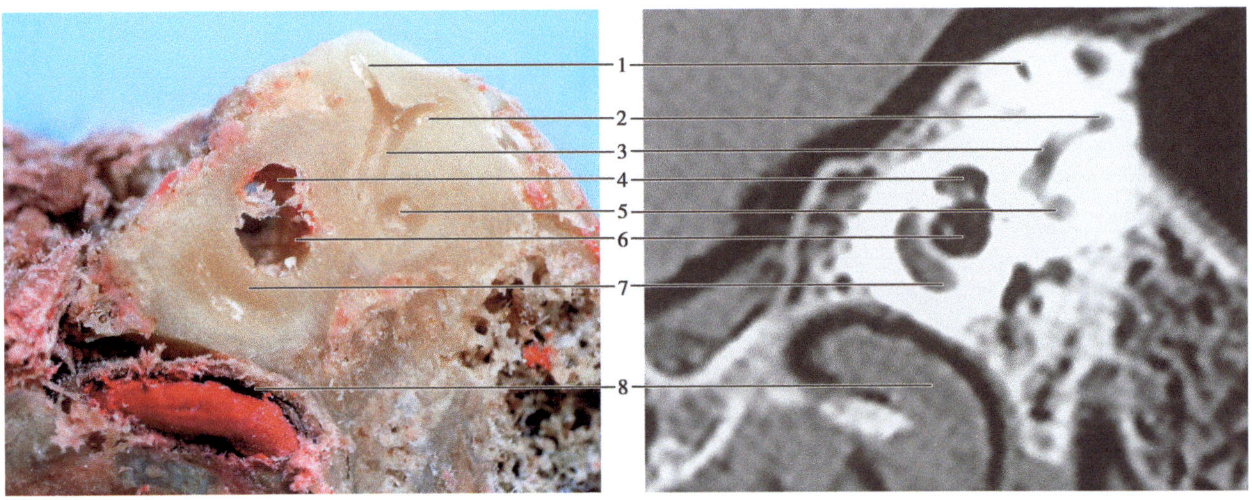

Fig. 2.47 Fundus of internal acoustic meatus and common crus plane (left). (1) Anterior semicircular canal. (2) Posterior semicircular canal. (3) Common crus of semicircular canal. (4) Superior area of fundus of internal acoustic meatus. (5) Ampulla of posterior semicircular canal. (6) Inferior area of internal acoustic meatus. (7) Cochlear canaliculus. (8) Carotid canal.

Note: The anterior semicircular canal and posterior semicircular canal share one crus (common crus) to the vestibule; The fundus of the internal acoustic meatus is divided into superior area (facial foramen area, superior vestibular foramen area), inferior area (cochlear foramen area, inferior vestibular foramen area, and single foramen by the transverse crest (Fig. 2.47)

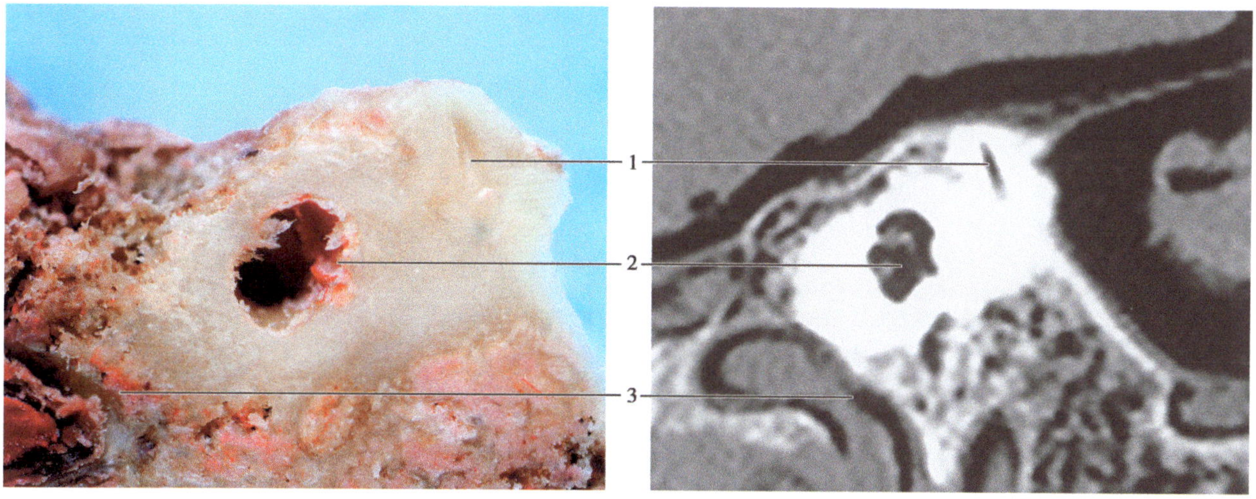

Fig. 2.48 Middle segment of internal acoustic meatus plane (left). (1) Anterior semicircular canal. (2) Internal acoustic meatus. (3) Carotid canal

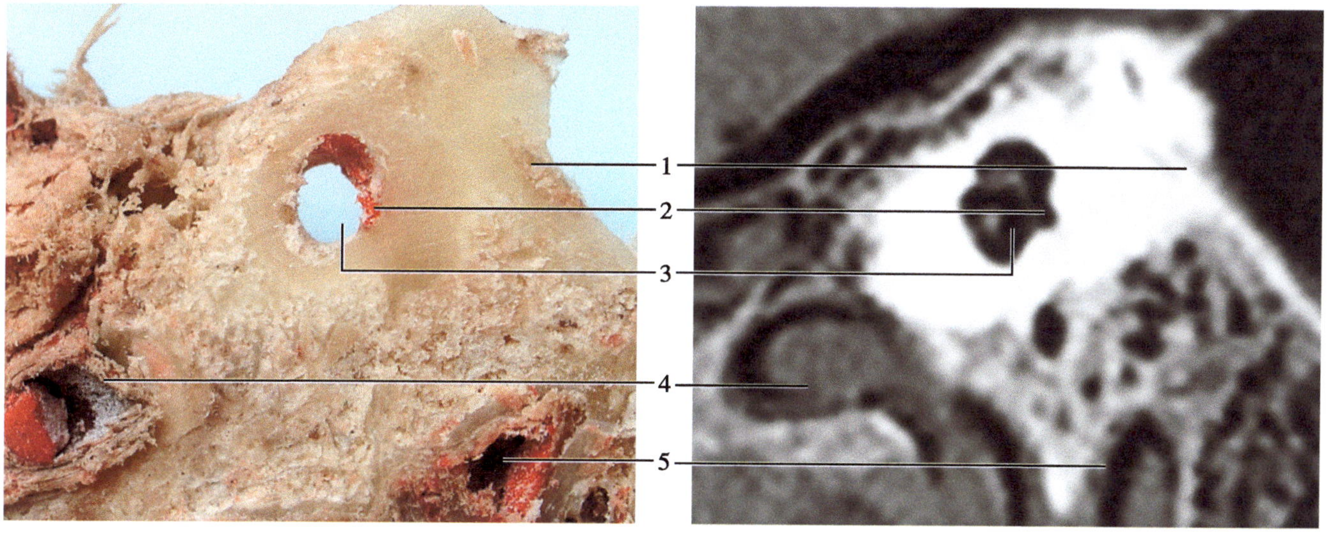

Fig. 2.49 Single foramen of internal acoustic meatus and endolymphatic sac plane (left). (1) Endolymphatic sac fissure. (2) Single foramen. (3) Internal acoustic meatus. (4) Carotid canal. (5) Jugular fossa.

Note: The four walls of the internal acoustic meatus can be displayed on sagittal view; The ampullary nerve of posterior semicircular canal runs through the single foramen, which is also one of the important landmarks of internal acoustic meatus in neurosurgery (Agirdir et al. 2001) (Fig. 2.49)

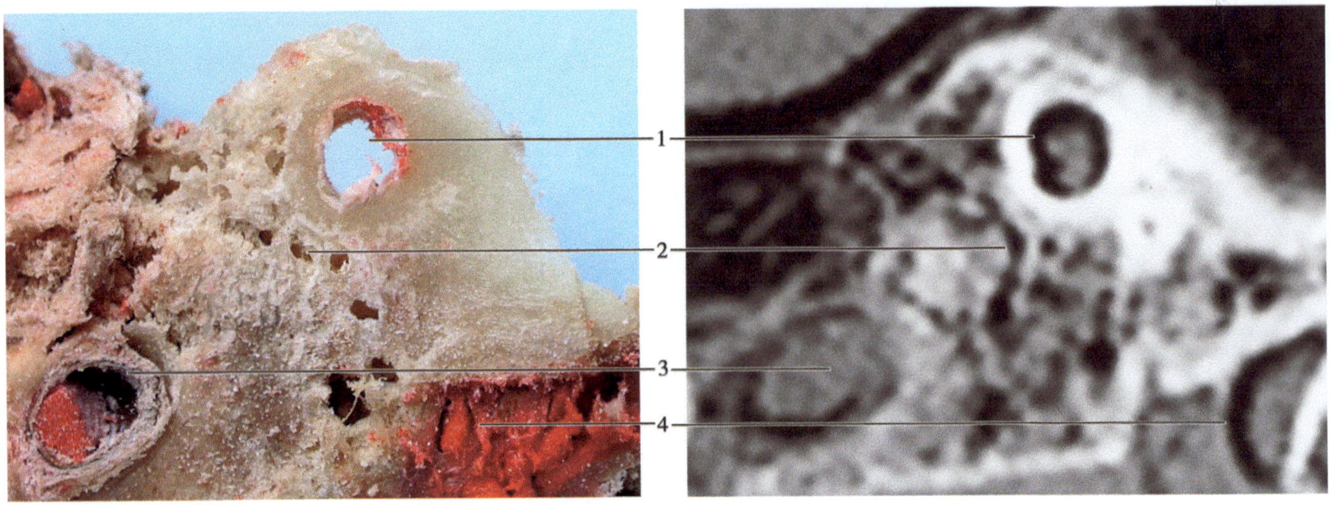

Fig. 2.50 Medial segment of internal acoustic meatus plane (left). (1) Internal acoustic meatus. (2) Cells of petrous apex. (3) Carotid canal. (4) Jugular fossa

3 Congenital Malformation and Anatomical Variation of Temporal Bone

Zilong Yu, Bentao Yang, and Haijiang Dai

The ear malformation can occur either alone or simultaneously with the maxillofacial region or other parts of the human body. The malformation of the external, middle, and inner ear can also occur alone or simultaneously. The diseases in this chapter are arranged according to the order of external auditory canal—middle ear—inner ear—petrous apex (including internal acoustic meatus).

3.1 Congenital Atresia/Stenosis of External Auditory Canal with Middle Ear Malformation and Postoperative Complications

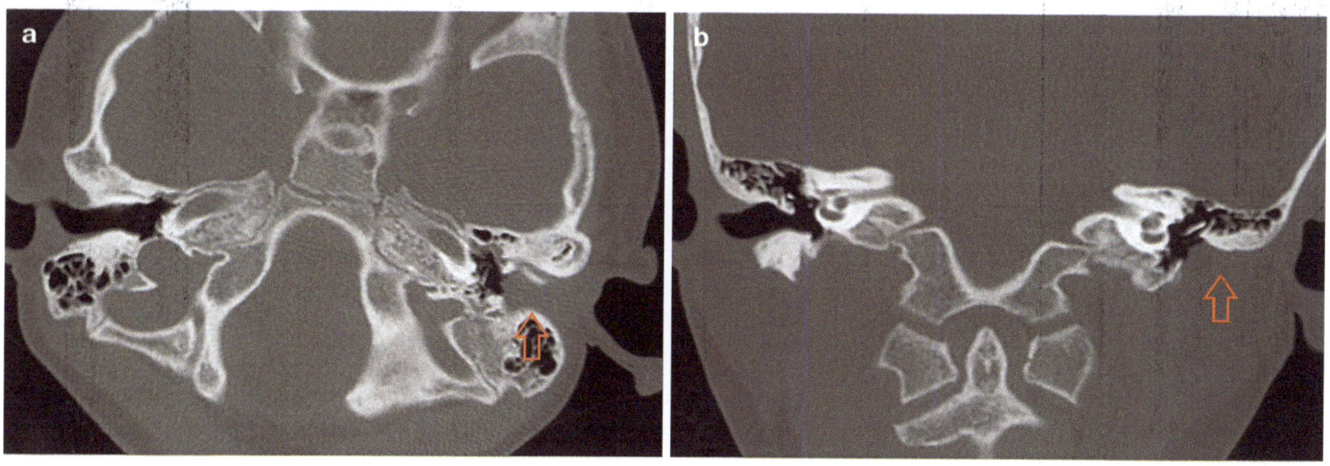

Congenital osseous atresia of external auditory canal in left ear. (**a**) Axial CT; (**b**) Coronal CT. Congenital osseous atresia of left external auditory canal, completely undeveloped tympanic portion of temporal bone, the position of external auditory canal was occupied by soft tissue (⇧), which was easily misdiagnosed as membranous atresia in axial view.

Z. Yu (✉) · H. Dai
Department of Otolaryngology Head and Neck Surgery, Beijing Tongren Hospital, Capital Medical University, Beijing, China

B. Yang
Department of Radiology, Beijing Tongren Hospital, Capital Medical University, Beijing, China

Z. Yu (ed.), *Ear Diseases and CT*, https://doi.org/10.1007/978-981-99-7220-3_3

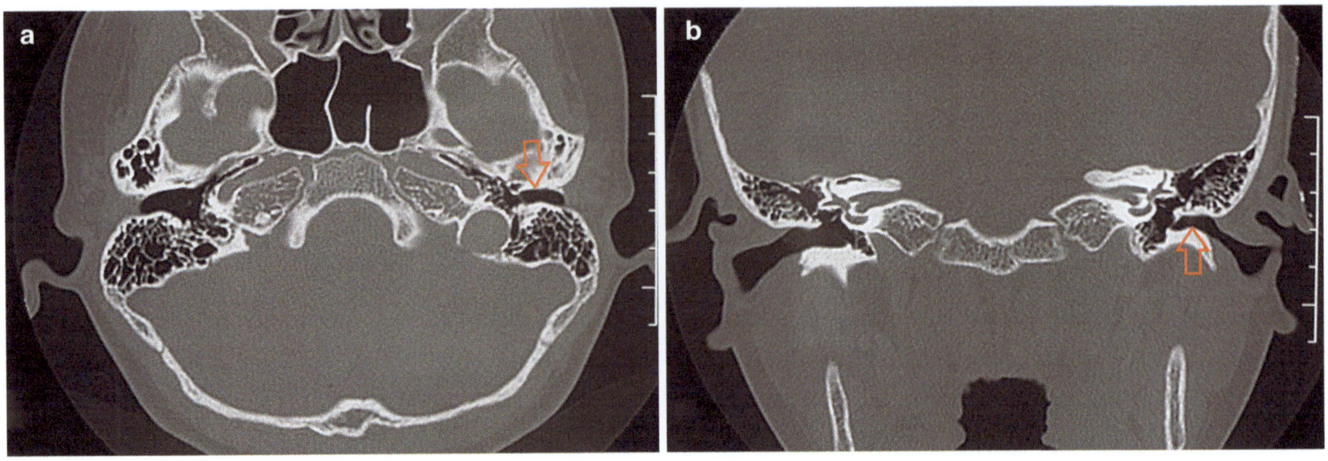

Congenital stenosis of external auditory canal in left ear. (**a**) Axial CT; (**b**) Coronal CT. Narrow external auditory canal (⇧).

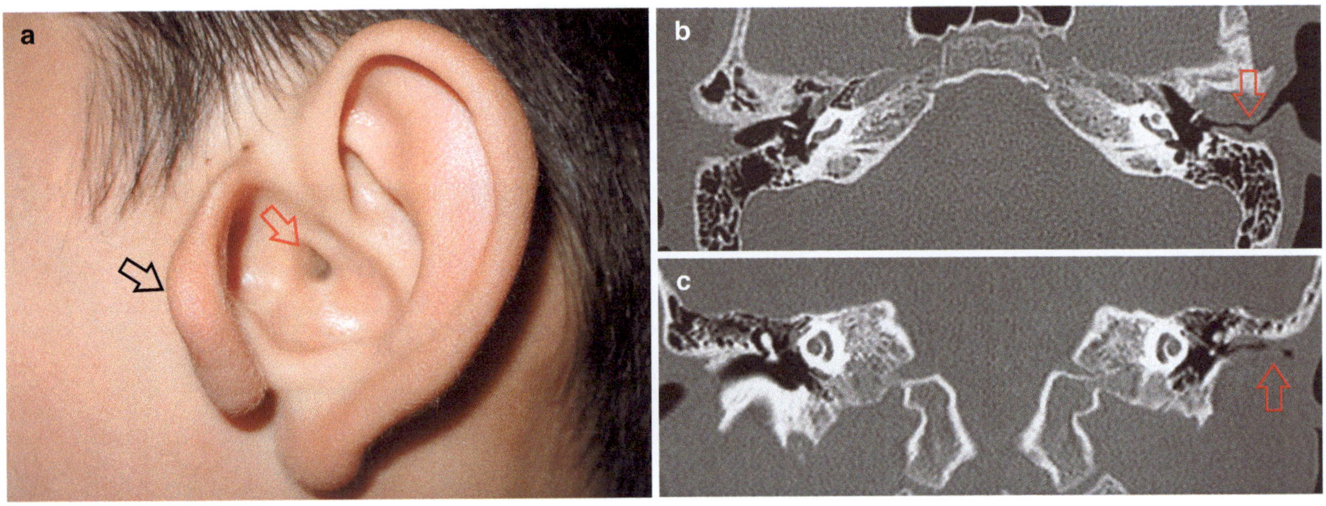

Congenital membranous stenosis of external auditory canal companying tragal malformation in left ear. (**a**) Lateral face of the patient; (**b**) Axial CT; (**c**) Coronal CT. Large and forwarded tragus (⇧) of left ear, membranous stenosis of external auditory canal (⇧).

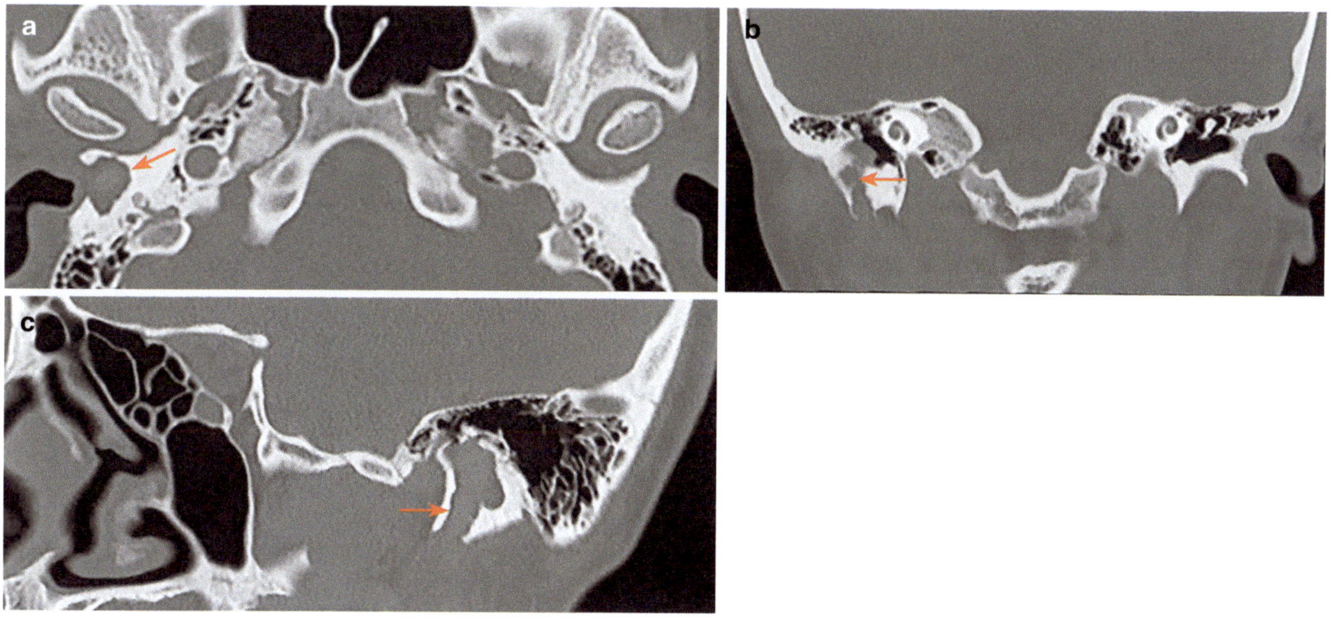

Fig. 3.1 Congenital branchial cleft fistula in right ear. (**a**) Axial CT; (**b**) Coronal CT; (**C**) Sagittal CT.

Note: This kind of congenital branchial fistula was easy to bet misdiagnosed as cholesteatoma of the external auditory canal only by horizontal observation. Combined with coronal and sagittal images, soft tissue of the external auditory canal (↑) could be seen through the inferior wall of the external auditory canal (tympanic bone), reaching the soft tissue of the deep neck (Fig. 3.1)

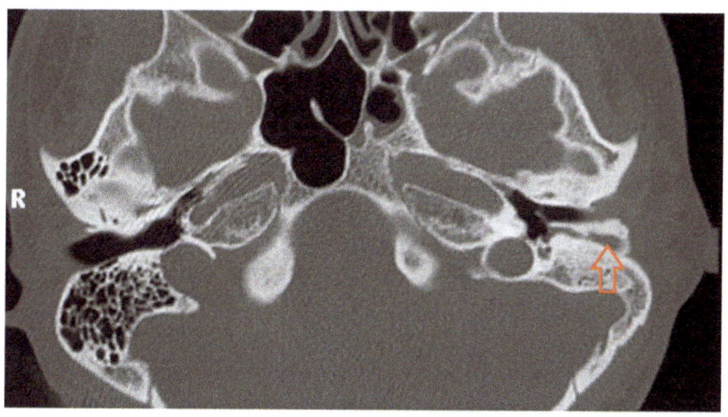

Fig. 3.2 Tympanomastoid fissure deformity of left ear on axial CT view. Tympanomastoid fissure of left ear (⇧) was enlarged, and external auditory canal was bony stenosis.

Note: Physical examination can show the stenosis of ipsilateral external auditory canal (Fig. 3.2)

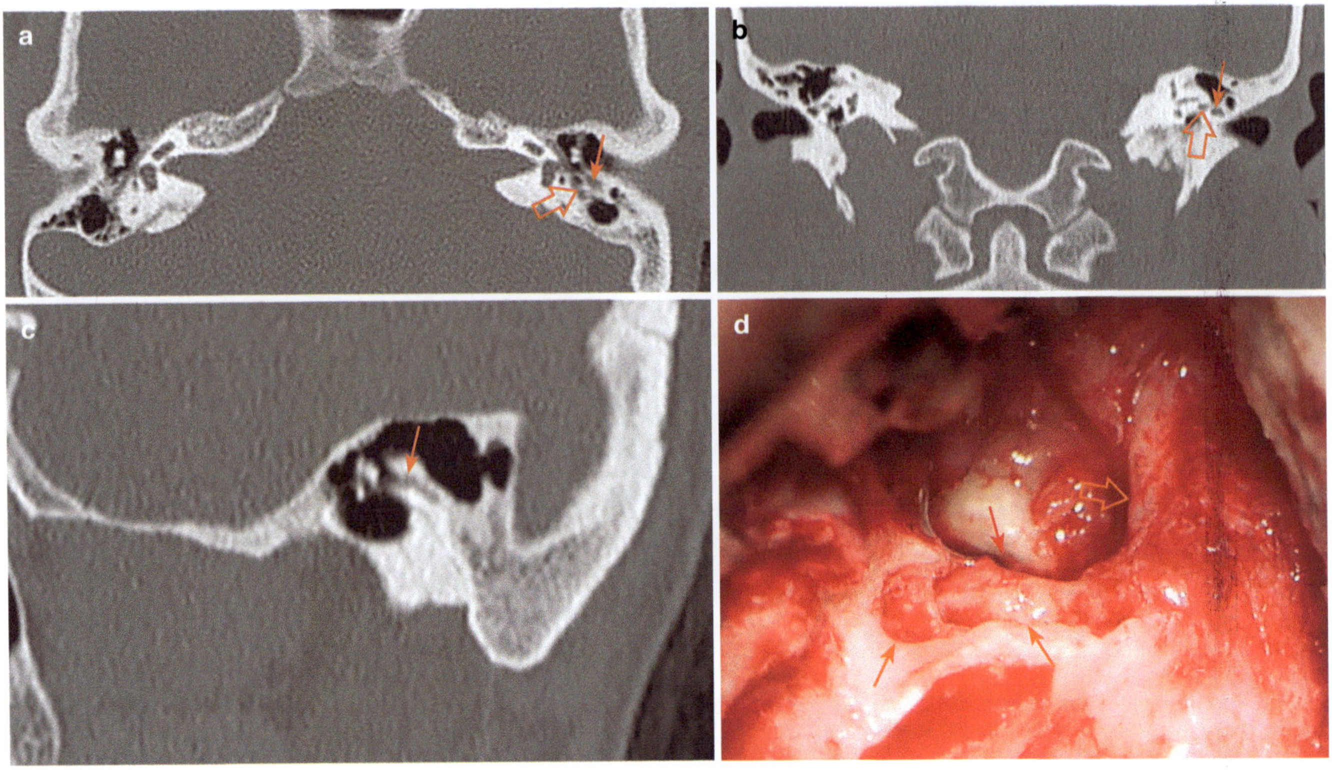

Fig. 3.3 Tubular cell in wall of retrotympanum. (**a**) Axial CT; (**b**) Coronal CT; (**c**) Sagittal CT; (**d**) Intraoperative finding**.** (**a**, **b**). Tubular cell (↑) located on lateral wall of second genu of facial nerve (⇧); (**c**) Tubular cell on sagittal view (↑); (**d**) Tubular cell (↑) in retrotympanic wall, tympanic segment of facial nerve (⇧), cochlear window niche (↑).

Note: This tubular cell might reach the inferior wall level of external auditory canal and had a similar course to vertical segment of facial nerve, drilled out this cell could lower the facial nerve ridge sufficiently. (Fig. 3.3)

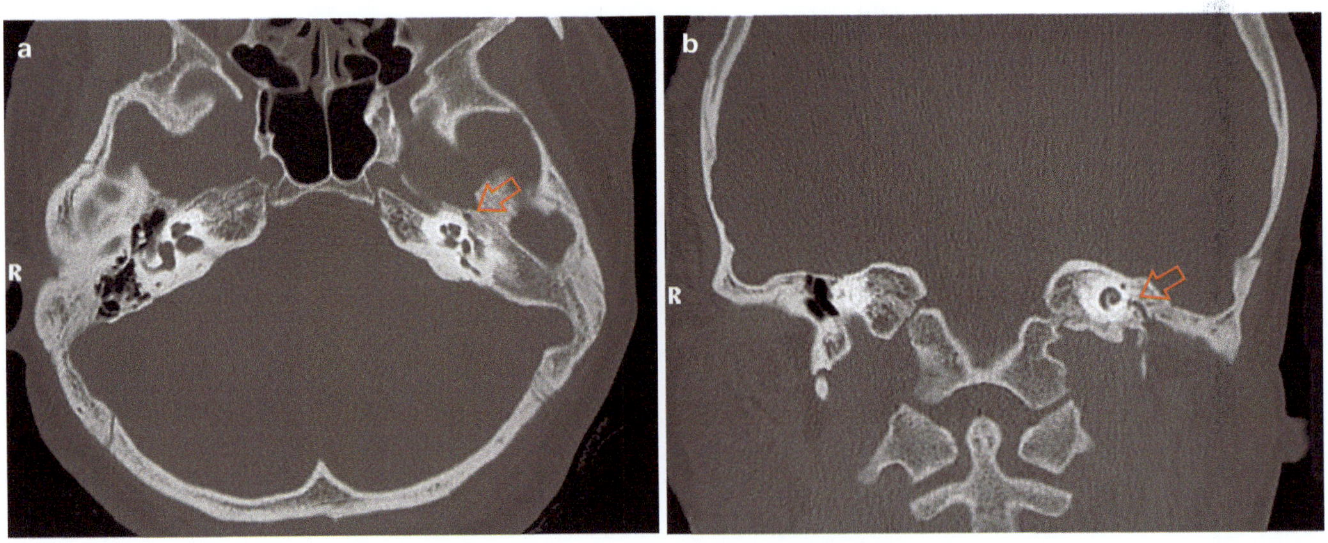

Congenital atresia of external auditory canal in left ear. (**a**) Axial CT; (**b**) Coronal CT. The vertical segment of facial nerve (⇧) moved forward to the level of the cochlea, the middle ear and tympanic sinus were not developed, and the middle cranial fossa was low.

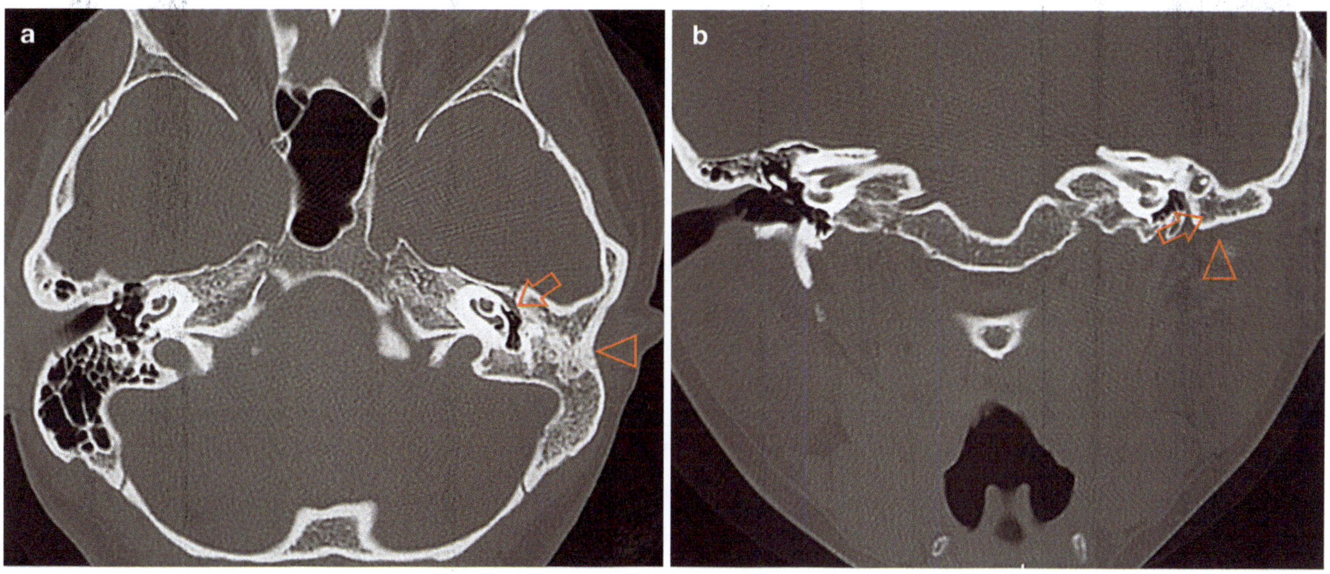

Congenital atresia of external auditory canal in left ear. (**a**) Axial CT; (**b**) Coronal CT. The vertical segment of facial nerve (⇧) moved forward on the cochlea level and was located on the medial side of the atresia plate (△)

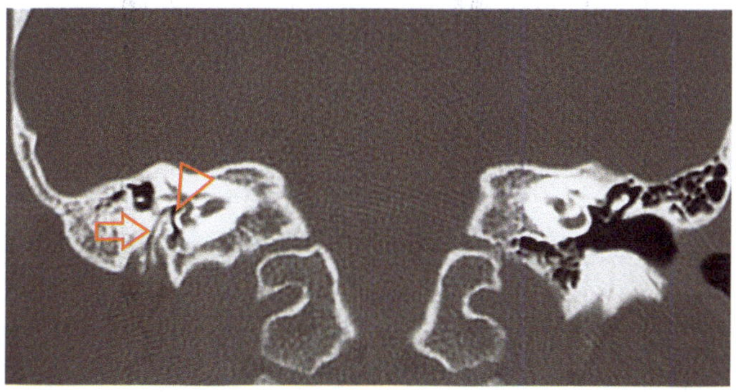

External auditory canal atresia in right ear on coronal CT view. The vertical segment of facial nerve (⇧) moved forward to the plane of vestibular window (△)

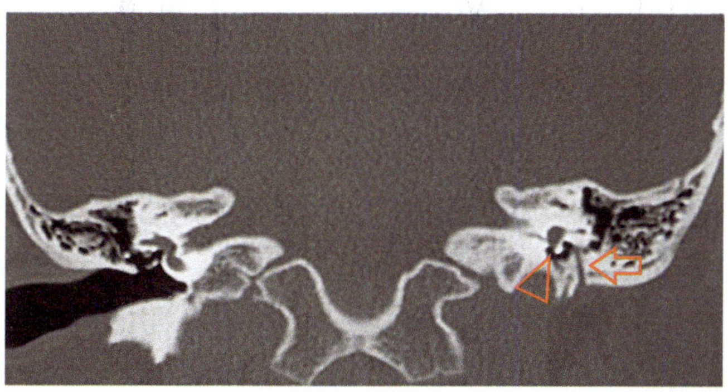

External auditory canal atresia in left ear on coronal CT view. The vertical segment of facial nerve (⇧) moved forward to the plane of cochlear vestibular window (△)

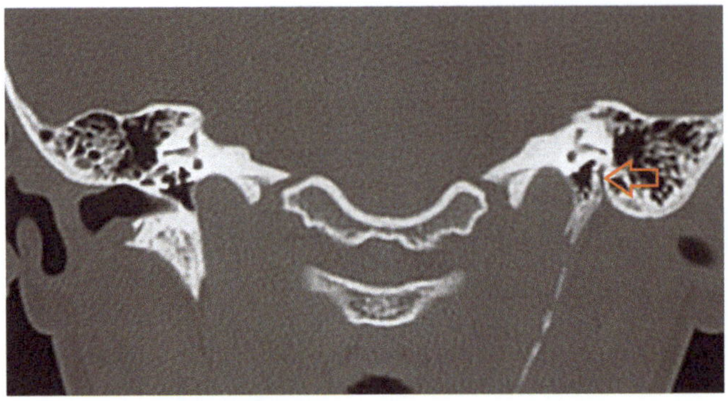

External auditory canal atresia of left ear on coronal CT view. The vertical segment of facial nerve (⇧) was located at the plane of posterior crus of lateral semicircular canal, without obvious forward position.

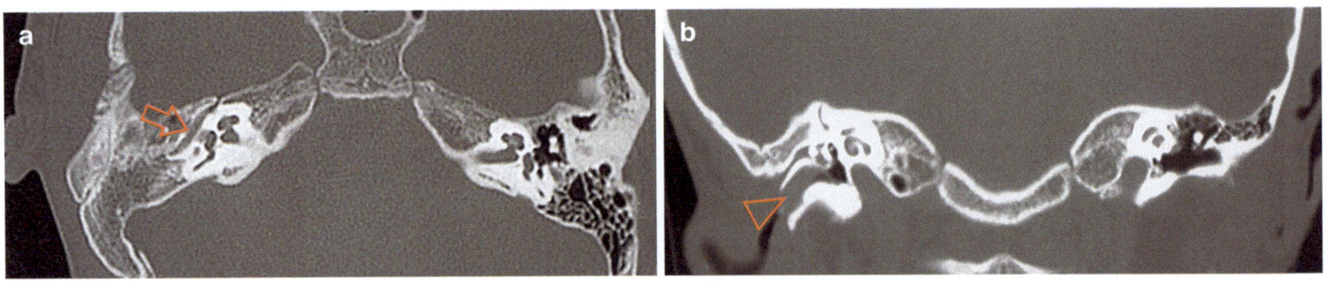

Right external auditory canal stenosis (**a**) Axial CT; (**b**) Coronal CT. The facial nerve canal was thick (⇧), external auditory canal was narrow and nearly vertical (△).

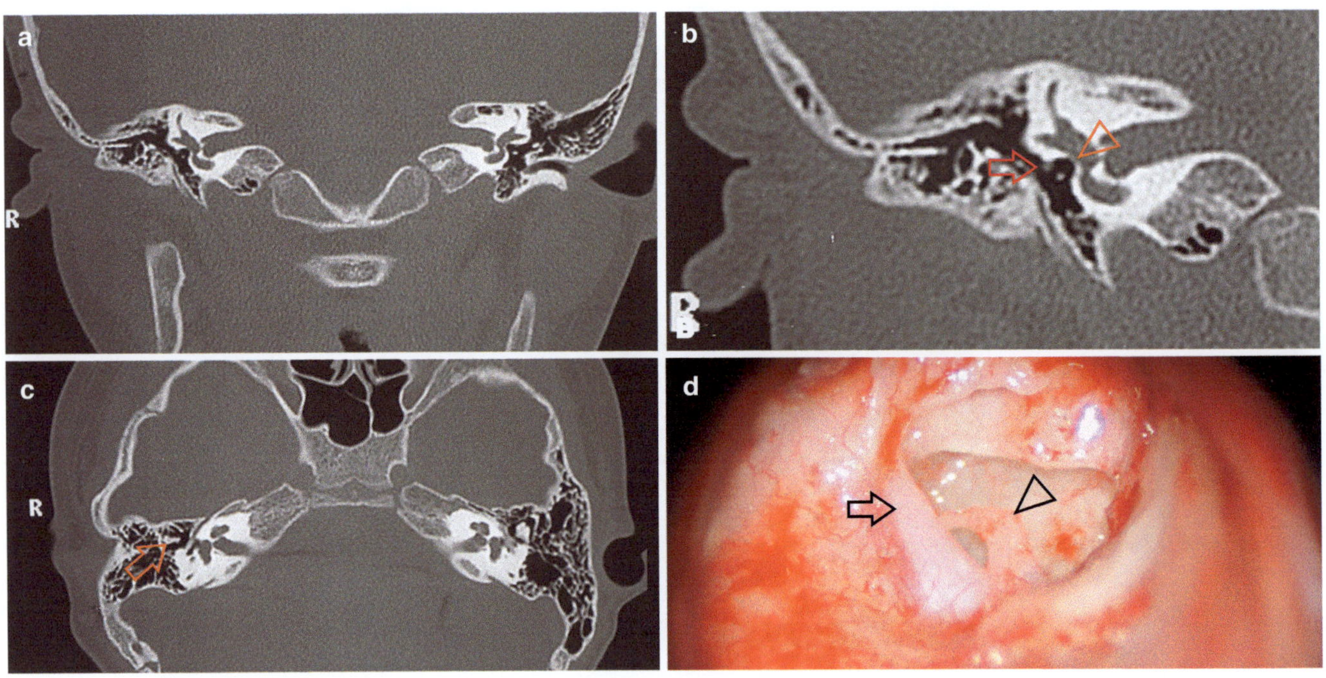

Congenital atresia of right external auditory canal. (**a**, **b**) Coronal CT; (**c**) Axial CT; (**d**) Intraoperative finding. (**a**) Right external auditory canal atresia, left external auditory canal stenosis; (**b**) Local magnification of right ear, horizontal segment of facial nerve (⇧) overlayed vestibular window (△); (**c**) Ossicles malformation of right ear (⇧); (**d**) Facial nerve (⇧) overlayed vestibular window, stapes deformity (△).

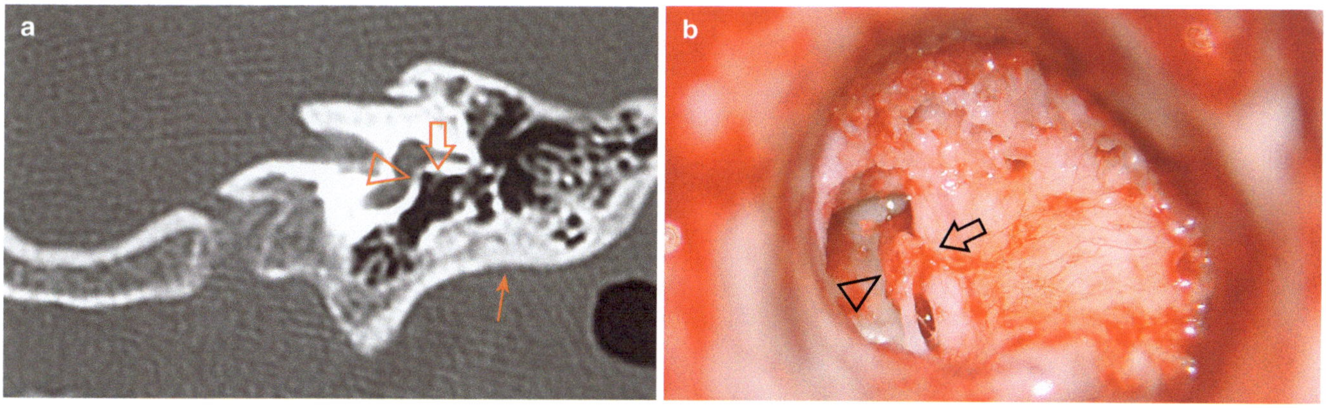

Congenital atresia of left external auditory canal. (**a**) Coronal CT; (**b**) Intraoperative finding. (**a**). External auditory canal atresia (↑) of left ear with horizontal segment of facial nerve (⇧) overlying vestibular window (△); (**b**) Incus and stapes were connected by soft tissue, the facial nerve (⇧) was seen to overlay vestibular window after the removal of the incus; the stapes (△).

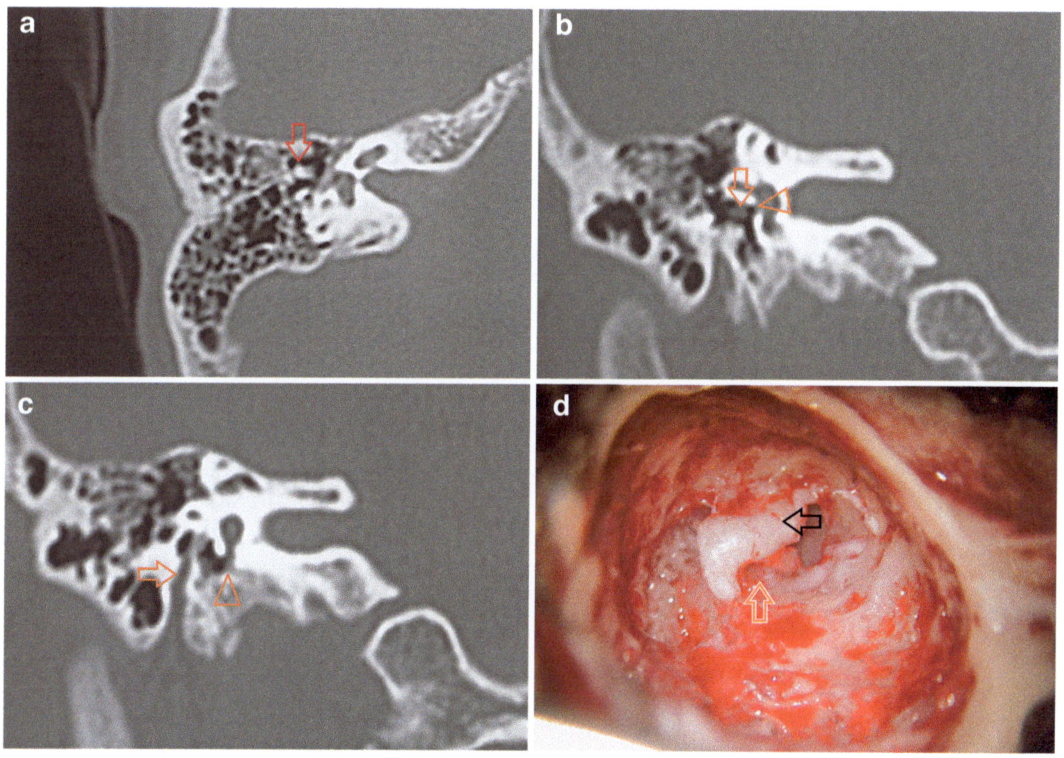

Congenital atresia of right external auditory canal. (**a**) Axial CT; (**b**, **c**) Coronal CT; (**d**) Intraoperative finding. (**a**) Abnormal ossicles (⇧) were fused with the atresia plate; (**b**) Horizontal segment of facial nerve (⇧) overlayed vestibular window (△); (**c**) Vertical segment of facial nerve (⇧) moved forward to the plane of cochlear window (△); (**d**) Facial nerve (⇧) was seen to overlay vestibular window and moved forward; deformed ossicles (⇧).

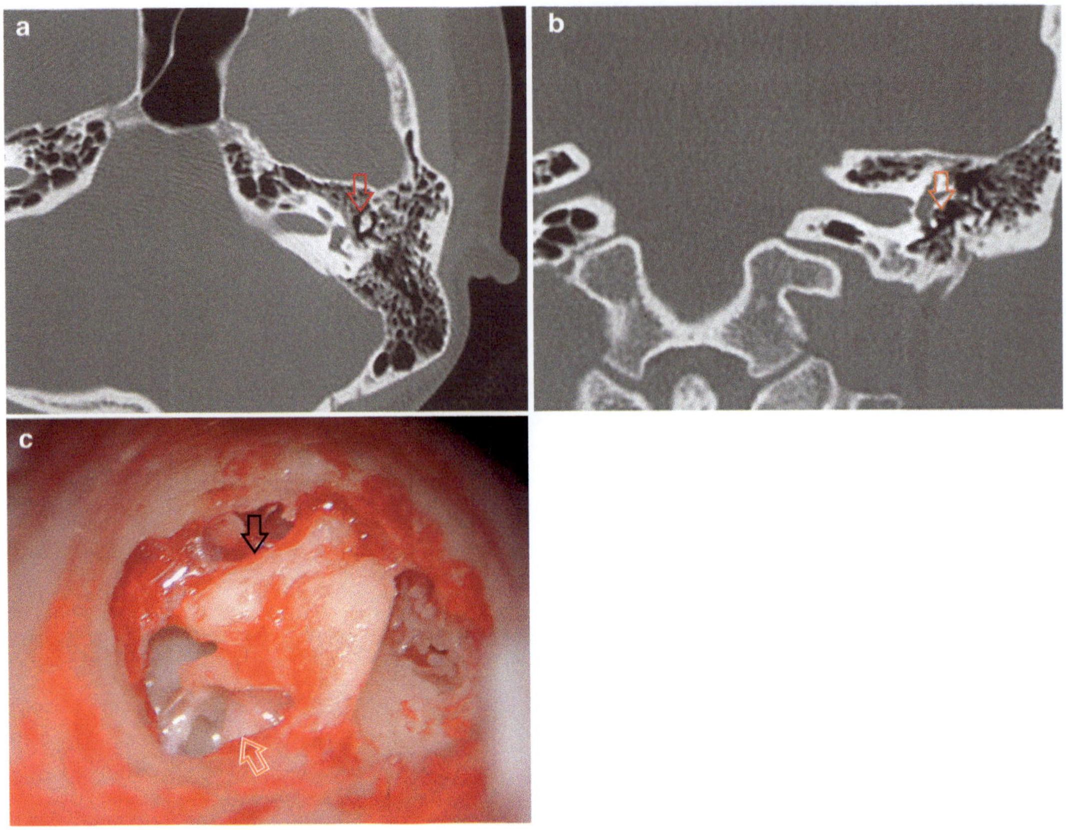

Atresia of left external auditory canal. (**a**). Axial CT; (**b**) Coronal CT; (**c**) Intraoperative finding. (**a**) Deformed ossicles (⇧); (**b**) Horizontal segment of facial nerve (⇧) mildly overlapped window; (**c**) Facial nerve (⇧) overlapped vestibular window partially; ossicular malformations (⇧).

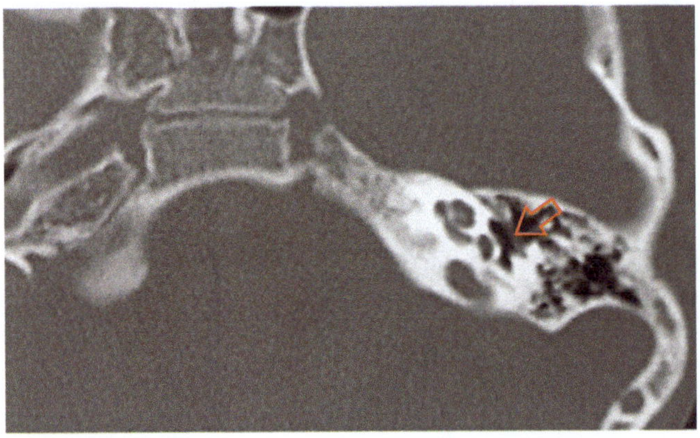

Atresia of left external auditory canal on axial CT view. The lower horizontal segment (⇧) of facial nerve was located between vestibular window and cochlear window.

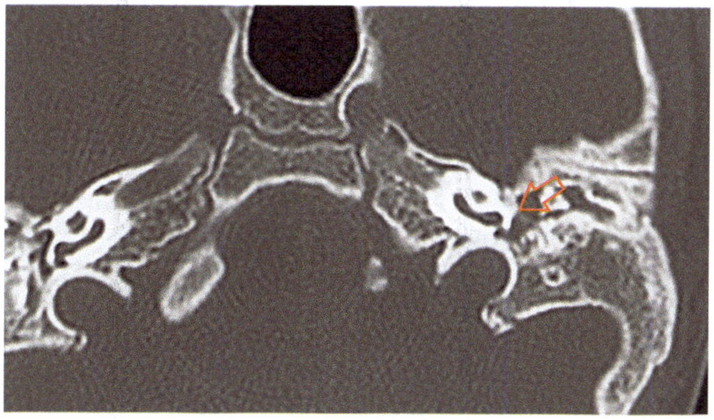

Atresia of left external auditory canal on axial CT view. The lower horizontal segment (⇧) of facial nerve was located at the plane of cochlear window.

Note: HRCT scanning is a necessary imaging examination for the surgical treatment of congenital atresia of the external auditory canal. It can accurately locate the facial nerve, understand the development of the vestibular window, the thickness of the atresia plate, the size of the tympanic cavity, et al. (Mayer et al. 1997; Yu et al. 2008).

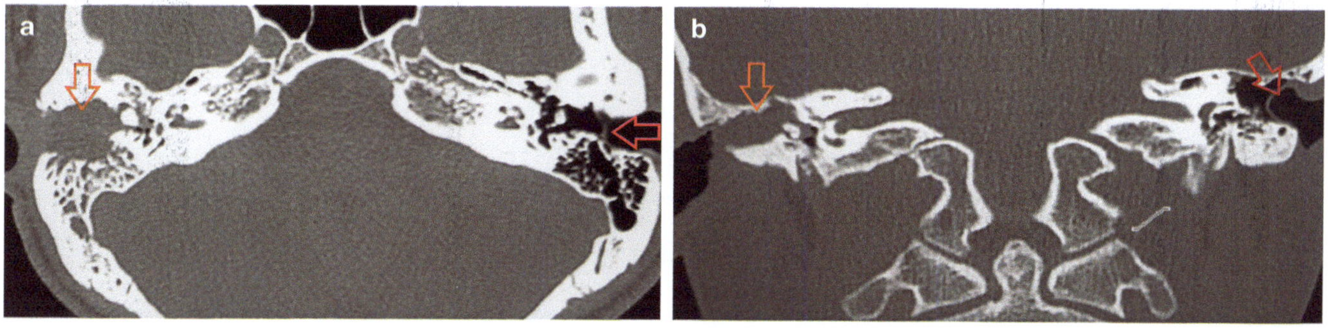

Postoperative complications of osseous atresia of external auditory canal (**a**) Axial CT; (**b**) Coronal CT. After reconstruction of bilateral external auditory canal atresia, lateralization of tympanic membrane (⇧) in left ear, membranous atresia (⇧) of external auditory canal in right ear.

3.2 Simple Middle Ear Malformation

See Figs. 3.4, 3.5, 3.6, 3.7, and 3.8.

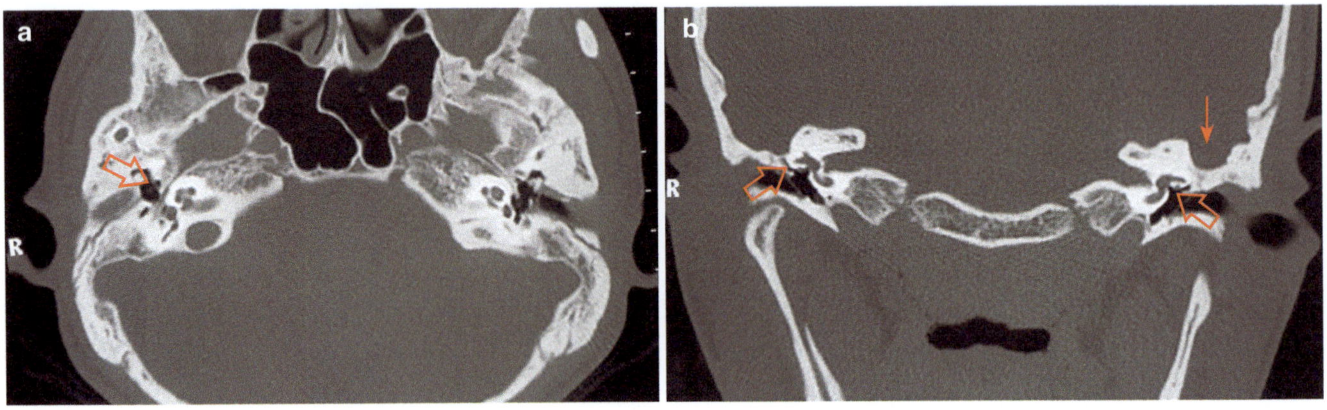

Fig. 3.4 Bilateral middle ear malformation. (**a**) Axial CT; (**b**) Coronal CT. Epitympanum (⇧) was small without ossicles, and middle cranial fossa was infradisplacement (↑)

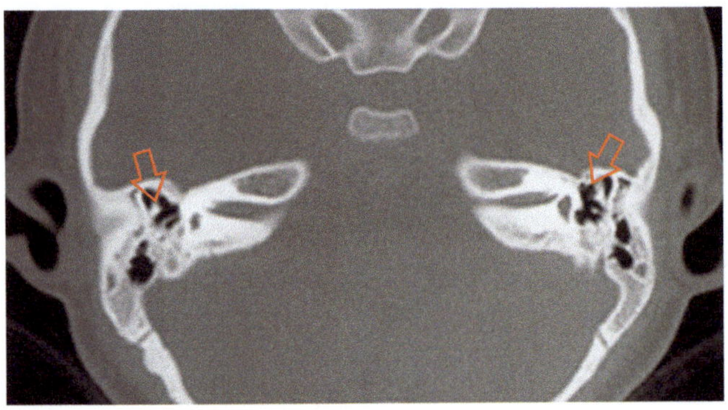

Fig. 3.5 Bilateral middle ear malformation on axial CT view. Ossicle malformation (⇧) in bilateral middle ear

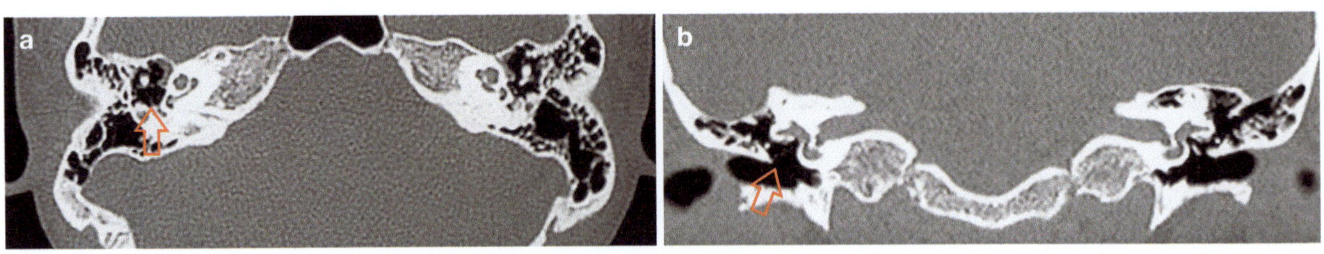

Fig. 3.6 Right congenital middle ear malformation (**a**) Axial CT; (**b**) Coronal CT. Incus and superstructure of stapes in right ear were not developed (⇧)

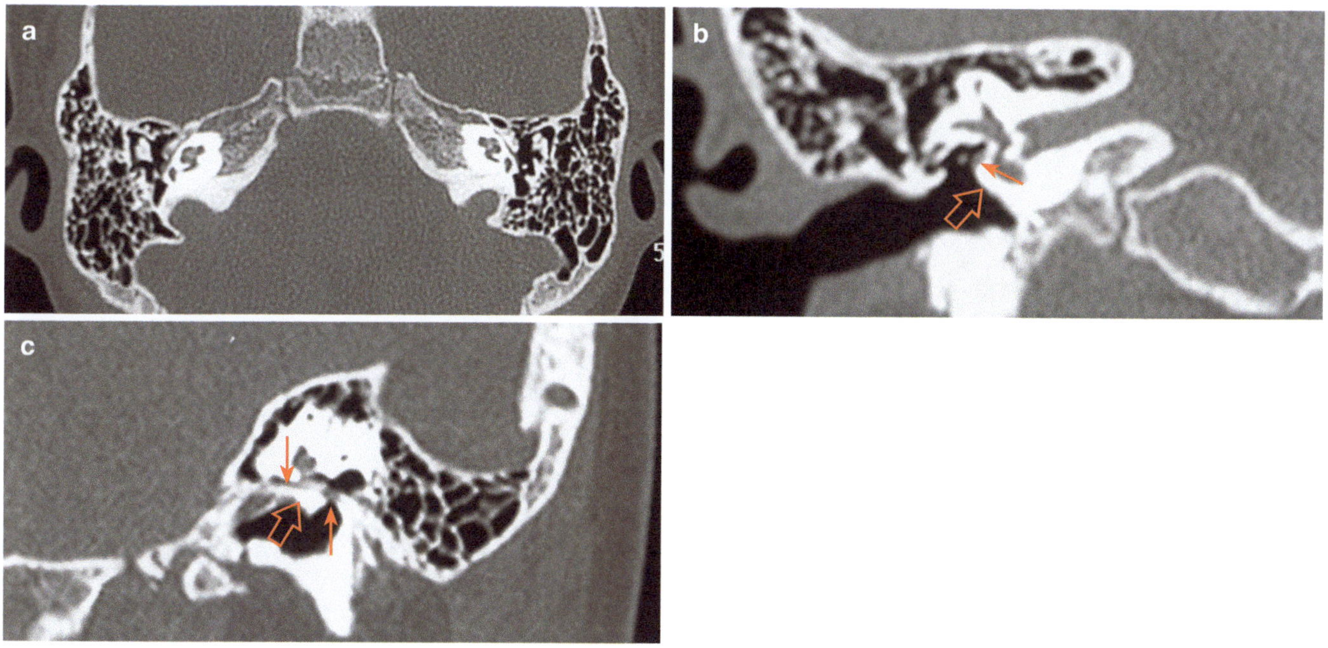

Fig. 3.7 Bilateral middle ear malformation with abnormal facial nerve course (**a**) Axial CT; (**b**) Coronal CT of right ear; (**c**) Sagittal CT of right ear. Horizontal (tympanic) segment of facial nerve (↑) was located at the inferior edge of vestibular window niche and the superior edge of promontory (⇧)

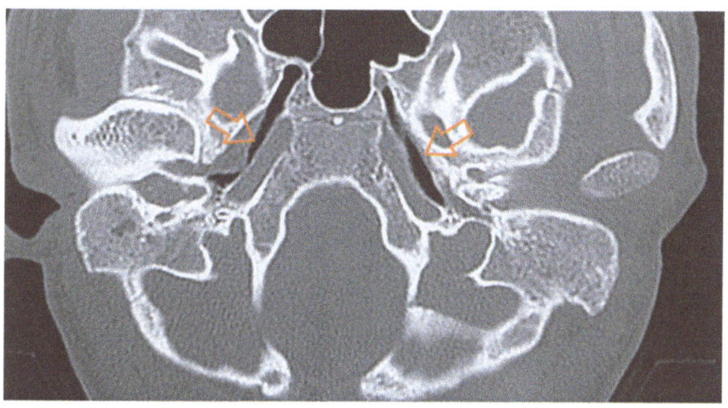

Fig. 3.8 Deformity of bilateral eustachian tube on axial CT view. Enlarged eustachian tube (⇧) in bilateral ears

3.3 Inner Ear Malformation

3.3.1 Vestibular Window Atresia

See Figs. 3.9 and 3.10.

3.3.2 Vestibule and Semicircular Canal Malformation

See Fig. 3.11.

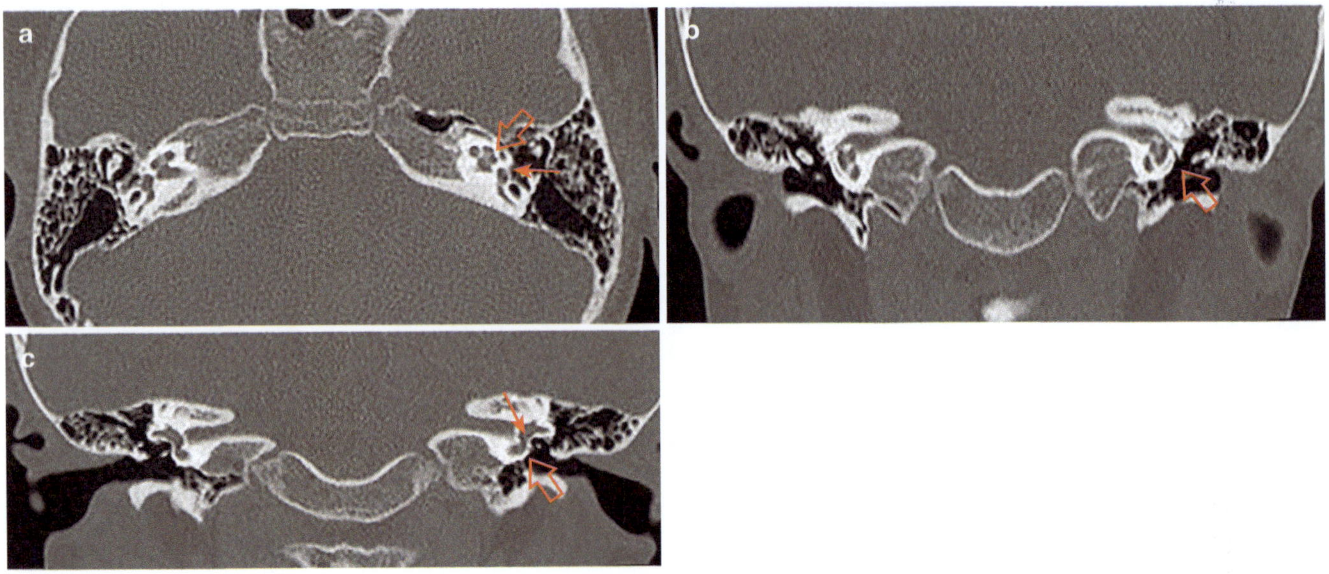

Fig. 3.9 Vestibular window atresia with facial nerve ectopia in left ear. (**a**) Axial CT; (**b**, **c**) Coronal CT. Facial nerve (⇧) walked on the surface of promontory, vestibular window (↑) was osseous atresia

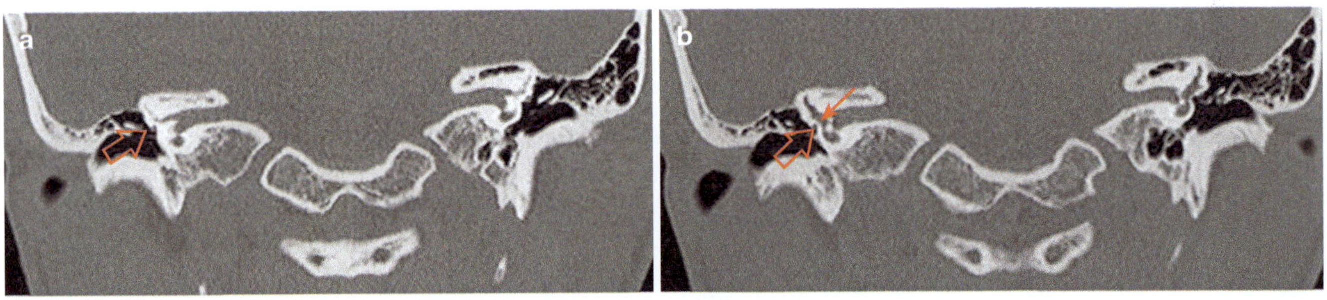

Fig. 3.10 Vestibular window atresia with facial nerve ectopia in right ear. (**a**, **b**) Coronal CT. Facial nerve (⇧) walked on the surface of vestibular window niche, vestibular window (↑) was osseous atresia

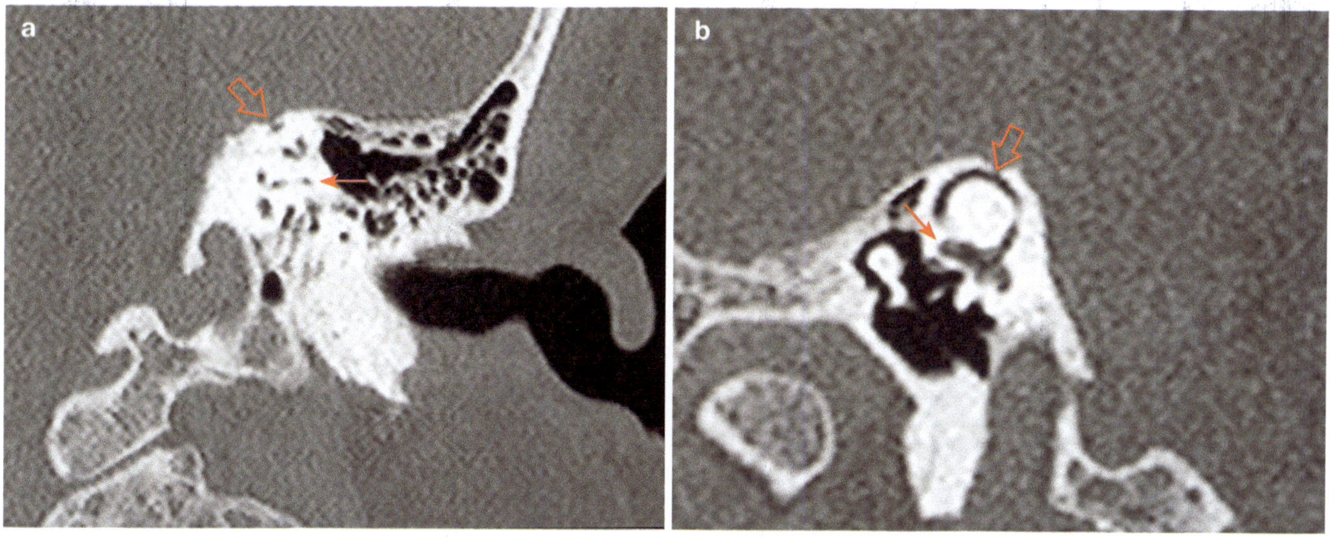

Fig. 3.11 Anterior semicircular canal dehiscence of left ear. (**a**) Coronal CT; (**b**) Oblique sagittal CT. Bone defect (⇧) of anterior semicircular canal arch, lateral semicircular canal (↑).

Note: Coronal CT view could show the bone defect at the anterior semicircular canal arch, but it was difficult to determine the size of the defect, oblique sagittal view (parallel scan with the plane of the anterior semicircular canal) could show the length and location of bone defect. Certainly, it should be differentiated from the thinning of the anterior semicircular canal bone when the superior petrosal sinus was deep and large (Juliano et al. 2018) [due to partial volume effect, thinning and defect were difficult to distinguish, however, the micro CT scan could clearly show the bone situation (Yu et al. 2021)]. Therefore, whether the anterior semicircular canal dehiscence syndrome existed or not, the clinical symptoms were very important. Horizontal position CT scanning had no advantage in the diagnosis of this disease.

Anterior semicircular canal dehiscence is characterized by lack of bony covering of anterior semicircular canal, resulting in a so called "third window", causing autophony, pseudo-conductive hearing loss, and Tullio phenomenon (sound-induced episodic vertigo and dysequilibrium (Carey et al. 2000; Minor et al. 1998 and 2005; Rajan et al. 2008; Yew et al. 2012), this is well assessed by CT scan (Eibenberger et al. 2014)

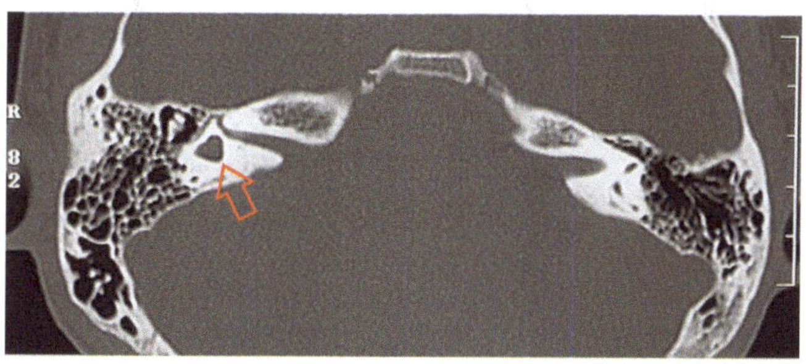

Lateral semicircular canal malformation of right ear on axial CT view. Lateral semicircular canal fusion (⇧).

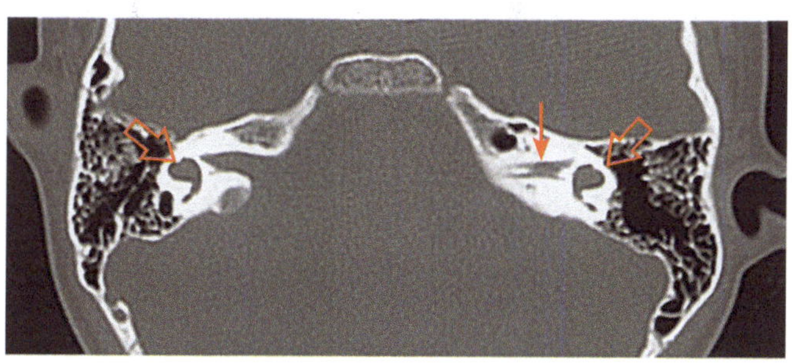

Bilateral external semicircular canal malformation on axial CT view. Lateral semicircular canal fusion (⇧), stenosis of internal auditory canal in left ear (↑).

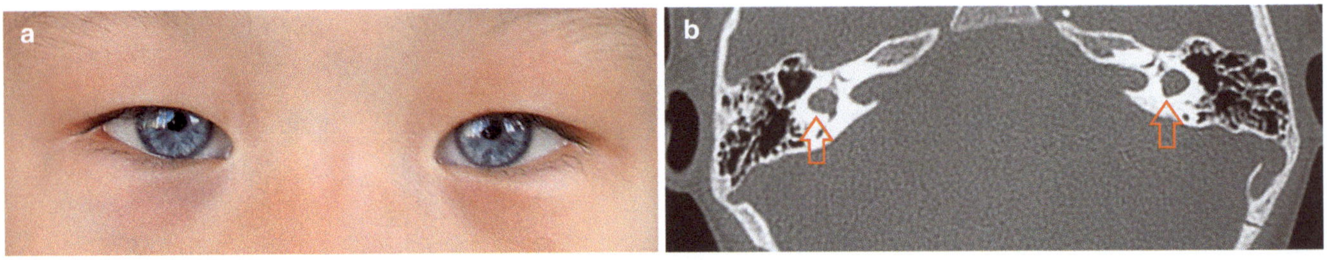

Waardenburg syndrome. (**a**) Appearance of the eyes; (**b**) Axial CT. (**a**) Abnormal iris pigment (deep gray) of bilateral eyes in children; (**b**) Bilateral lateral semicircular canal malformation (⇧).

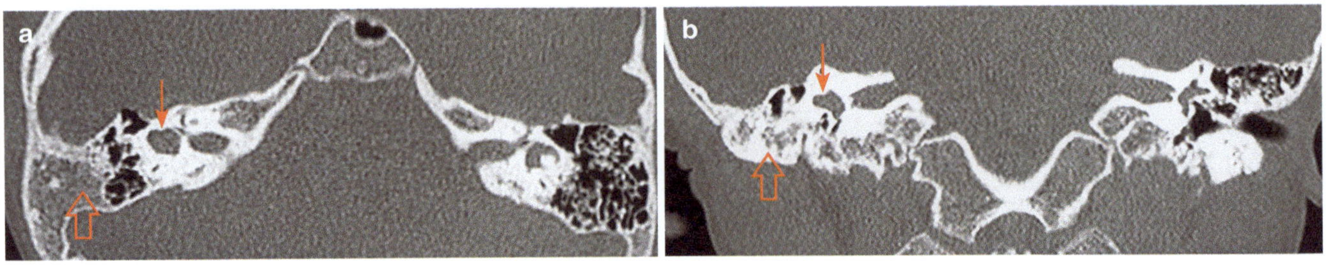

Congenital atresia of external auditory canal with lateral semicircular canal malformation in right ear. (**a**) Axial CT; (**b**) Coronal CT. Right atresic external auditory canal (⇧), short and thick lateral semicircular canal (↑).

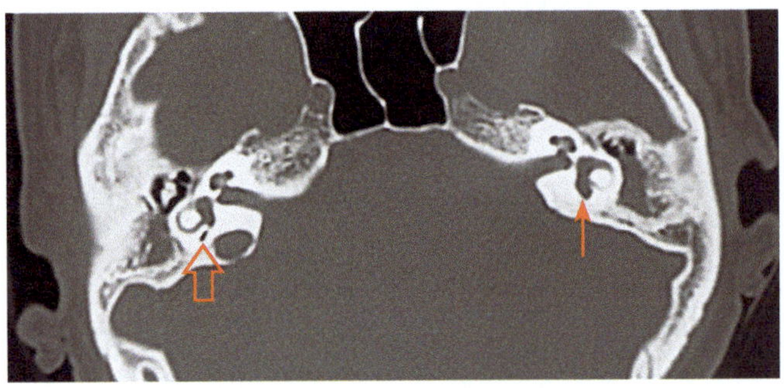

Bilateral posterior semicircular canal dysplasia on axial CT view. Right semicircular canal is short and small (⇧), left semicircular canal is short and thick (↑).

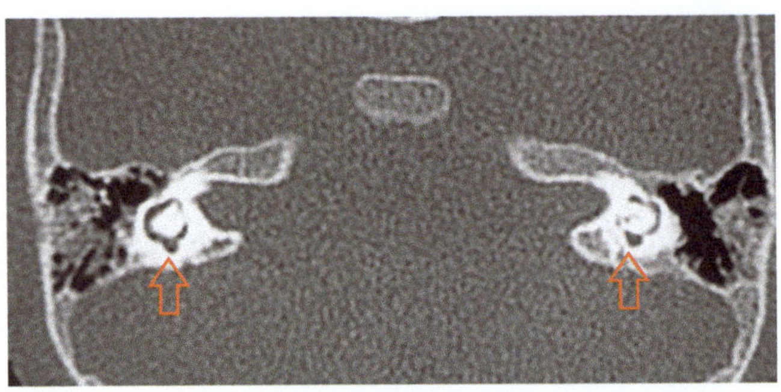

Bilateral posterior semicircular canal malformation on axial CT view. There were only remnants of the posterior semicircular canal of bilateral ears (⇧).

3.3.3 Vestibular Aqueduct Malformation

See Figs. 3.12, 3.13, 3.14 and 3.15.

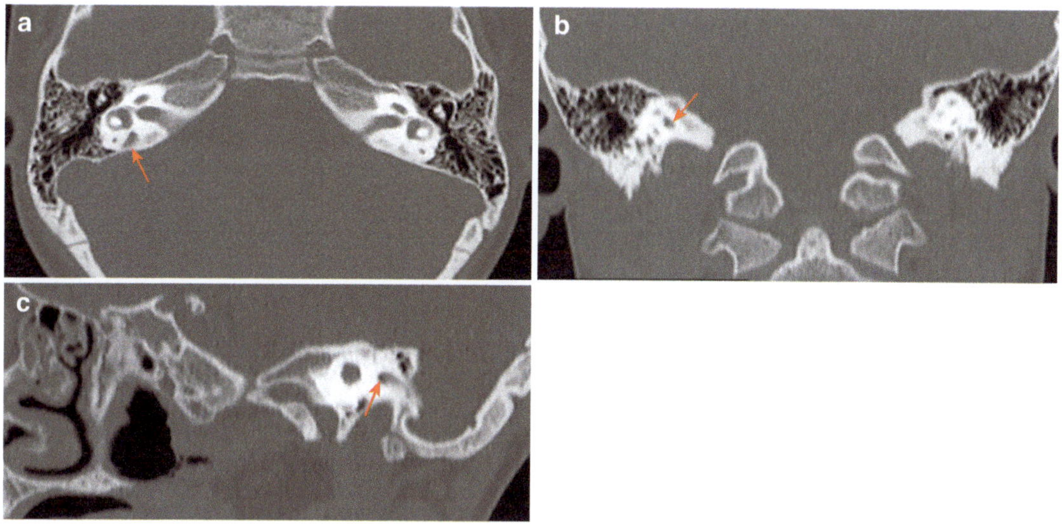

Fig. 3.12 Vestibular aqueduct enlargement of right ear. (**a**) Axial CT; (**b**) Coronal CT; (**c**) Sagittal CT. Unilateral vestibular aqueduct enlargement (↑) is relatively rare

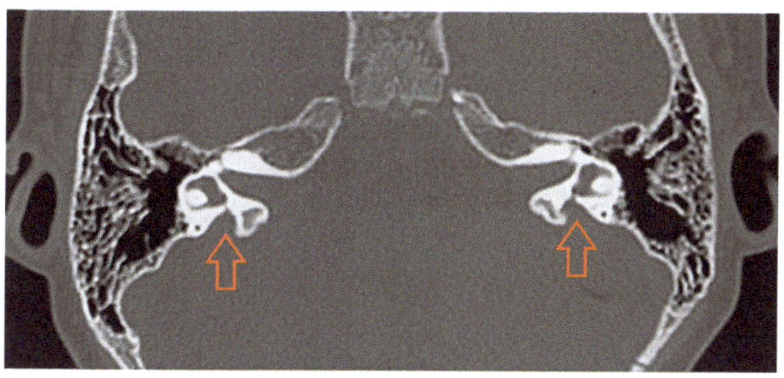

Fig. 3.13 Bilateral vestibular aqueduct enlargement on axial CT view. Conical enlargement of bilateral vestibular aqueducts (⇧)

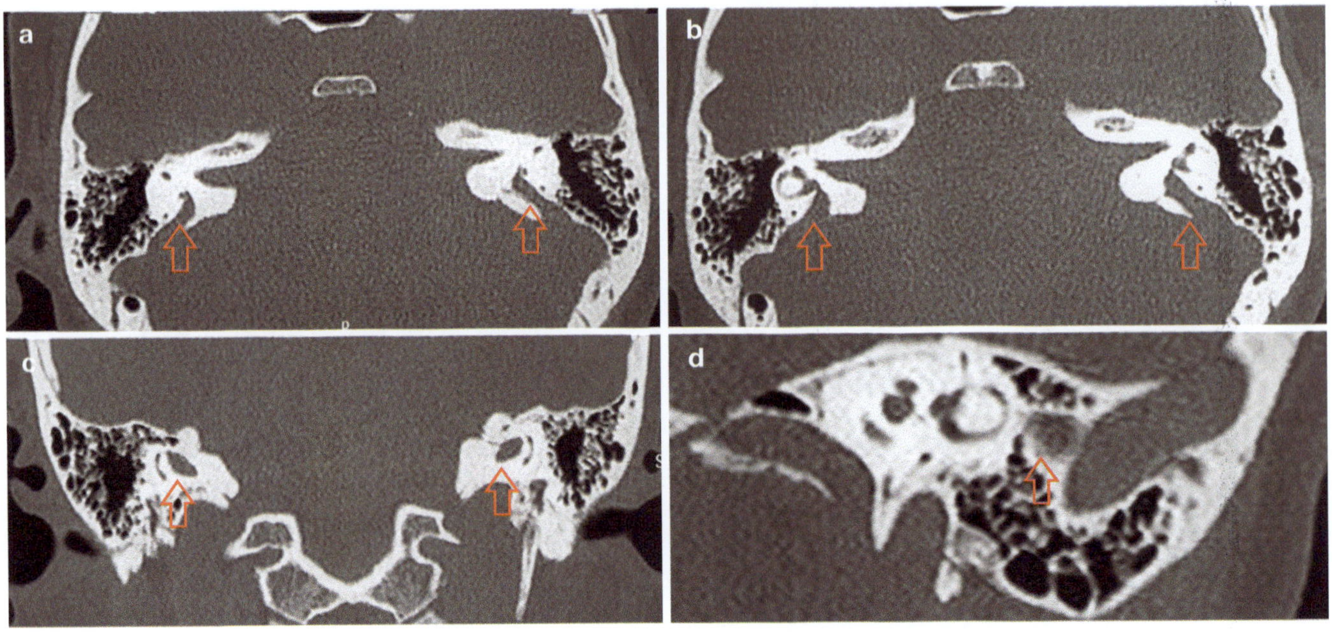

Fig. 3.14 Enlarged vestibular aqueduct in bilateral ears. (**a**, **b**). Axial CT; (**c**) Coronal CT; (**d**) Sagittal CT. Different view positions showed enlarged flat tubular vestibular aqueduct (⇧)

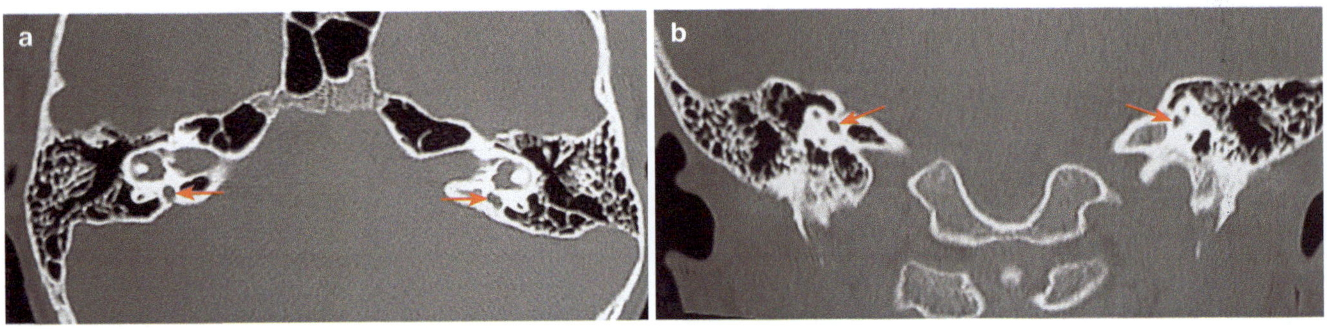

Fig. 3.15 Enlarged bilateral vestibular aqueduct. (**a**) Axial CT; (**b**) Coronal CT. Middle segment of vestibular aqueduct was enlarged (⇧).

Note: Large vestibular aqueduct (LVA) is the most common inner ear anomaly with sensorineural hearing loss (Dewan et al. 2009)

3.3.4 Cochlear Malformation

See Figs. 3.16 and 3.17.

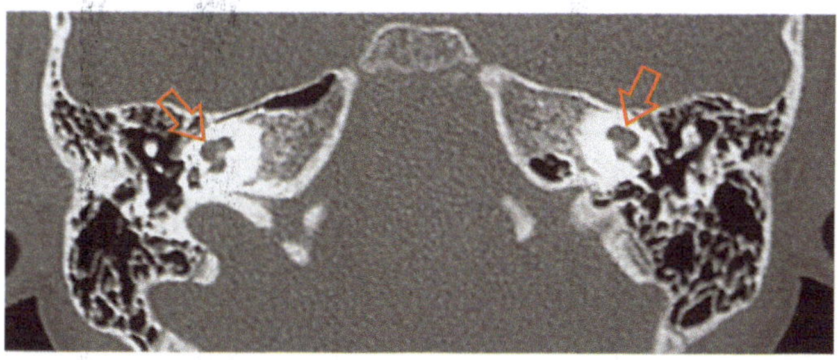

Fig. 3.16 Mondini malformation of bilateral cochleae on axial CT view. Cochlear fusion in the second and third turns (⇧)

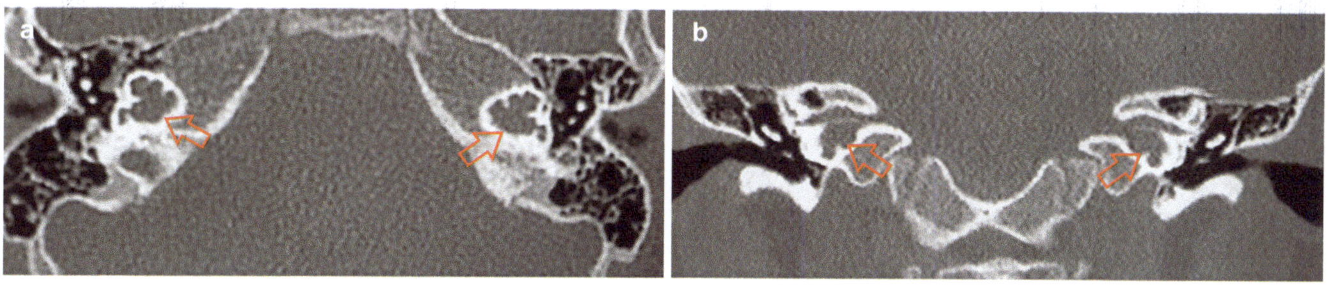

Fig. 3.17 Cochlear malformation of bilateral cochleae (**a**) Axial CT; (**b**) Coronal CT. Modiolus of bilateral cochleae disappeared and was sac-shaped (⇧), fused with the internal acoustic meatus

3.3.5 Malformation of Internal Acoustic Meatus and Foramen of Cochlear Nerve

See Figs. 3.18, 3.19 and 3.20.

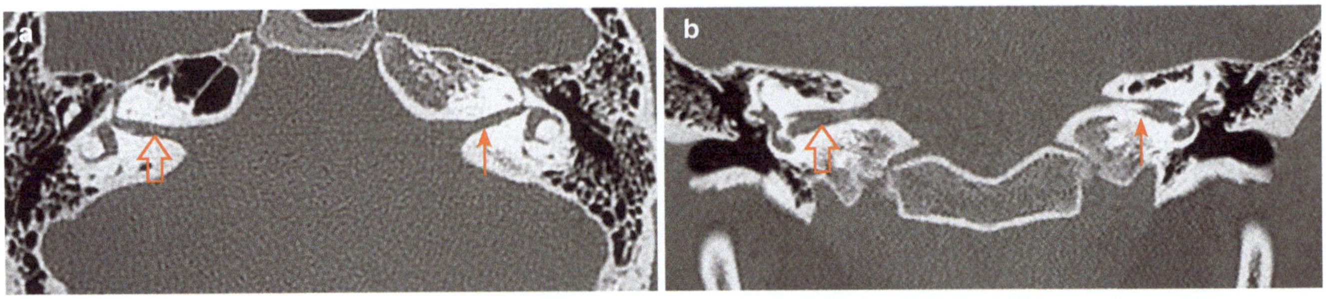

Fig. 3.18 Bilateral internal acoustic meatus stenosis. (**a**) Axial CT; (**b**) Coronal CT. Bilateral internal auditory canal stenosis, right ear (⇧), left ear (↑)

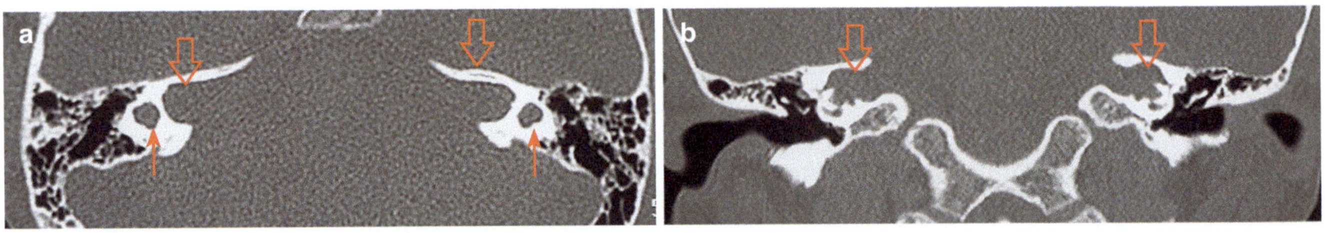

Fig. 3.19 Bilateral inner ear and internal acoustic meatus malformation. (**a**) Axial CT; (**b**) Coronal CT. Ampullary enlargement of bilateral internal acoustic meatus (⇧), bilateral lateral semicircular canal malformation (↑)

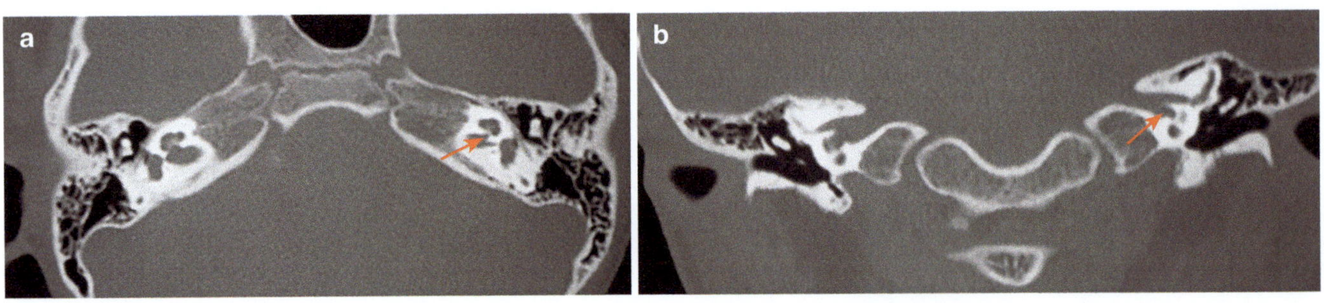

Fig. 3.20 Stenosis of cochlear foramen in left ear. (**a**) Axial CT; (**b**) Coronal CT. Narrow cochlear foramen (↑)

3.3.6 Complex Malformations of Inner Ear

See Figs. 3.21 and 3.22.

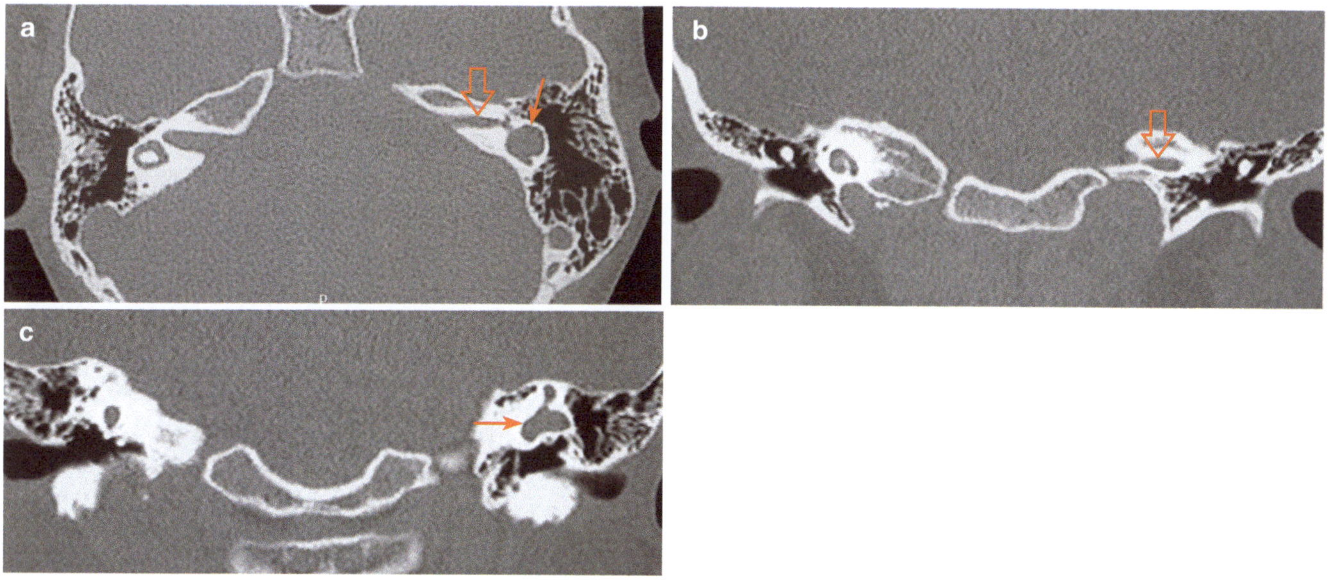

Fig. 3.21 Malformation of internal acoustic meatus and vestibular & cochlea in left ear. (**a**) Axial CT; (**b**, **c**) Coronal CT. Internal acoustic meatus stenosis (⇧), lateral semicircular canal fusion (↑), no cochlear development

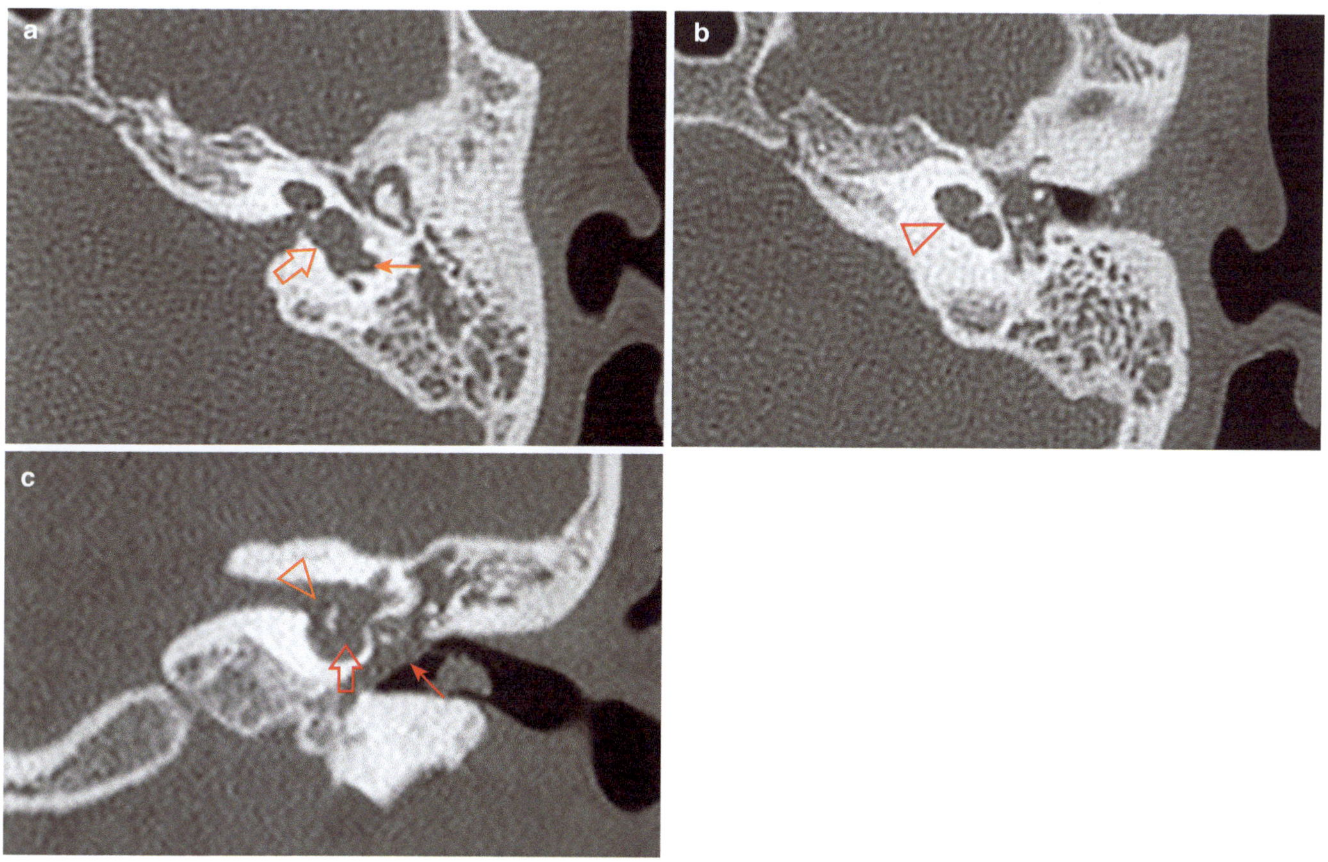

Fig. 3.22 Common cavity malformation with cerebrospinal fluid otorrhea in left ear. (**a**, **b**) Axial CT; (**c**) Coronal CT. Expanded vestibule (⇧), lateral semicircular canal (↑) and cochlear duct (△) were fused into one body, fundus of internal acoustic meatus was also hypoplasia, tympanomastoid cavity was full of soft tissue shadow (↑).

Note: The patient had suffered from ipsilateral suppurative meningitis for several times, the hearing of ipsilateral ear had lost completely, MR hydrography was needed for the diagnosis of cerebrospinal fluid otorrhea

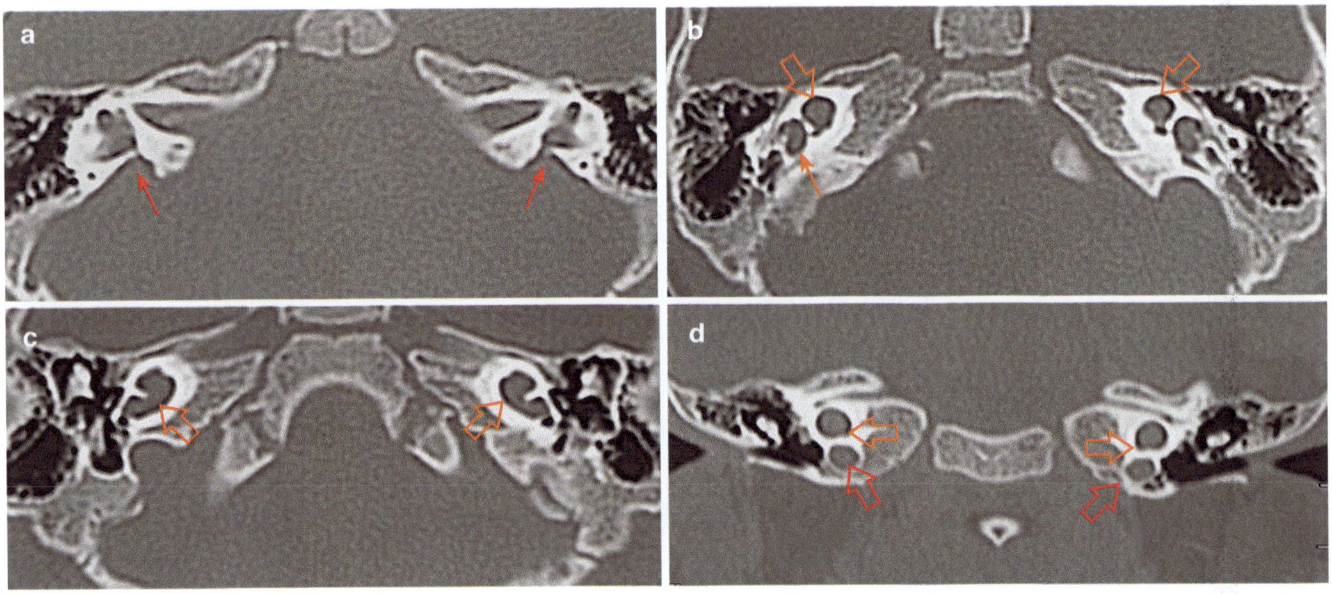

Complex malformations of bilateral inner ear. (**a–c**). Axial CT; (**d**). Coronal CT. Bilateral sacculated cochleae (⇧), enlarged vestibular (↑) and vestibular aqueduct (↑); carotid artery canal (⇧).

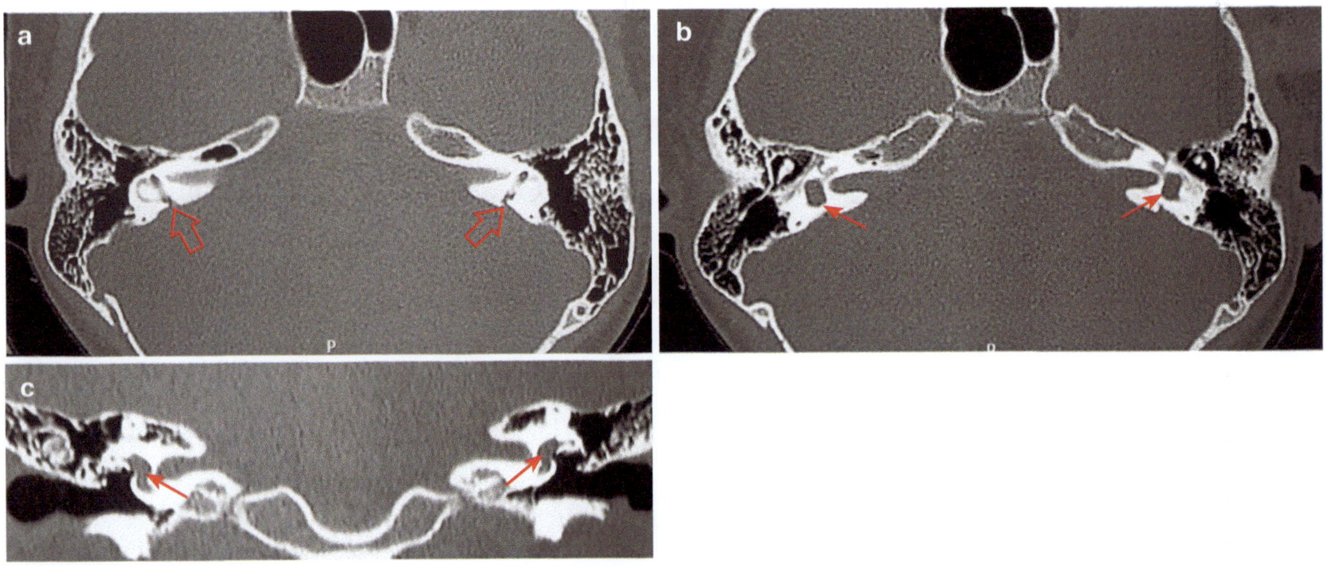

Enlarged vestibule and vestibular aqueduct. (**a**, **b**). Axial CT; (**c**) Coronal CT. A short and enlarged vestibular aqueducts (⇧) and enlarged vestibule (↑).

3.3.7 Complete Labyrinthine Aplasia

See Figs. 3.23, 3.24 and 3.25.

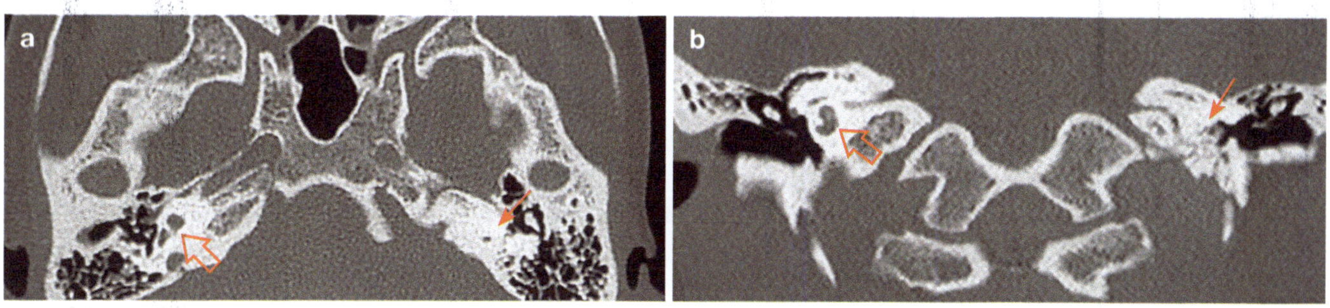

Fig. 3.23 Mondini and Michel aplasia. (**a**) Axial CT; (**b**) Coronal CT. Right Mondini aplasia -the cochlea (⇧) only had 1½ turns, left inner ear (↑) was completely aplasia -Michel aplasia

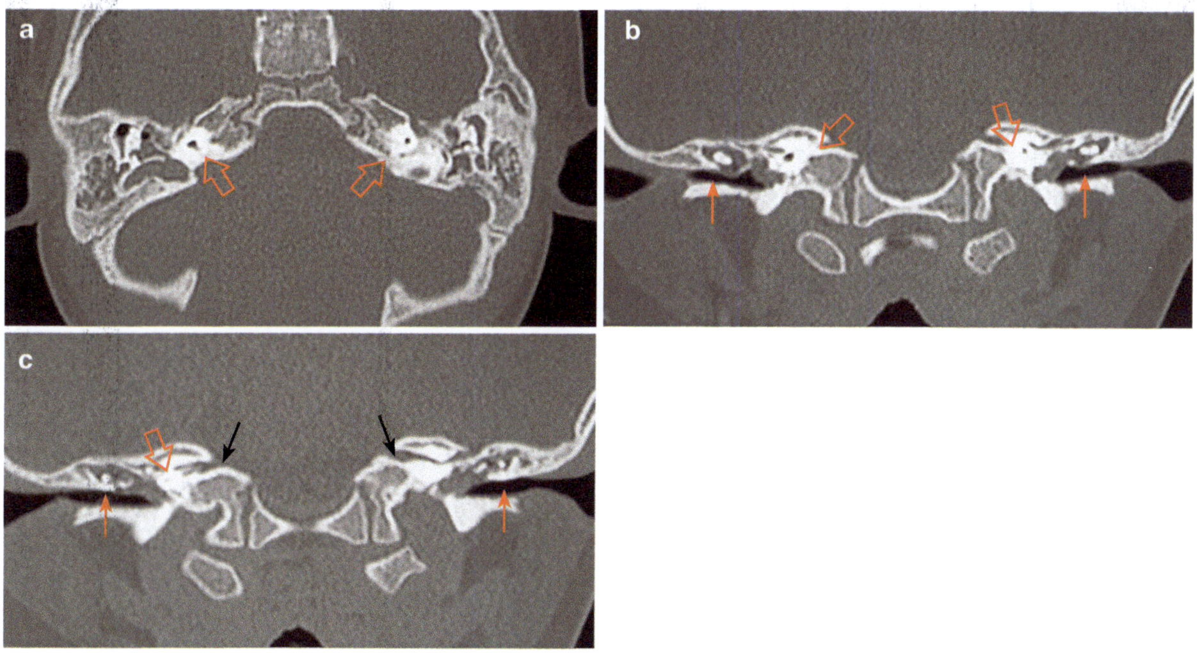

Fig. 3.24 Bilateral Michel aplasia. (**a**) Axial CT; (**b**, **c**) Coronal CT. Bilateral inner ear (⇧) were completely aplasia-Michel aplasia; Stenosis of external auditory canal (↑) and internal acoustic meatus (↑) with tympanic soft tissue shadow

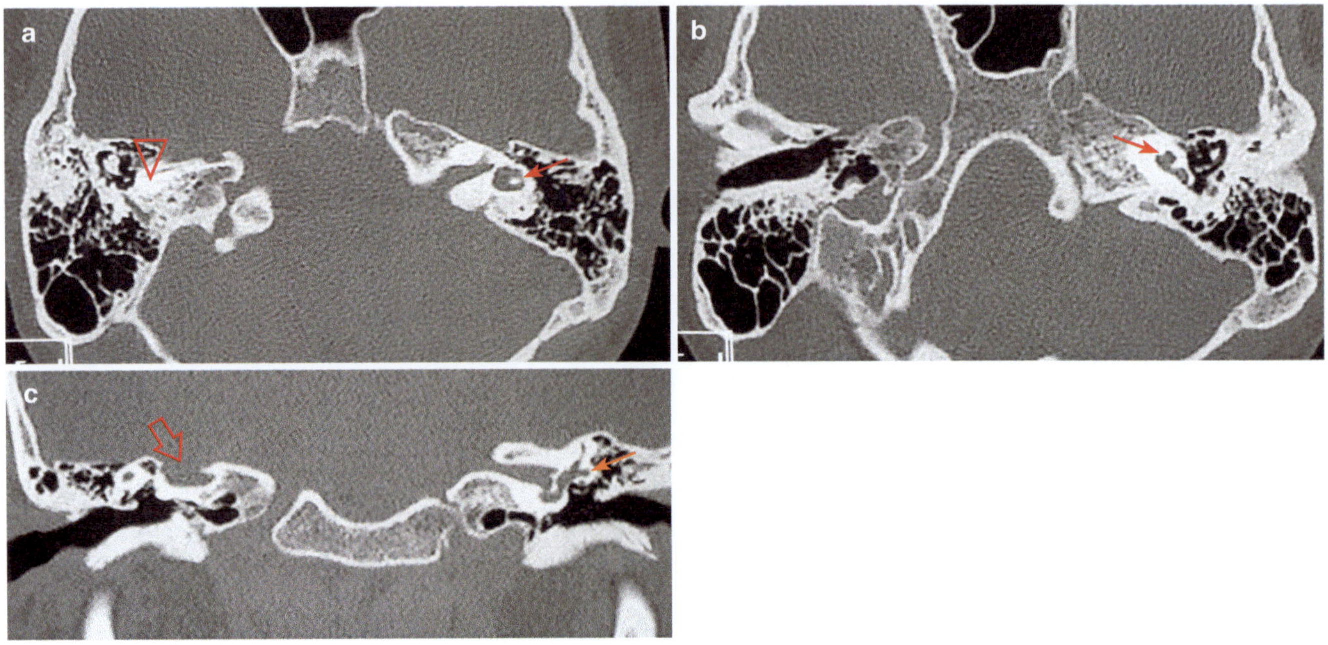

Fig. 3.25 Inner ear aplasia in right deformed petrous portion of temporal bone. (**a**, **b**). Axial CT; (**c**) Coronal CT. Aplasia state (△) of right inner ear and internal acoustic meatus; Petrous apex hypoplasia with deep depression (⇧). Mondini malformation of left cochlea (↑) with short and thick lateral semicircular canal (↑)

3.4 Congenital Anatomical Variation of Temporal Bone

3.4.1 Hypoposition of Middle Cranial Fossa

See Figs. 3.26 and 3.27.

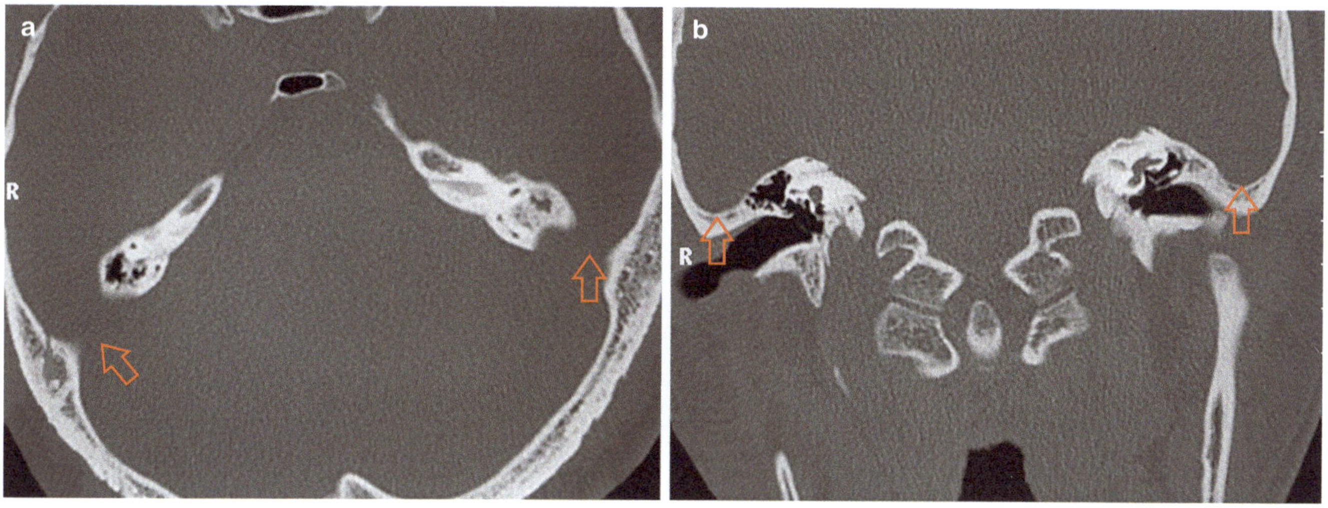

Fig. 3.26 Hypoposition of bilateral middle cranial fossa. (**a**) Axial CT; (**b**) Coronal CT. (**a**) Discontinuities between the petrous and squamous portion of bilateral temporal bones at this level (⇧); (**b**) Lower position of bilateral middle cranial fossa (⇧)

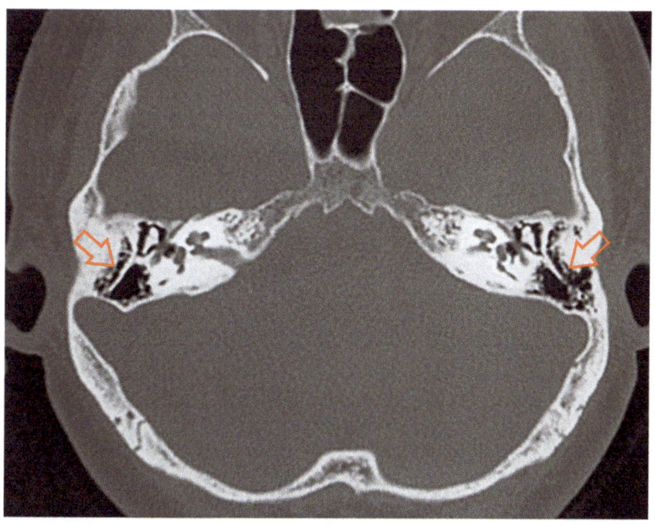

Fig. 3.27 Bilateral Korner septum on axial CT view. Korner septum (⇧) divided the mastoid cavity into the inner and the outer parts

3.4.2 Anteposition of Sigmoid Sinus

See Figs. 3.28 and 3.29.

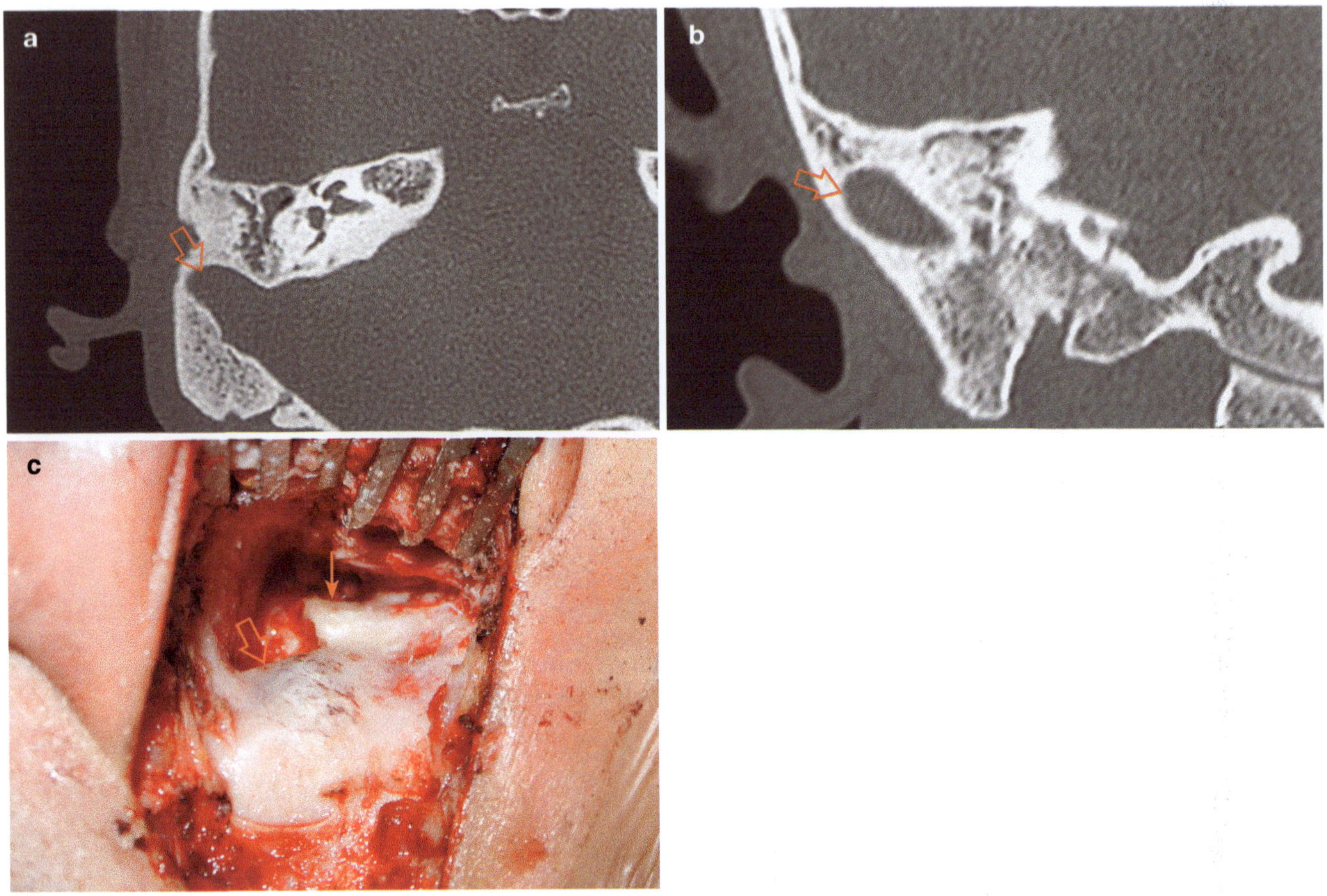

Fig. 3.28 Anteposition of right sigmoid sinus. (**a**) Axial CT; (**b**) Coronal CT; (**c**) Intraoperative finding. (**a**) Sigmoid sinus moved forward at the plane of epitympanum) (⇧); (**b**) Soft tissue shadow with smooth edges could be seen in the sclerotic mastoid cavity (⇧); (**c**) Anteriorly moved sigmoid sinus wall (⇧) and posterior wall of the external auditory canal (↑)

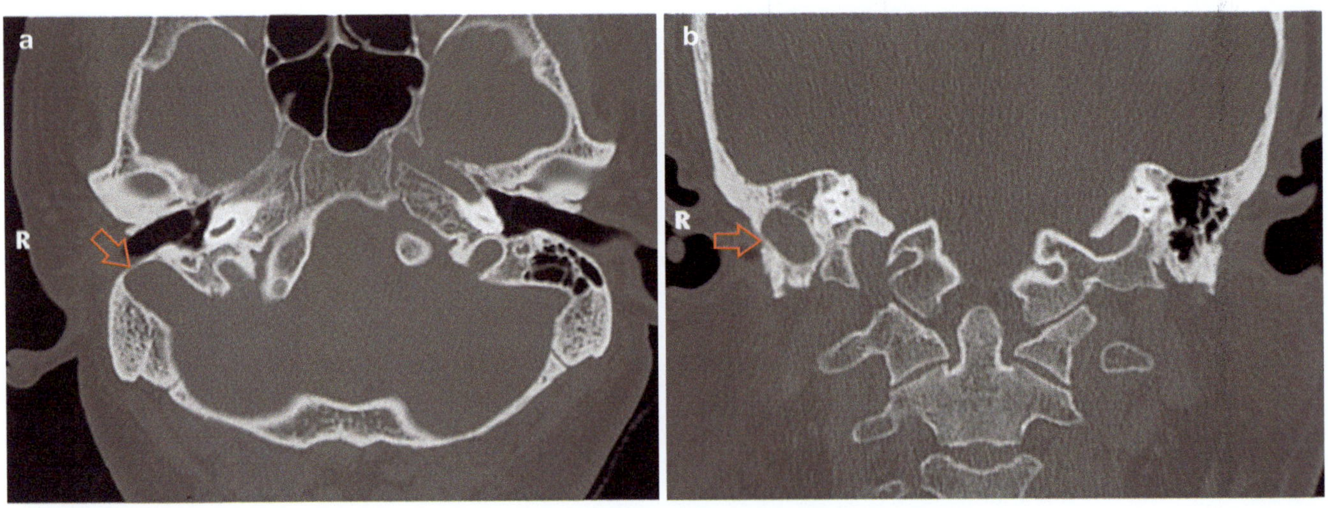

Fig. 3.29 Anteposition of right sigmoid sinus (**a**). Axial CT; (**B**) Coronal CT. (**a**).There is only a thin layer of bone plate (⇧) between sigmoid sinus and posterior wall of external auditory canal;(**b**) Soft tissue shadow with smooth oval edge can be seen in position of mastoid cavity (⇧)

3.4.3 Hyperposition or Nakedness of Jugular Bulb, Carotid Canal, Sigmoid Sinus and so on

Figs. 3.30, 3.31, 3.32, 3.33, 3.34, 3.35, and 3.36.

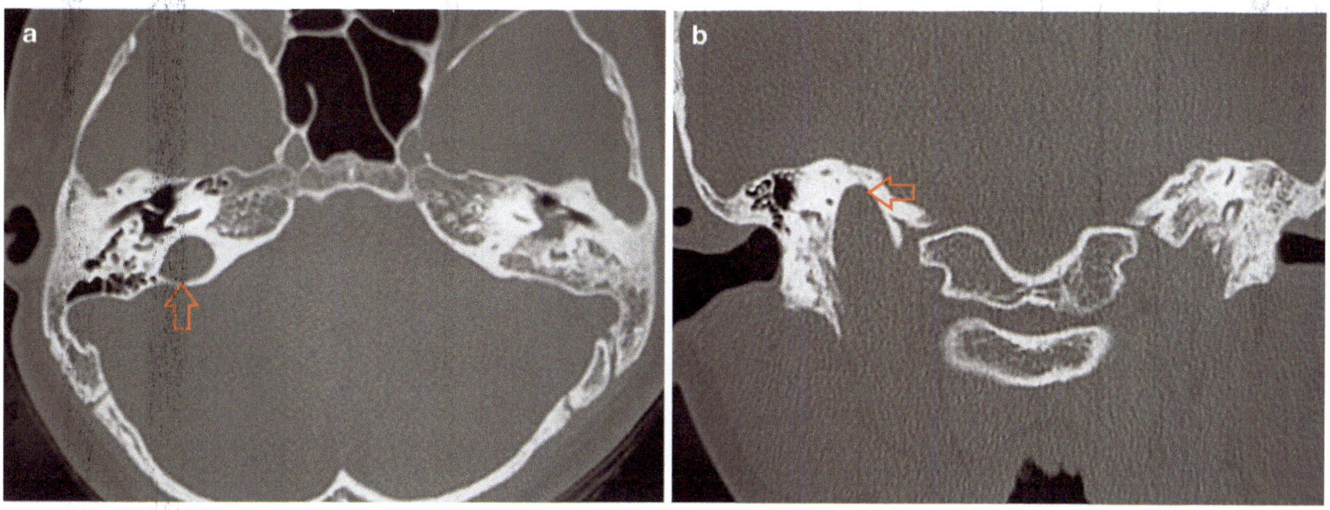

Fig. 3.30 Hyperposition of jugular bulb (fossa) in right ear. (**a**) Axial CT; (**b**) Coronal CT. (**a**) Jugular bulb (⇧) was higher over the level of round window niche; (**b**) Jugular bulb (⇧) was located between the superior and inferior crura of posterior semicircular canal

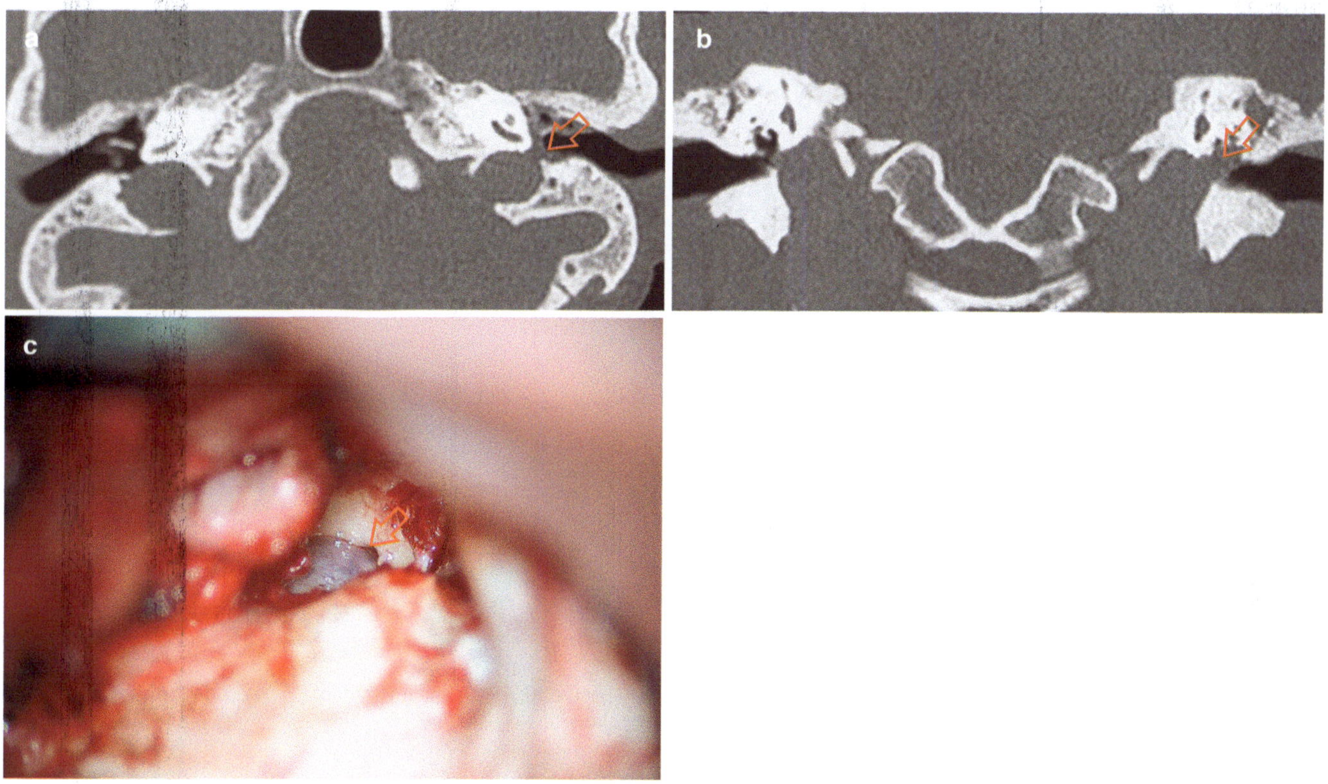

Fig. 3.31 Hyperposition and nakedness of jugular bulb in left ear. (**a**) Axial CT; (**b**) Coronal CT; (**c**) Intraoperative finding. (**a**) Jugular bulb (⇧) protruded into posterior inferior tympanum; (**b**) High located jugular bulb (⇧) was collusion with inferior tympanum; (**c**) Light blue high jugular bulb (⇧) was located at the cochlear window niche

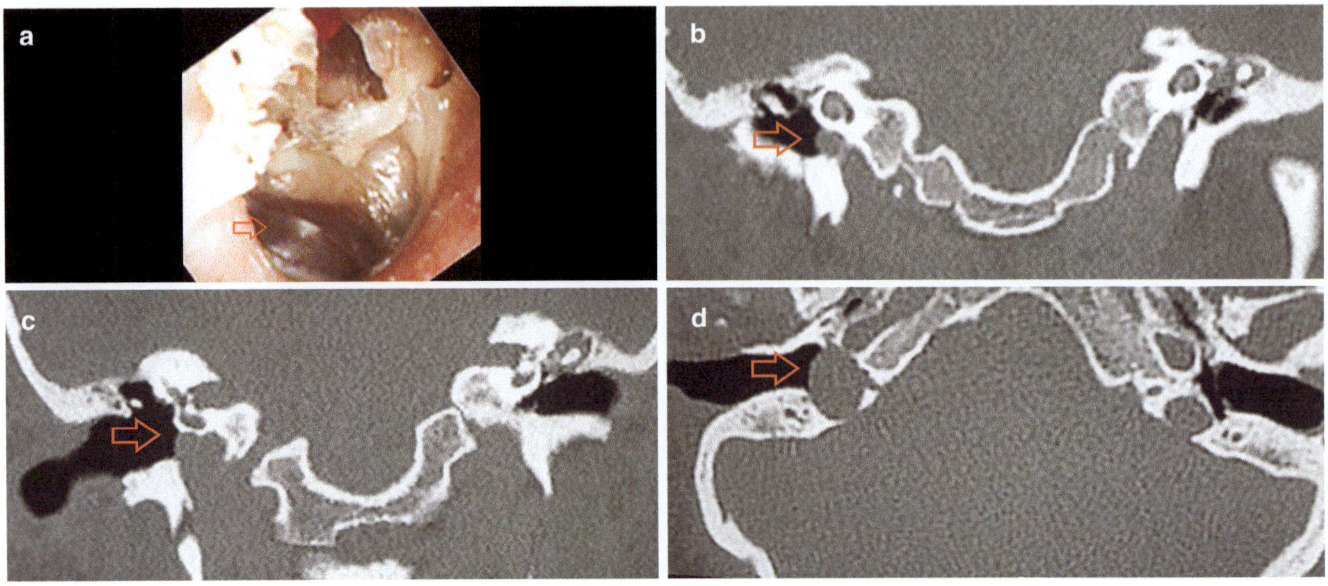

Fig. 3.32 Hyperposition and nakedness of jugular bulb in right ear with adhesive otitis media. (**a**) Endoscopic view; (**b**, **c**). Coronal CT; (**d**). Axial CT. (**a**) Dark jugular bulb in posteroinferior tympanum was seen via ear endoscope (pulsation was visible under dynamic observation), the surface of jugular bulb was covered with the invaginated tympanic membrane (⇧); (**b**–**d**). Spherical soft tissue shadow (⇧) could be seen in hypotympanum, there was no osseous tissue on its surface

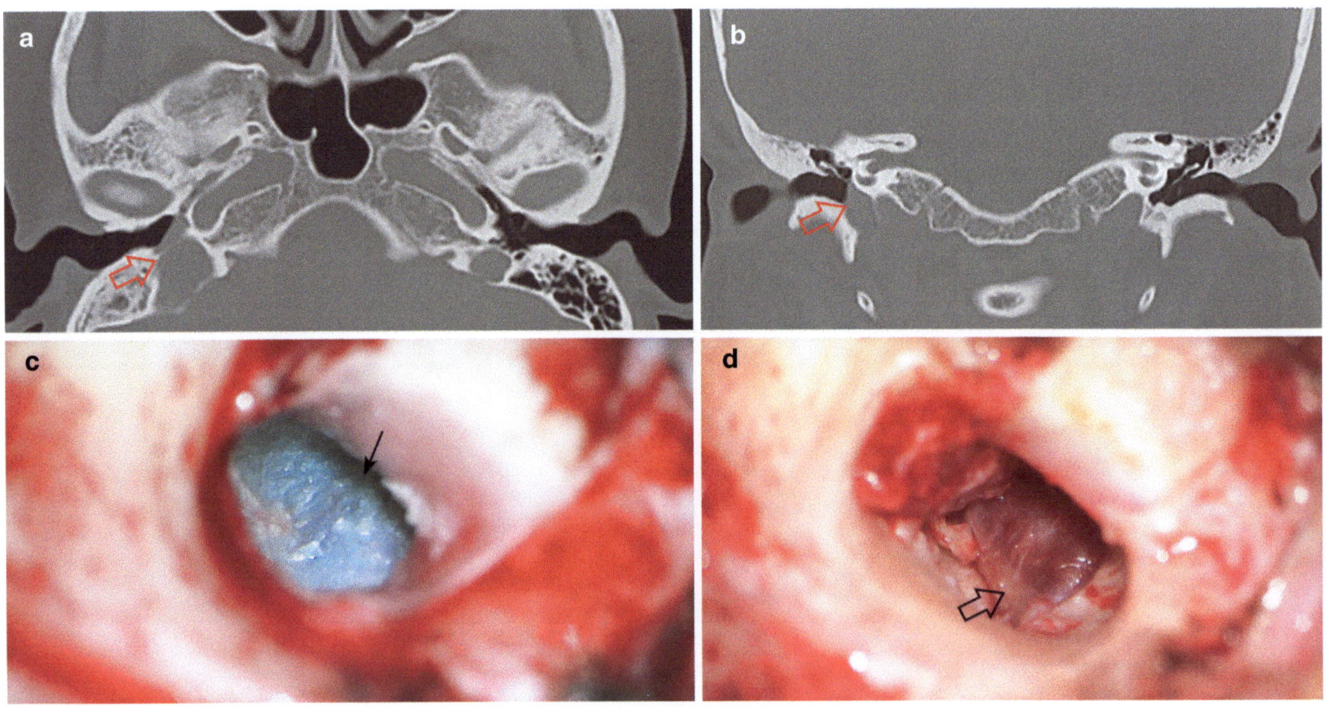

Fig. 3.33 Hyperposition and nakedness of jugular bulb in right ear. (**a**). Axial CT; (**b**) Coronal CT; (**c**, **d**) Intraoperative finding. (**a**, **b**). High located and exposed jugular bulb (⇧) protruded into posteroinferior tympanum; (**c**) Tympanic membrane (↑) was dark blue; (**d**) Exposed jugular bulb was dark red (⇧)

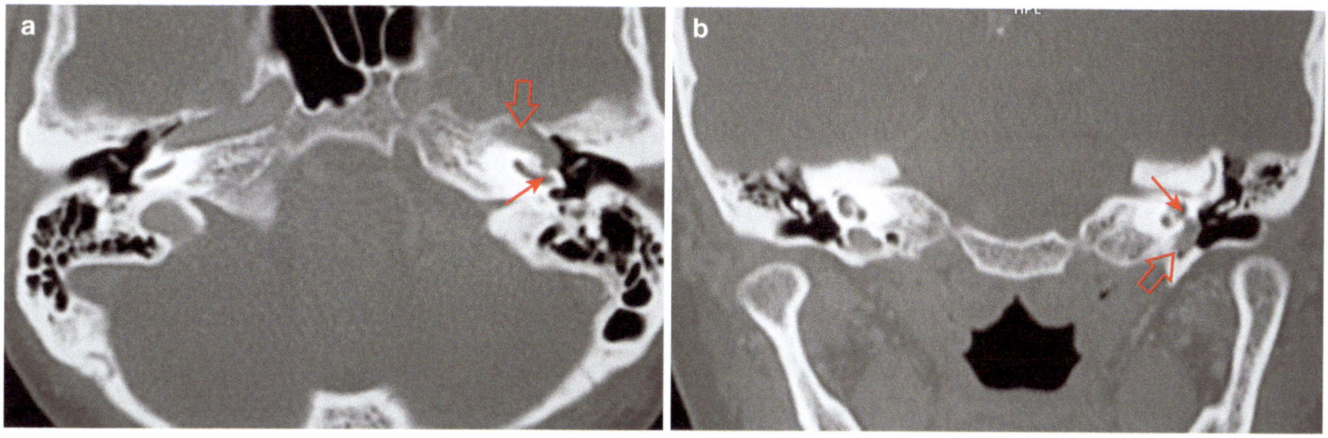

Fig. 3.34 Hyperposition of carotid artery with partial absence of cochlear bone. (**a**) Axial CT; (**b**) Coronal CT. High positional carotid artery (⇧) was attached to cochlear duct with partial bone absence of cochlea(↑)

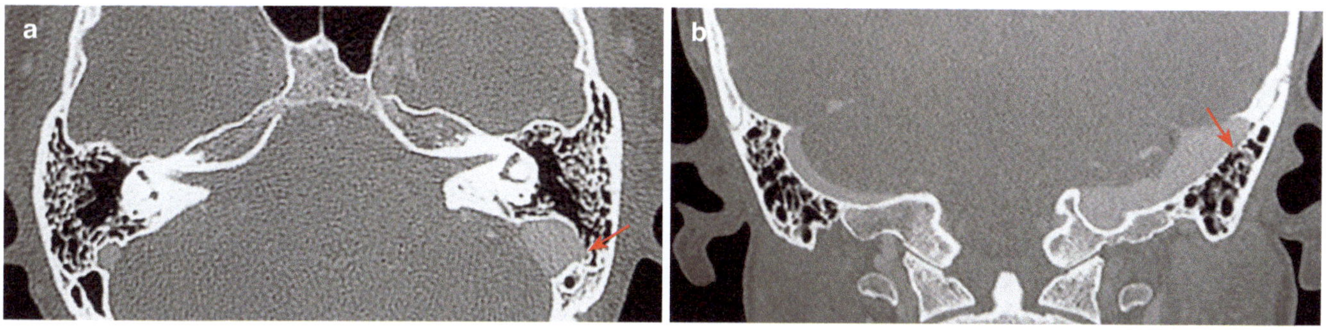

Fig. 3.35 Bony absence of sigmoid sulcus in left ear with ipsilateral pulsatile tinnitus. (**a**) Axial CT; (**b**) Coronal CT. Bone plate of sigmoid sulcus was discontinuous (↑) in left ear

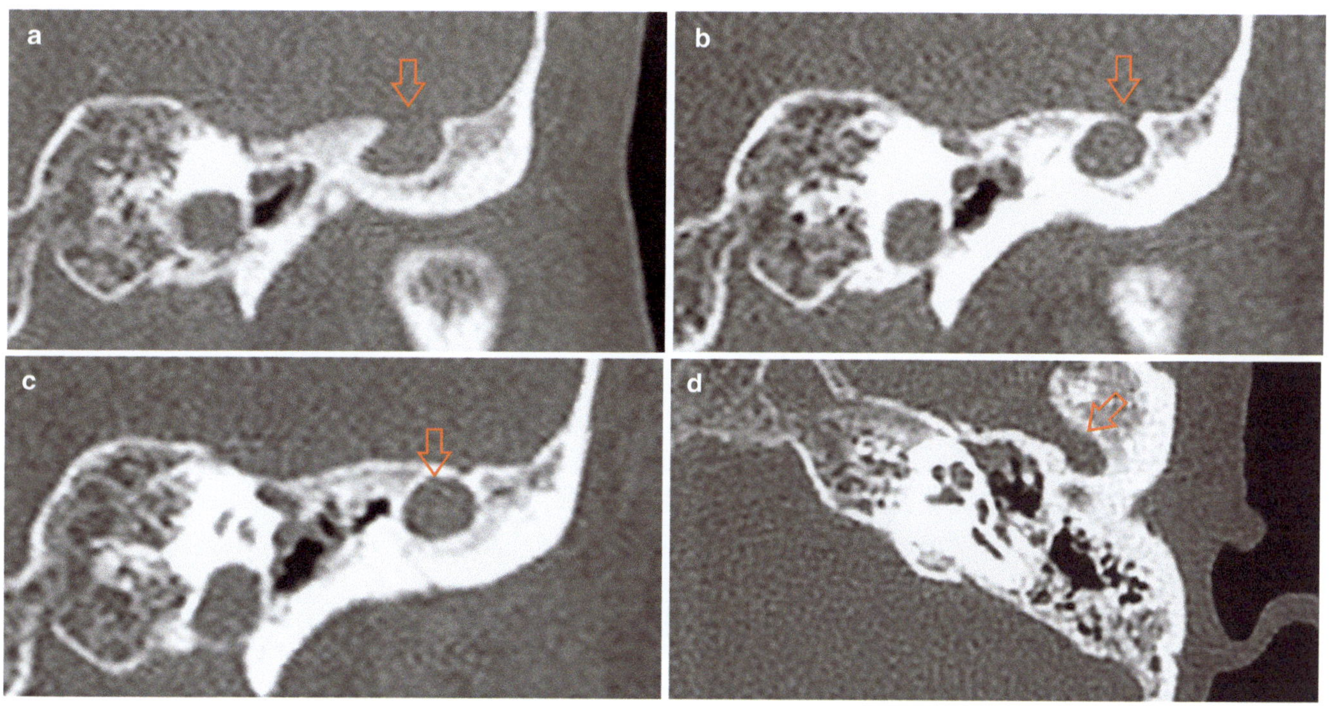

Fig. 3.36 Abnormal venous sinus in basal wall of middle cranial fossa (left). (**a**–**c**) Coronal CT; (**d**) Axial CT. Deep osseous depression (⇧) or tubular osseous canal (⇧) in basal wall of middle cranial fossa

3.4.4 Excessive Pneumatization of Temporal Bone

See Figs. 3.37 and 3.38.

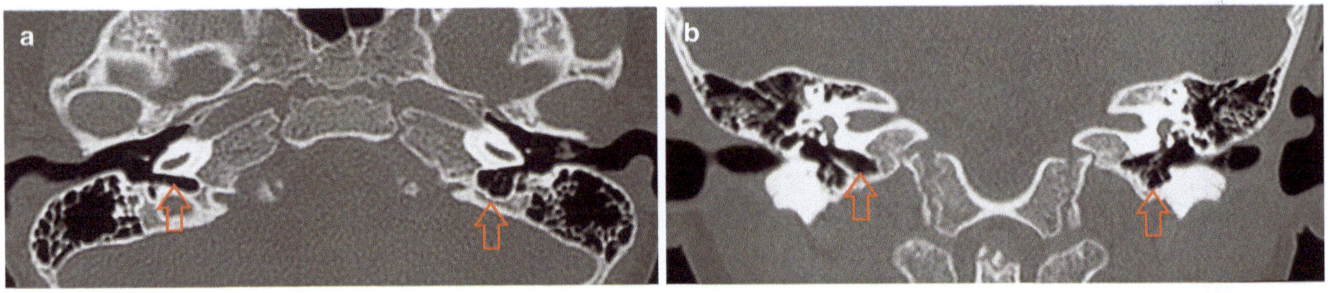

Fig. 3.37 Posteroinferior cells of labyrinth in bilateral ears. (**a**) Axial CT; (**b**) Coronal CT. Temporal bones were excessively pneumatized, deep and large air cells (⇧) were located in posteroinferior region of labyrinth

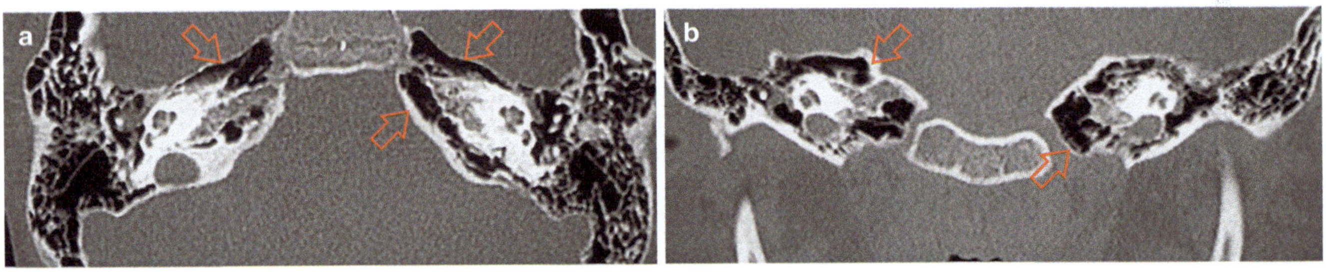

Fig. 3.38 Excessive pneumatization in whole temporal bone. (**a**) Axial CT; (**b**) Coronal CT. Whole temporal bone (including the petrous apex) (⇧) was excessive pneumatized

Trauma of Ear

4

Zilong Yu, Bentao Yang, and Xiping Li

The ear is located on both sides of the skull and mainly consists of temporal bone, which is one of the important structures forming the lateral skull base. Trauma of ear is usually a part of craniocerebral trauma. While paying attention to craniocerebral trauma, we should notice if it is accompanying the temporal bone injury. Intracranial complications can also occur if temporal bone trauma is not treated in time. Transverse fractures of temporal bone are more commonly associated with facial nerve paralysis (approx. up to 50%) than longitudinal fractures (approx. up to 20%) (Aguilar et al. 1987; Cannon et al. 1983), but the longitudinal fracture is more common, accounting for about 70%–80% of temporal bone fracture (Raghavan et al. 2009). There are two weak areas in the temporal bone, which are prone to form transverse fractures. The first is internal acoustic meatus where the fractures can cause facial nerve injury and cochlear fracture; the second is the cochlear canaliculus where the fracture can result in cochlear fracture.

4.1 Transverse Fracture of Temporal Bone

See Fig. 4.1.

Z. Yu (✉)
Department of Otolaryngology Head and Neck Surgery, Beijing Tongren Hospital, Capital Medical University, Beijing, China

B. Yang
Department of Radiology, Beijing Tongren Hospital, Capital Medical University, Beijing, China

X. Li
Department of Otolaryngology Head and Neck Surgery, Beijing Anzhen Hospital, Capital Medical University, Beijing, China

Z. Yu (ed.), *Ear Diseases and CT*, https://doi.org/10.1007/978-981-99-7220-3_4

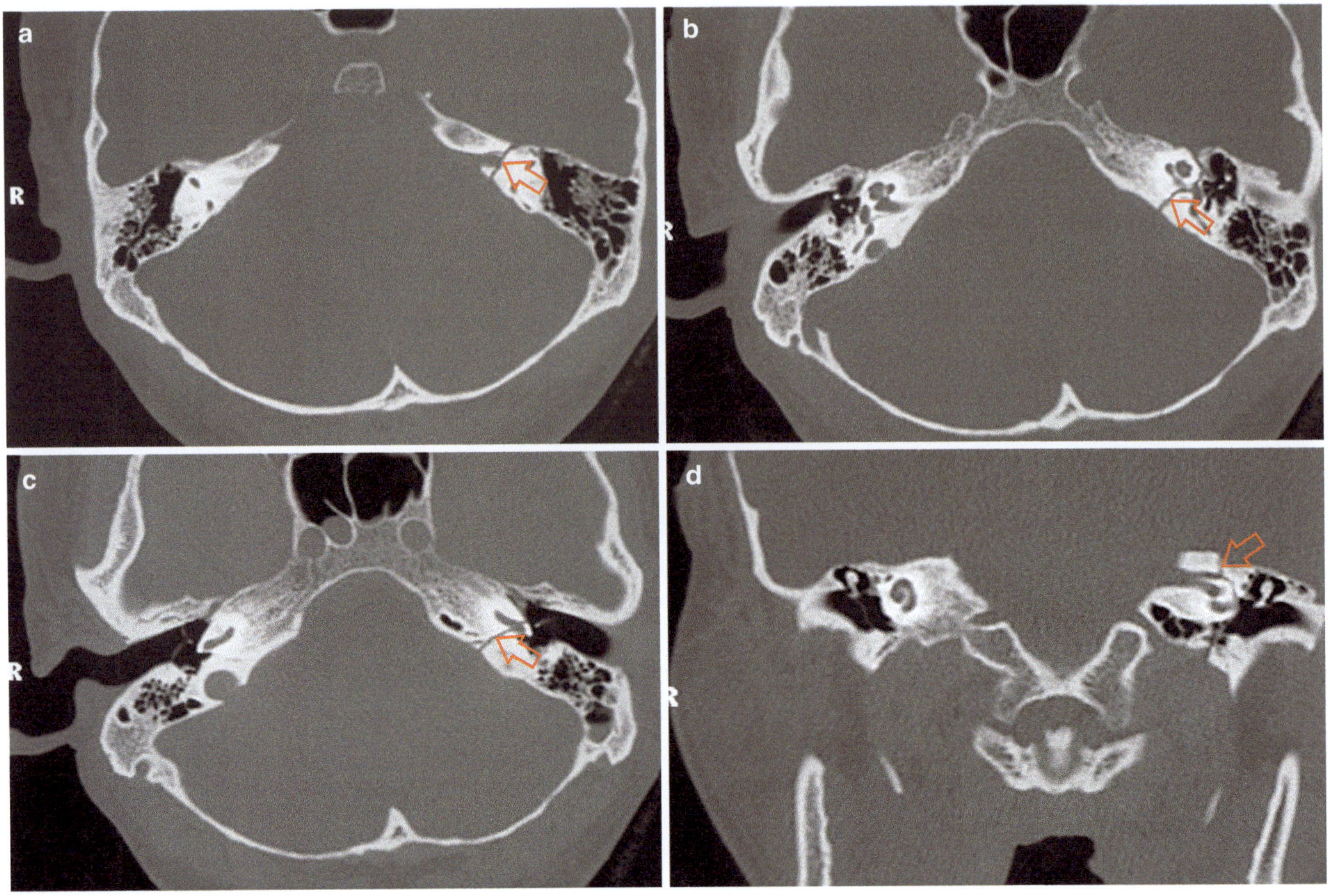

Fig. 4.1 Transverse fracture of left temporal bone. (**a–c**) Axial CT; (**d**) Coronal CT. (**a** and **d**). Fracture line (⇧) traversed fundus of internal acoustic meatus; (**b**) Fracture line ran through vestibular window (⇧); (**c**) Fracture line (⇧) traversed the cochlear canaliculus and cochlea

4.2 Longitudinal Fracture of Temporal Bone

See Fig. 4.2.

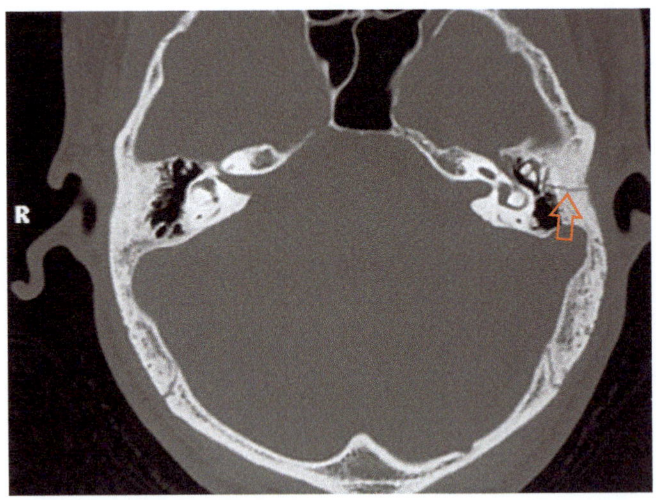

Fig. 4.2 Longitudinal fracture of left temporal bone on axial CT view. Fracture line (⇧) passed through the top wall of external auditory canal

4.3 Multiple and Comminuted Fractures of Temporal Bone

See Figs. 4.3, 4.4, 4.5, 4.6 and 4.7.

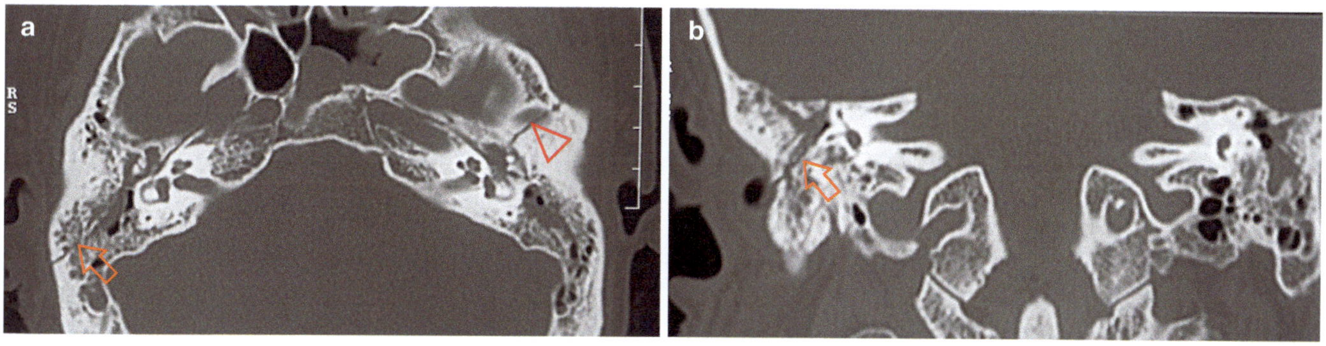

Fig. 4.3 Bilateral temporal bone fracture. (**a**) Axial CT; (**b**) Coronal CT. (**a**) Right ear longitudinal fracture line (⇧) crossed mastoid process, middle ear cavity and petrous portion of temporal bone, left ear fracture line (⇧) crossed temporomandibular joint; (**b**) Right fracture line obliquely crossed skull base of middle cranial fossa (⇧)

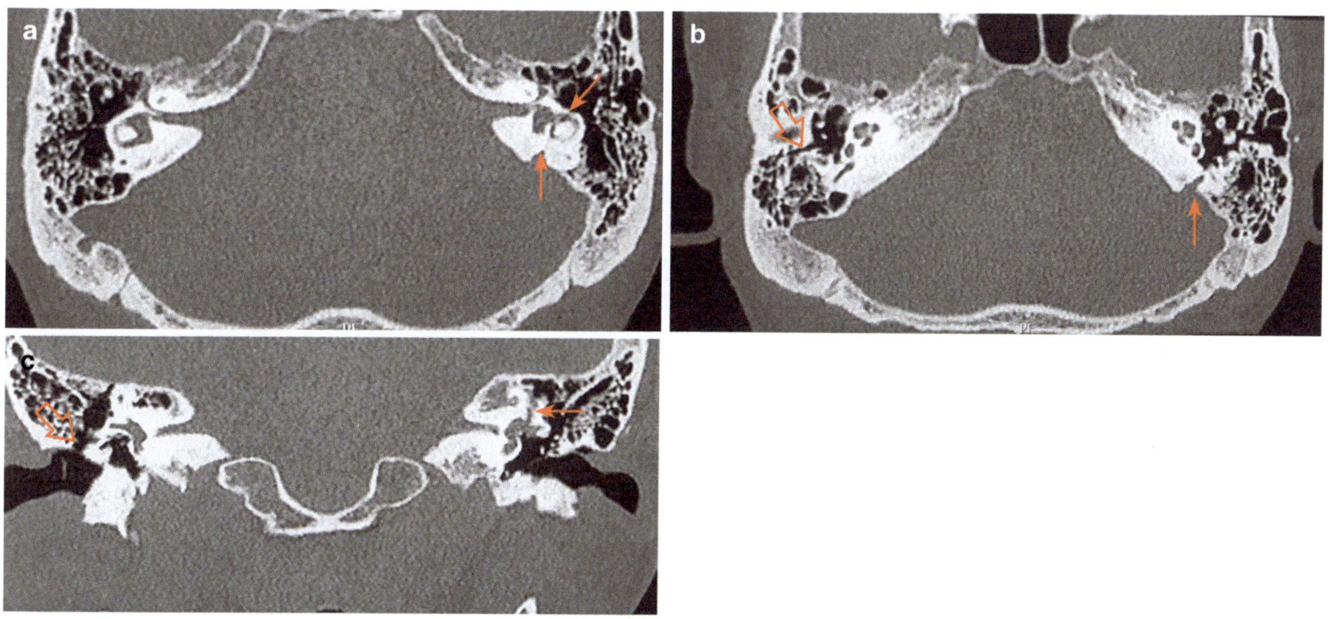

Fig. 4.4 Bilateral temporal bone fracture. (**a**, **b**) Axial CT; (**c**) Coronal CT. (**a**) Fracture line crossed lateral semicircular canal of left ear (↑); (**b**) Fracture line crossed superior wall of right external auditory canal (⇧), the long axis of left petrous portion was broken and displacement (↑); (**c**) Fracture line crossed the skull base of right middle cranial fossa (⇧) and fracture line passed through anterior semicircular canal of left ear (↑)

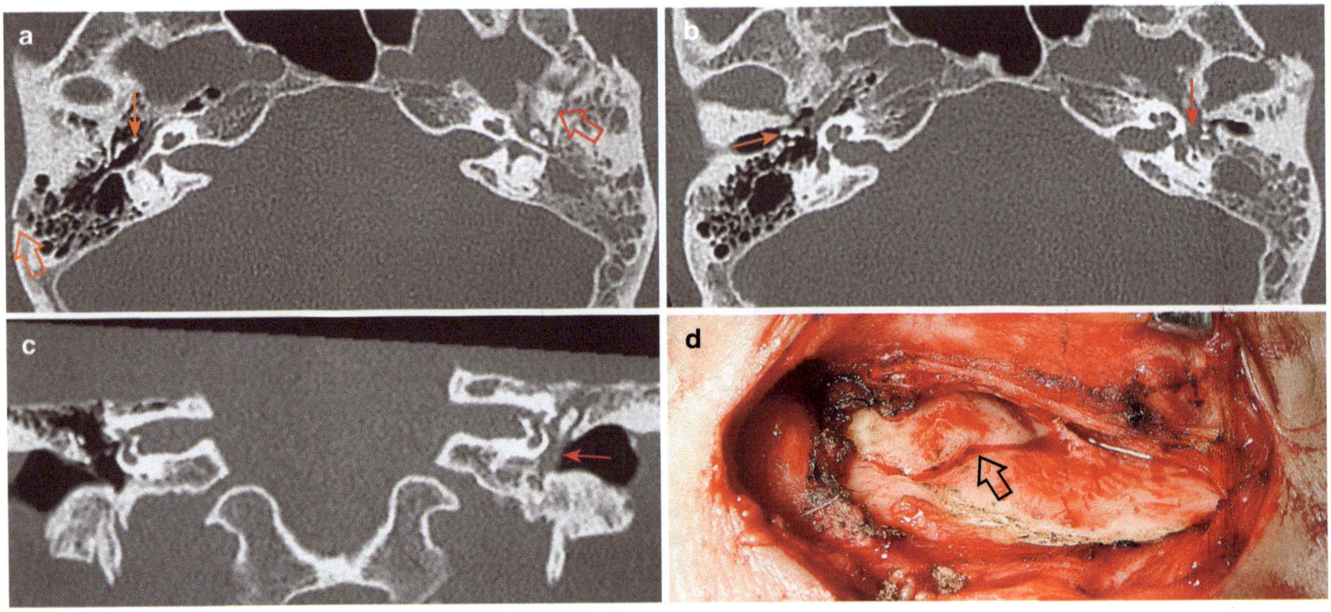

Fig. 4.5 Bilateral temporal bone fracture. (**a, b**) Axial CT; (**c**) Coronal CT; (**d**) Intraoperative finding. (**a**) Right ear longitudinal fracture (⇧) and malleus displacement (↑), left transverse fracture (⇧); (**b**) Right ear malleus lying horizontally in tympanum (↑), soft tissue shadow (↑) in left ear mastoid tympanum; (**c**) Left ear tympanum effusion (cerebrospinal fluid to be excluded) (↑); (**d**) Fracture line (⇧) crossed bone cortex of mastoid in right ear

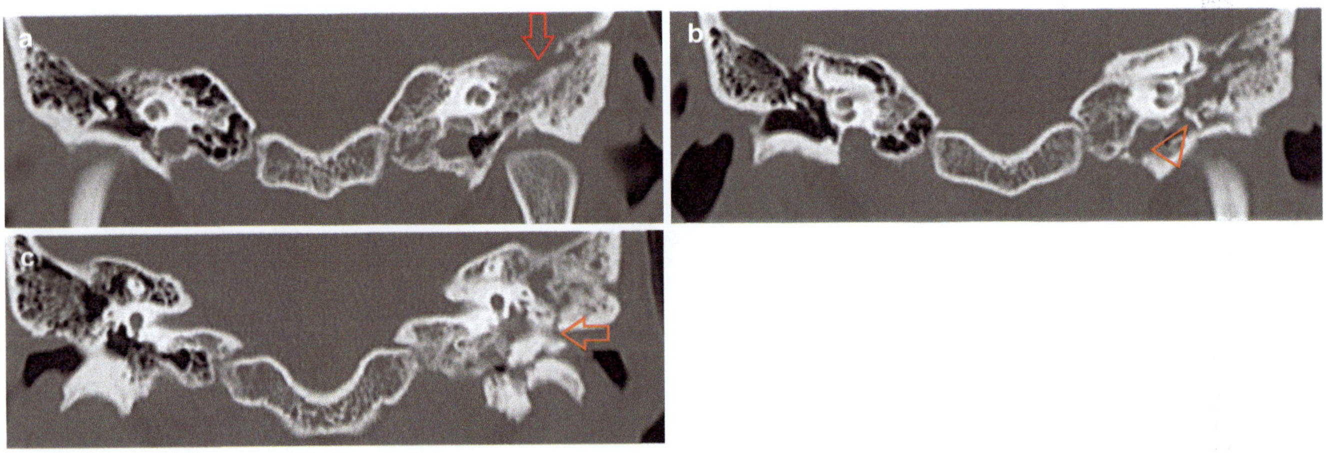

Fig. 4.6 Left temporal bone comminuted fracture. (**a–c**) Coronal CT. (**a**) Fracture of middle cranial fossa base (⇧) in left, middle ear mastoid effusion, eustachian tube contained air; (**b**) Middle ear mastoid effusion (cerebrospinal fluid-confirmed by intraoperative finding), and the displaced malleus and incus (△) blocked tympanic orifice of eustachian tube; (**c**) External auditory canal was obstructed by broken bones (⇧) came from squamous portion and tympanic portion of temporal bone, resulting in external auditory canal atresia, therefor the patient's cerebrospinal fluid did not overflow through external auditory canal or nasopharynx.

Note: When cerebrospinal fluid otorrhea is suspected, MR hydrography examination is needed

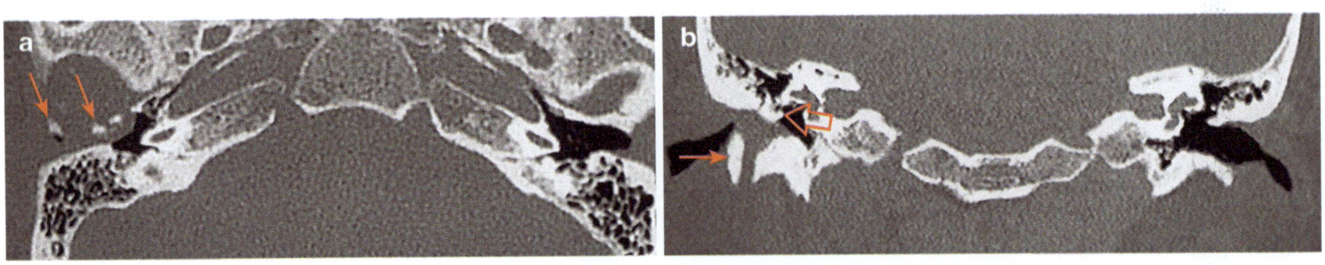

Fig. 4.7 Right temporal bone fracture. (**a**) Axial CT; (**b**) Coronal CT. (**a**) Posterior wall (↑) of right temporomandibular joint (anterior part of tympanic portion) comminuted fracture; (**b**) Inferior wall (↑) of external auditory canal and tympanic scutum fracture (⇧)

4.4 Traumatic Membranous Atresia of External Auditory Canal

See Fig. 4.8.

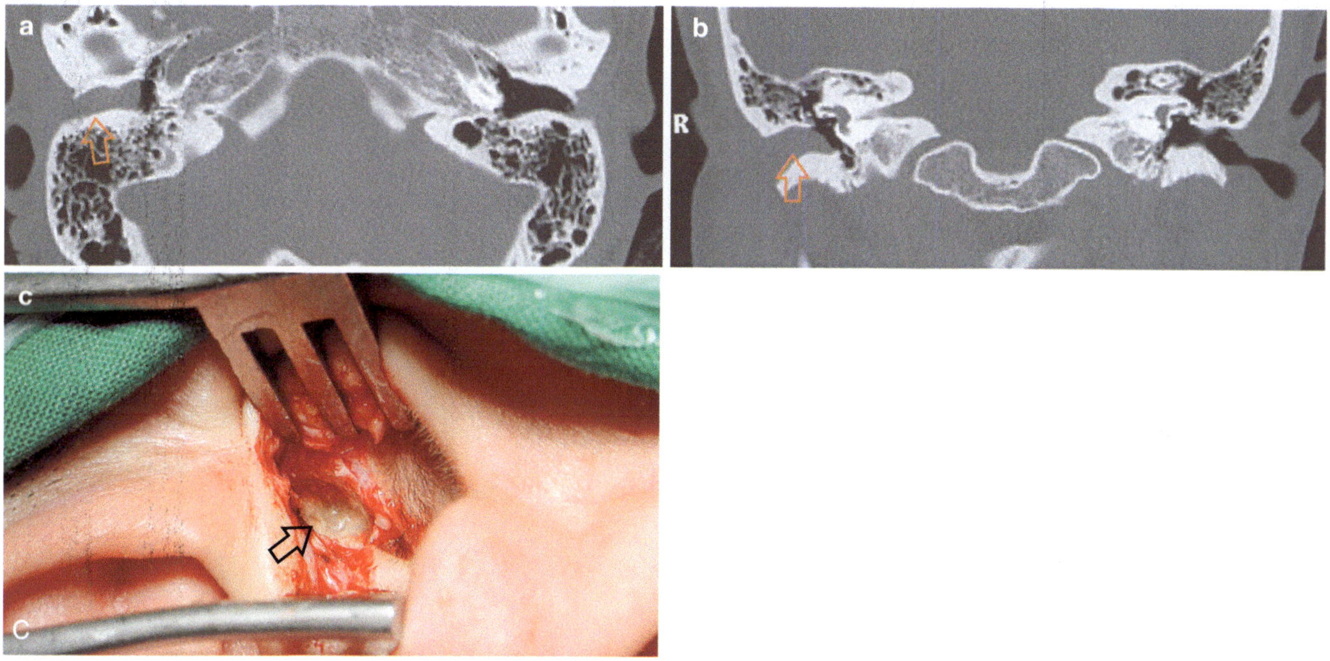

Fig. 4.8 Traumatic membranous atresia of right external auditory canal with formation of cholesteatoma. (**a**) Axial CT; (**b**) Coronal CT; (**c**) Intraoperative finding. (**a**, **b**) Showed soft tissue shadow in right external auditory canal (⇧); (**c**) Right external auditory canal was filled with Cheese-like substance after incision of atresia membrane (⇧).

Note: Membranous atresia of the external auditory canal has a complete bony external auditory canal

4.5 Traumatic Dislocation of Ossicular Chain

Figs. 4.9, 4.10, 4.11, 4.12 and 4.13.

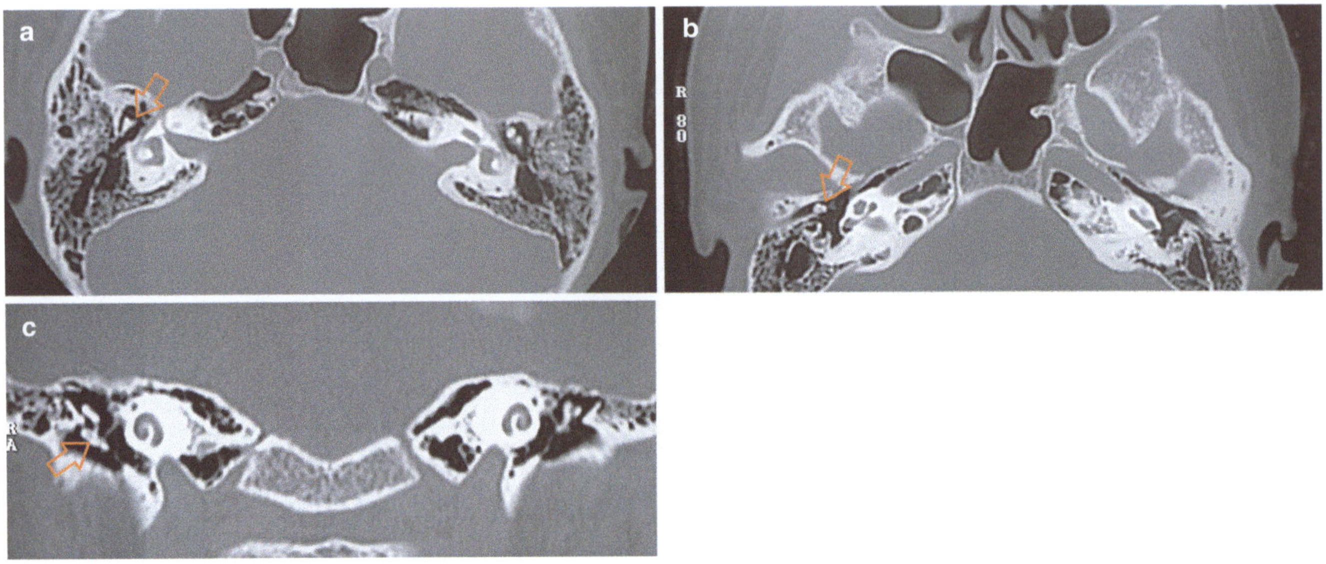

Fig. 4.9 Right ear ossicular chain dislocation. (**a, b**) Axial CT; (**c**) Coronal CT. (**a**) Malleus fell off (⇧); (**b**) Malleus (⇧) moved to the middle tympanum; (**c**) Malleus (⇧) fell off to below the incus

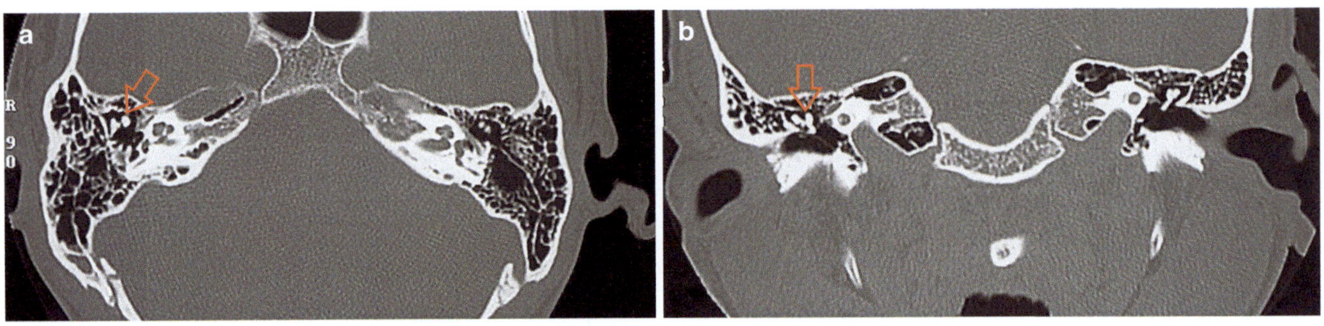

Fig. 4.10 Dislocation of the incudomalleolar articulation in right ear. (**a**) Axial CT; (**b**) Coronal CT. The malleus (⇧) moved to the anteromedial side of incus

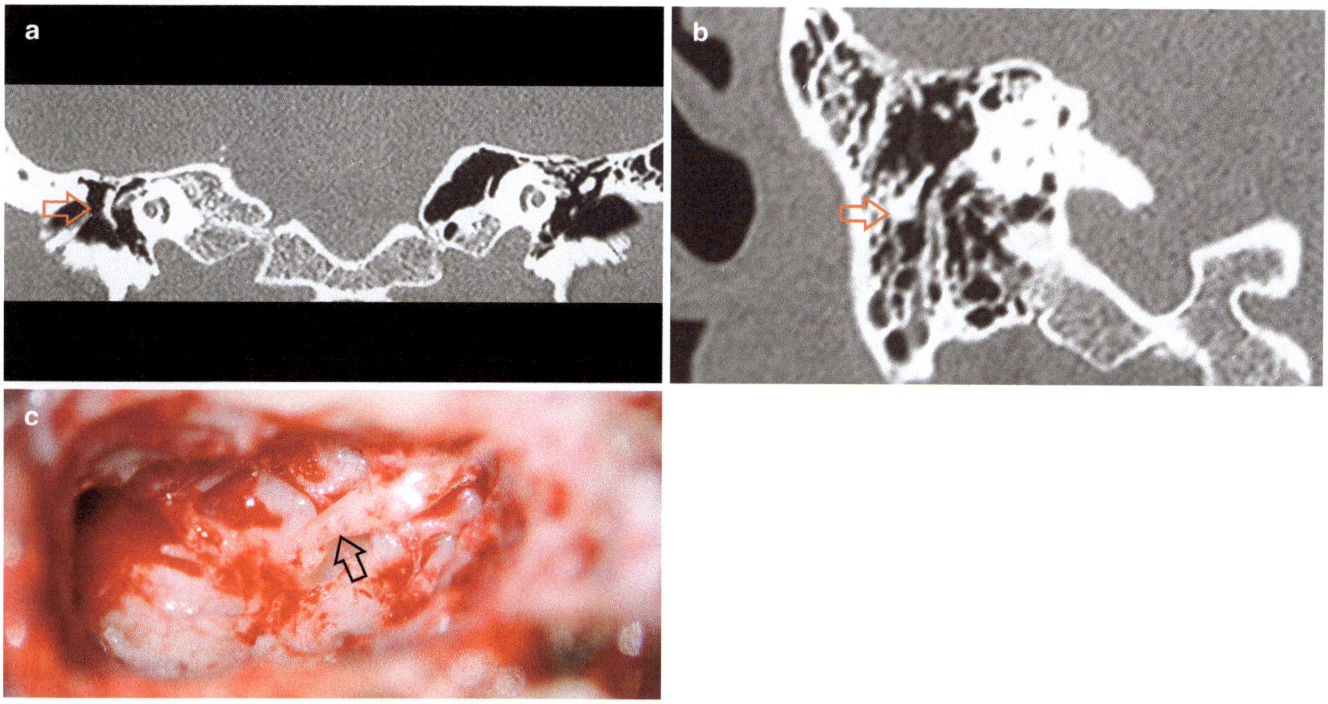

Fig. 4.11 Dislocation of the incus. (**a**, **b**) Coronal CT; (**c**) Intraoperative finding. (**a**) Loss of the incus (⇧); (**b**) Body of incus moved into mastoid cavity (⇧); (**c**) Residual incus in mastoid cavity (⇧)

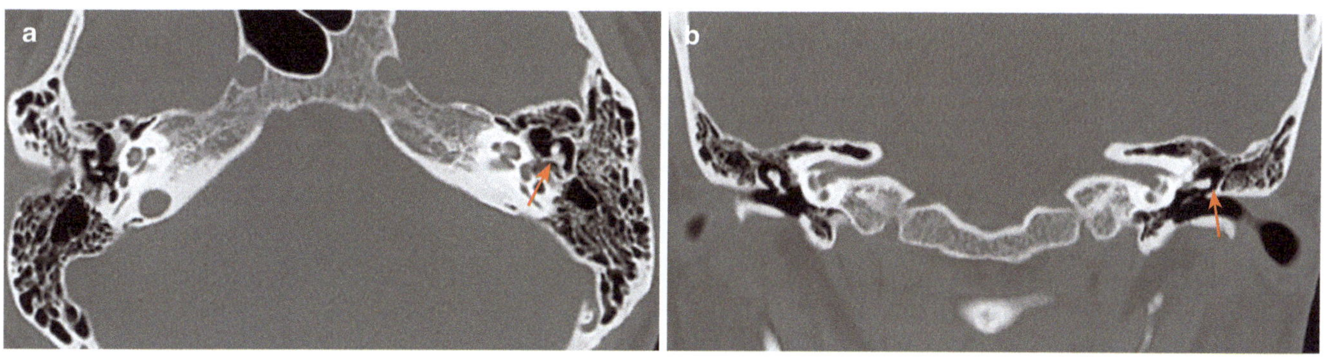

Fig. 4.12 Dislocation of incus in left ear. (**a**) Axial CT; (**b**) Coronal CT. (**a**) Displaced long crus (↑) of incus; (**b**) Long crus of incus (↑) had fused with facial nerve canal

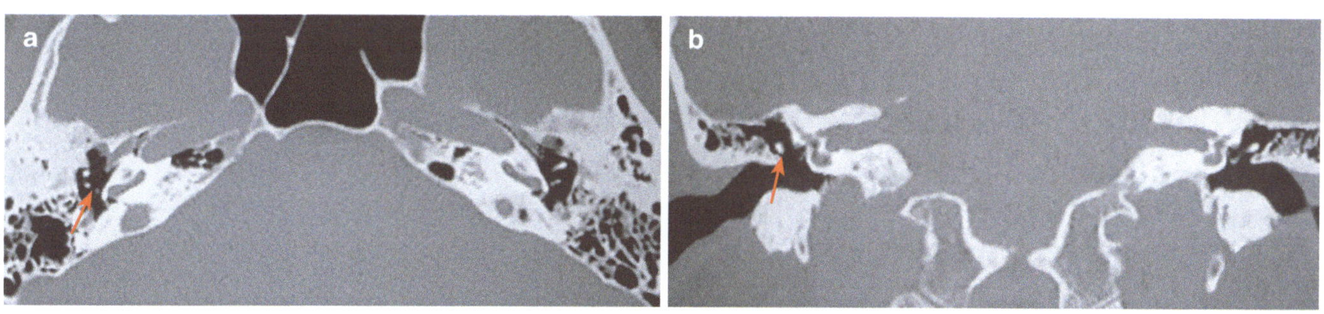

Fig. 4.13 Dislocation of incudostapedial articulation in right ear. (**a**) Axial CT; (**b**) Coronal CT. (**a**) Lenticular process (↑) of incus was not present in incudostapedial articulation; (**b**) Displaced long crus of incus (↑).

Note: The most common injury to the ossicular chain is incudostapedial articulation dislocation, due to the thin and fragile articulation between two axes of rotation, and/or simultaneous tetanic contractions of both the tensor tympani tendon which causes sudden incus retraction medially and the stapedius tendon which causes stapes retraction posteriorly) (Swartz et al. 1989) (Fig. 4.13)

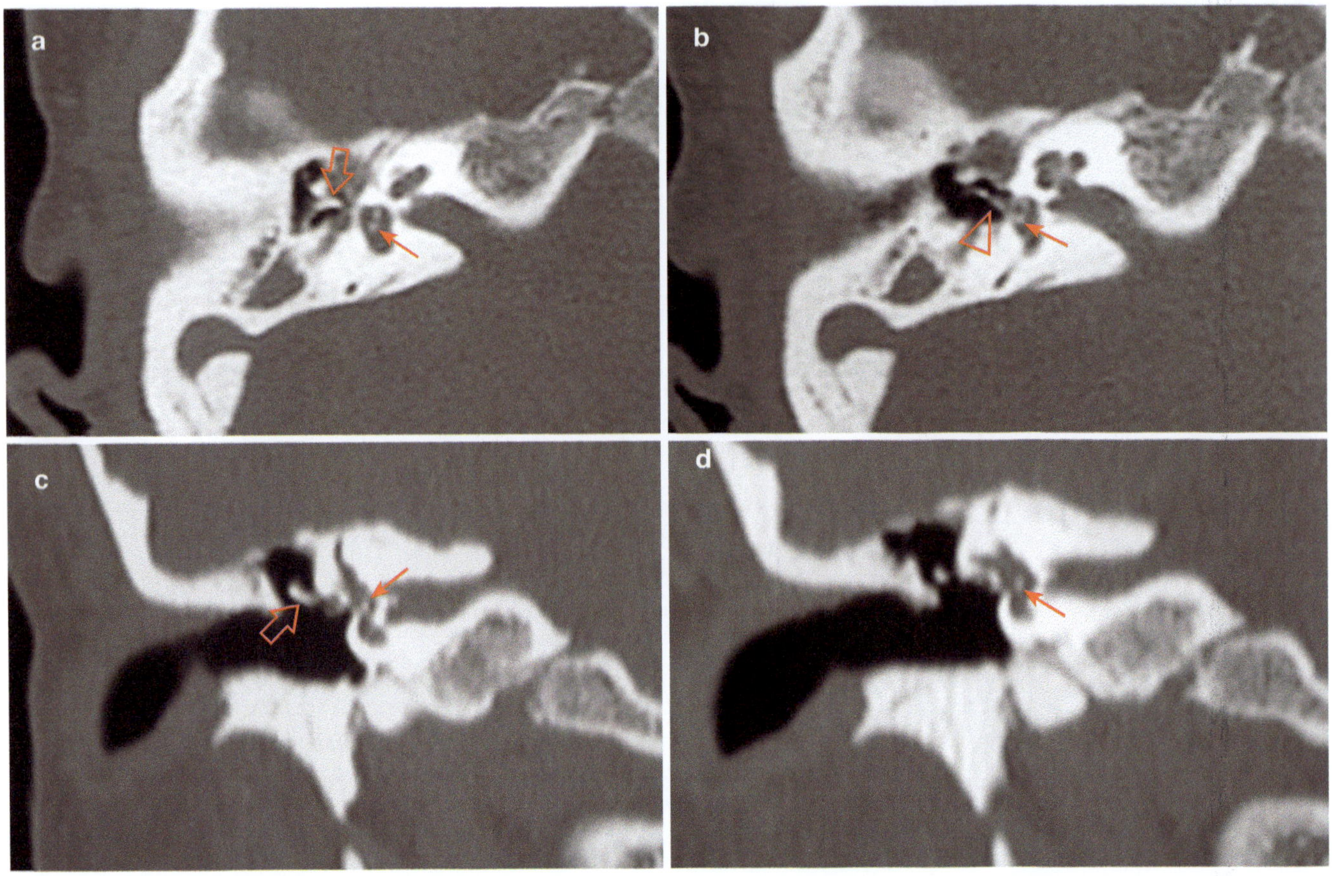

Stapes falling into vestibule in right ear. (**a**, **b**). Axial CT; (**c**, **d**). Coronal CT. (**a**, **d**). Long crus of incus (⇧) in abnormal position; (**a**–**d**). Footplate (↑) of stapes fallen into the vestibule; (**b**) Incudostapedial articulation (△) was dislocated.

Note: The patient had persistent dizziness and severe sensorineural hearing loss.

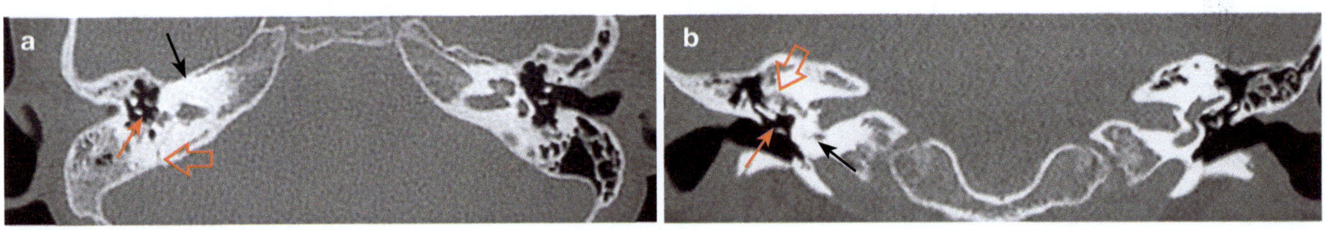

Traumatic labyrinthitis. (**a**) Axial CT; (**b**) Coronal CT. Old fracture line (⇧), dislocation of incudostapedial articulation (↑), ossified cochlea (↑).

4.6 Traumatic Stenosis of Eustachian Tube

See Fig. 4.14.

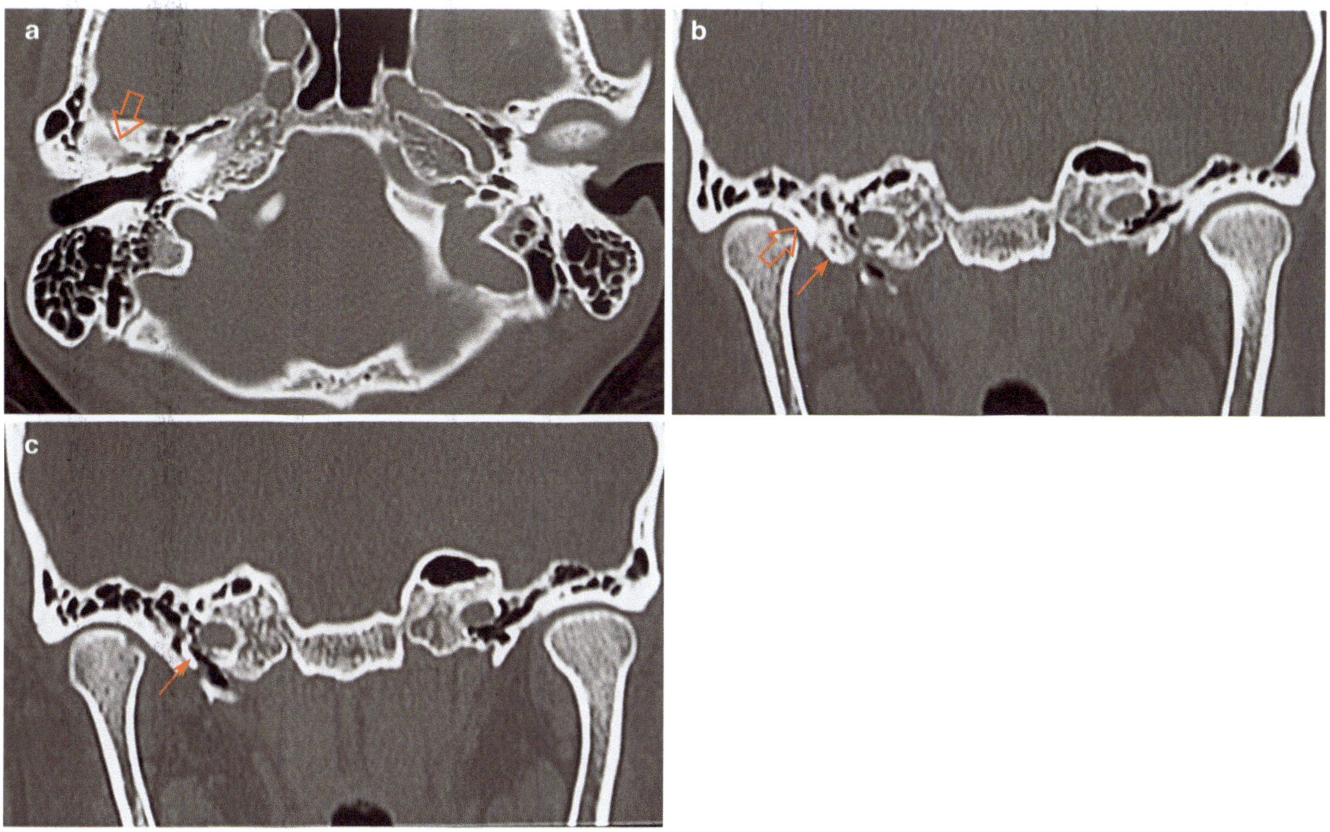

Fig. 4.14 Fracture of outer wall of eustachian tube and stenosis of eustachian tube. (**a**) Axial CT; (**b**, **c**). Coronal CT. (**a**, **b**). Fracture of medial-superior wall (⇧) of temporomandibular joint (outer wall of eustachian tube); (**b**, **c**). Fracture of outer wall of eustachian tube (↑)

4.7 Intra- and Extra-Cranial Complications Caused by Temporal Bone Fracture

The temporal bone (skull base) fracture can cause cranny or even bone loss at the skull base, and then may cause cerebrospinal fluid otorrhea (Fig. 4.6), intracranial infection, and encephalomalacia. Therefore, the larger skull base bone loss should be repaired in time to avoid the occurrence of sequelae (Fig. 4.15).

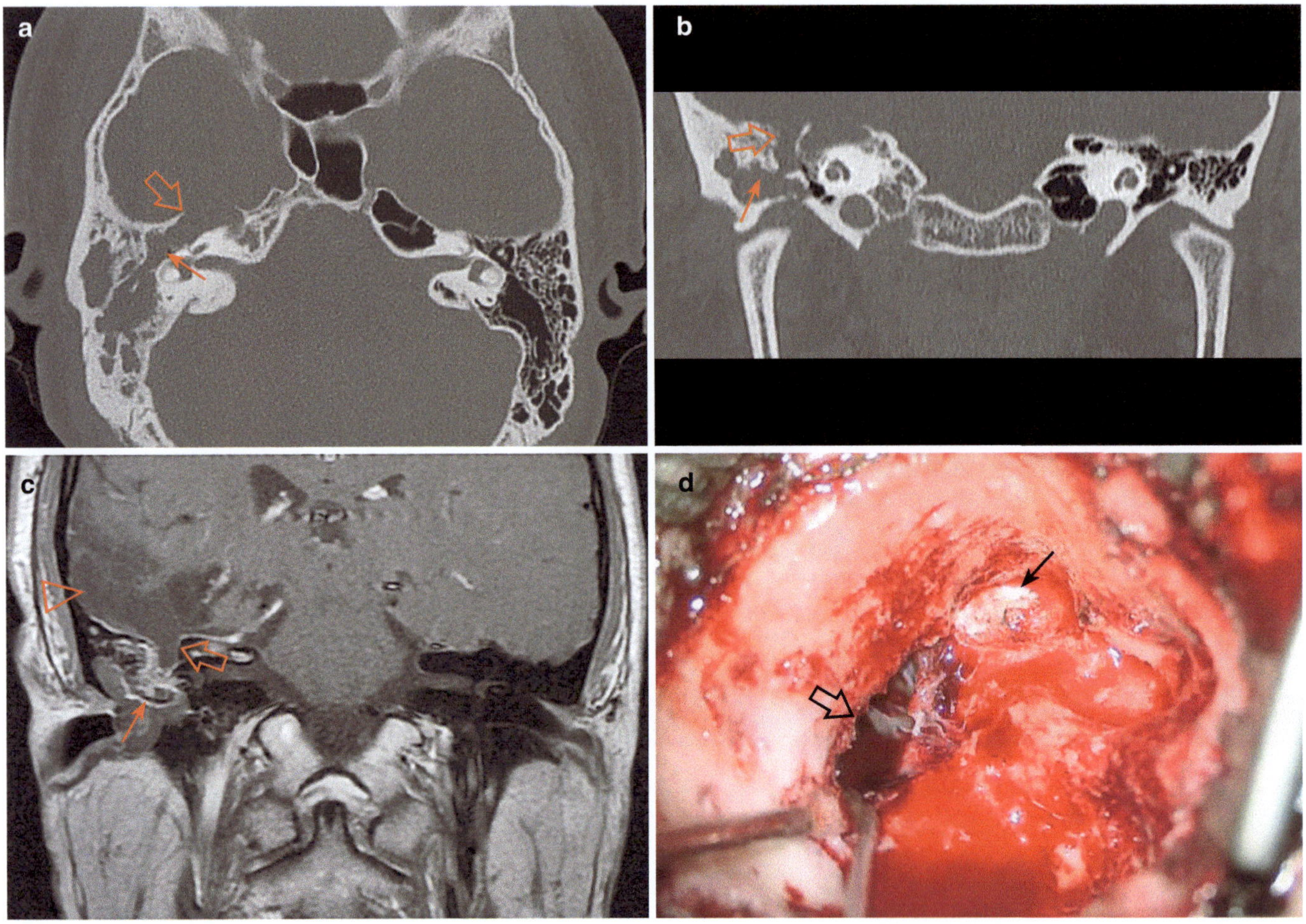

Fig. 4.15 Right traumatic skull base fracture (**a**). Axial CT; (**b**) Coronal CT; (**c**) Coronal MRI T_1WI postgadolinium; (**d**) Intraoperative finding. (**a–c**) Meningoencephalocele (⇧); (**a–d**) Temporal bone cholesteatoma (↑); (**c**) Ipsilateral encephalodialysis (△); (**d**) Tore dura (⇧) and cholesteatoma epithelium (↑).

Note: Seven years after cranial trauma, the patient saw doctor for ear discharge and blooding in the right ear and ipsilateral headache (Fig. 4.15)

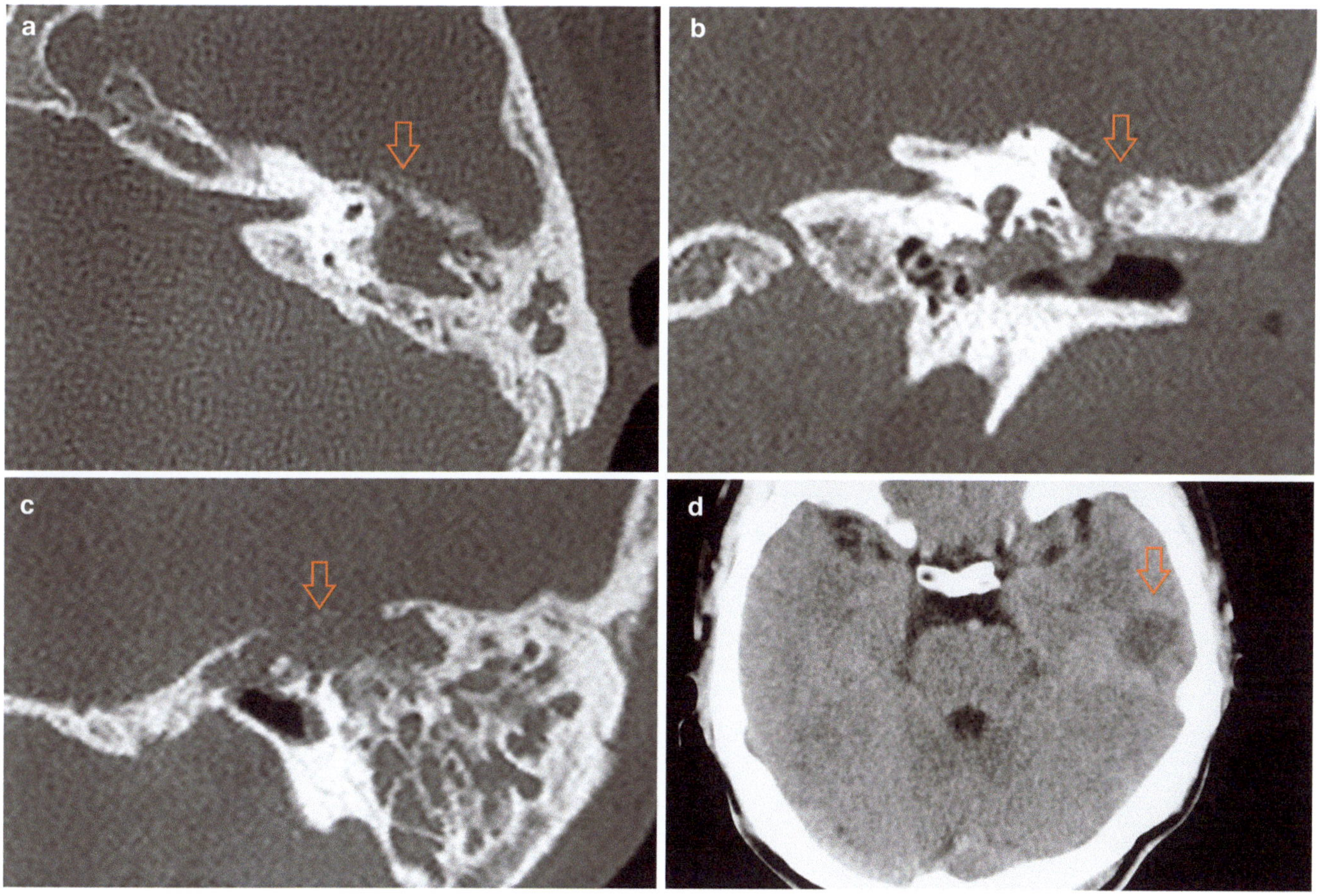

Brain abscess formation after temporal bone (skull base) fracture (left) (**a**) Axial CT; (**b**) Coronal CT; (**c**) Sagittal CT; (**d**) Cranial CT. (**a–c**). Fractures of tegmens of tympanic cavity and tympanic antrum (⇧); (**b**) Fracture of skull base communicating brain with external auditory canal (⇧); (**d**) Soft tissue window of cranial CT showed round hypodensity shadow in same temporal lobe of brain (⇧).

Note: Four years later after temporal bone fracture, the patient saw doctor for ear discharge of left ear, fever and ipsilateral headache for 2 days.

5 Inflammatory Diseases and Cholesteatoma of Ear

Zilong Yu, Shubin Chen, Jie Wang, and Bentao Yang

As a common and frequently-occurring disease in otolaryngology, inflammatory diseases of the ear can be not only divided into non-specific inflammation (aseptic, suppurative, etc.), specific inflammation (tuberculosis, syphilis, etc.), but also divided into acute and chronic inflammation.

Cholesteatoma of the middle ear and mastoid process is also one of the common diseases in otology. It can occur alone or simultaneously with infection. It is concerned for its destructive, recurrent nature, and can cause intracranial and extracranial complications.

CT or/and MR is a meticulous and reliable imaging modality for related examinations of ear disease and plays a very important role in the diagnosis and judgement of prognosis of ear disease. In this book, the ear diseases are arranged according to the primary sites from the external auditory canal to the internal acoustic meatus.

5.1 Non-specific Inflammatory Diseases of Ear

5.1.1 Otitis Externa

See Figs. 5.1 and 5.2.

Z. Yu (✉) · S. Chen · J. Wang
Department of Otolaryngology Head and Neck Surgery, Beijing Tongren Hospital, Capital Medical University, Beijing, China

B. Yang
Department of Radiology, Beijing Tongren Hospital, Capital Medical University, Beijing, China

Z. Yu (ed.), *Ear Diseases and CT*, https://doi.org/10.1007/978-981-99-7220-3_5

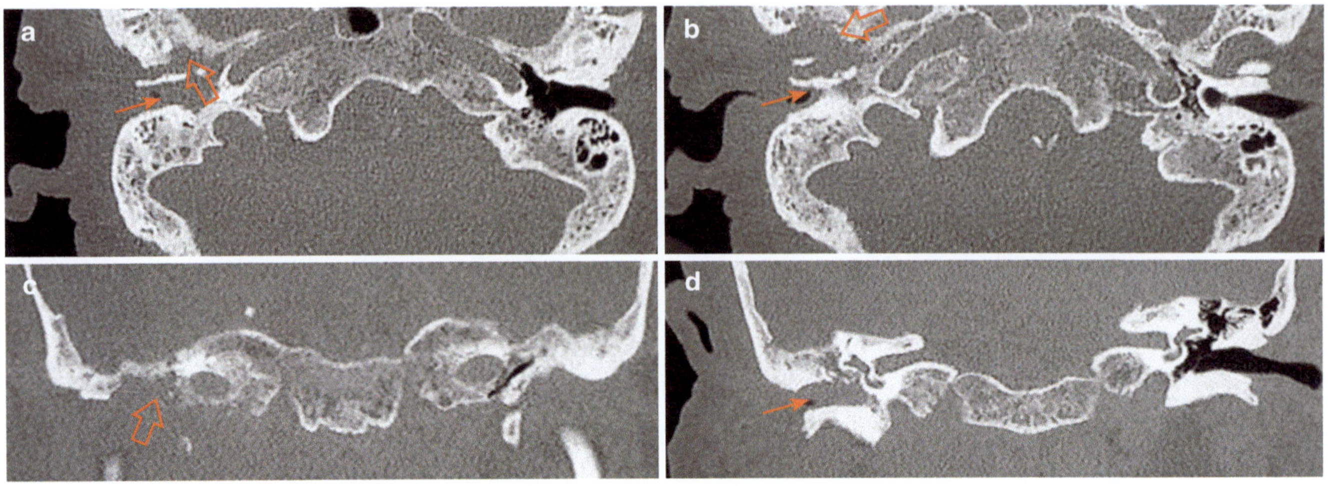

Fig. 5.1 Necrotizing otitis externa in right ear. (**a**, **b**) Axial CT; (**c**, **d**). Coronal CT. (**a**–**c**) Osteocortical destruction and absorption of mandibular fossa (⇧); (**a**–**d**). Soft tissue shadow in external auditory canal and middle ear and mastoid process (↑), bone cortex of external auditory canal was rough.

Note: Necrotic otitis externa is also known as malignant otitis externa, which is characterized by severe otalgia, discharge, and hearing loss. In severe cases, it can be accompanied by bone destruction at the skull base and invasion of cranial nerves. Most patients are older and have a history of diabetes. The secretion culture of ear might show pseudomonas aeruginosa, and pathology is mostly inflammatory granulation

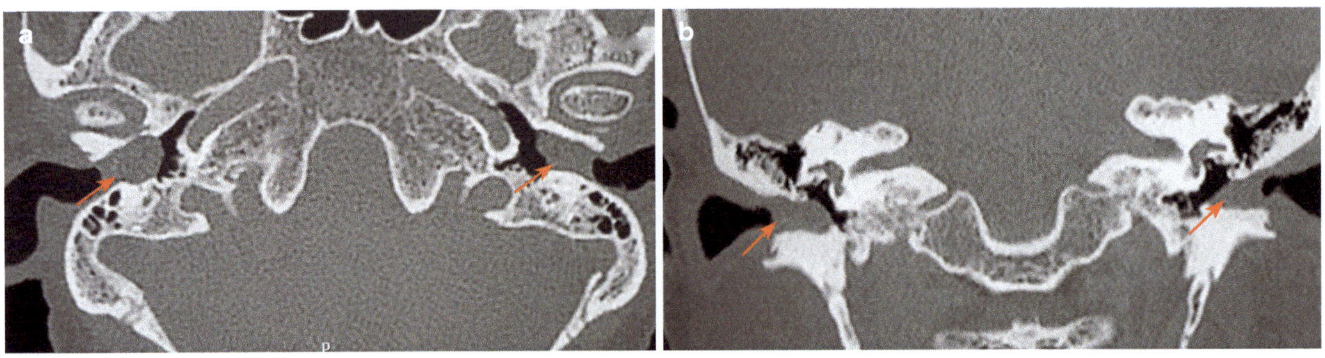

Fig. 5.2 Membranous atresia of bilateral external auditory canal. (**a**) Axial CT; (**b**) Coronal CT. Bilateral external auditory canals were full of tissue shadow (↑) without clear history of trauma, it should be further examined to eliminate rheumatic immune disease

5.1.2 Acute Suppurative Otitis Media and Mastoiditis

See Fig. 5.3.

5.1.3 Non-suppurative Otitis Media and Mastoiditis

See Figs. 5.4, 5.5, and 5.6.

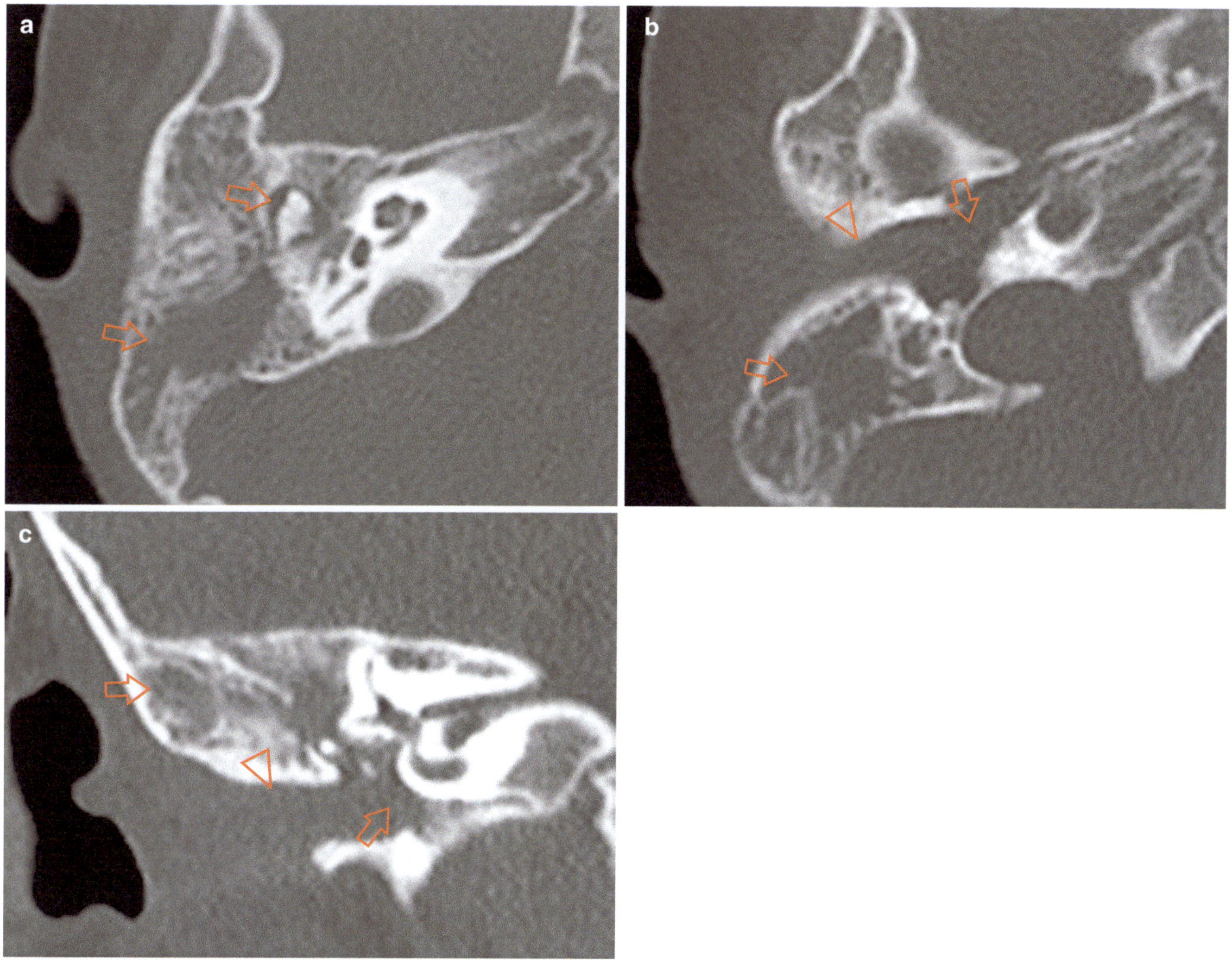

Fig. 5.3 Acute suppurative otitis media and mastoiditis. (**a**, **b**). Axial CT; (**c**) Coronal CT. External auditory canal (△), mastoid process (⇧), and tympanic cavity (⇧) were full of soft tissue shadow; temporal bone was intact.

Note: Acute suppurative otitis media is common in infants and young children. After ear discharge, the body temperature drops rapidly, and other symptoms are also relieved quickly. If the symptoms such as fever are still not relieved after regular treatment, the possibility of complications should be considered, and radiologic examination is really necessary

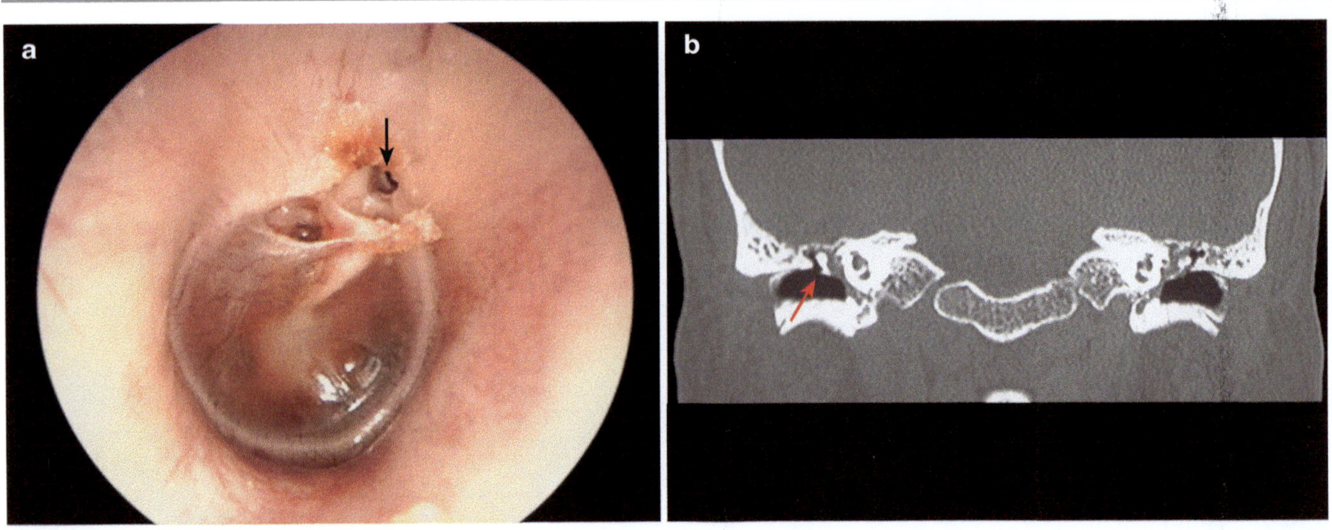

Fig. 5.4 Secretory otitis media in bilateral ears. (**a**) Endoscopic view of tympanic membrane; (**b**) Coronal CT. (**a**) Pars tensa of tympanic membrane was turbid, which was amber or orange, pars flaccida (Prussak space) was invaginated (otoscope) (↑); (**b**) Pars flaccida (↑) was invaginated, soft tissue was full of tympanomastoid cavity on bilateral ears, there was no bone destruction.

Note: Diagnosis and treatment of secretory otitis media seems simple, but in fact, misdiagnosis and mistreatment are not rare. It can be caused by acute otitis media, it can also be result of non-bacterial inflammation of eustachian tube dysfunction, and it can also be caused by the invasion of adjacent diseases into the temporal bone. More importantly, it may be the manifestation of cerebrospinal fluid otorrhea, allergy and rheumatic immune diseases in the ear. Therefore, clinical medical history, physical and hearing examination, and imaging examination are all necessary

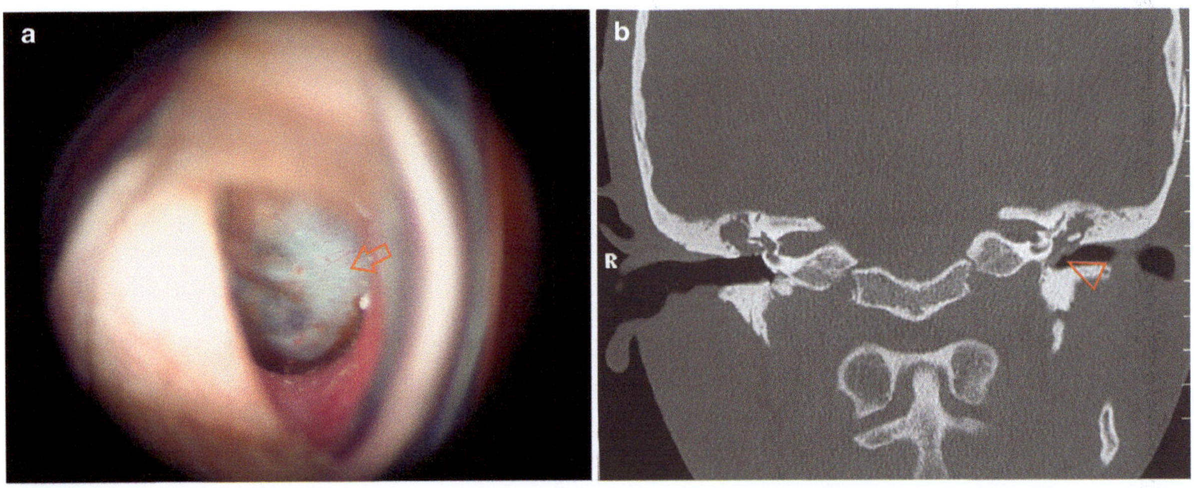

Fig. 5.5 Cholesterol granuloma in left ear. (**a**) Endoscopic view of tympanic membrane; (**b**) Coronal CT. (**a**) Tympanic membrane of left ear was blue; (**b**) Soft tissue shadow was full of left tympanic cavity and the tympanic membrane was swollen (⇧)

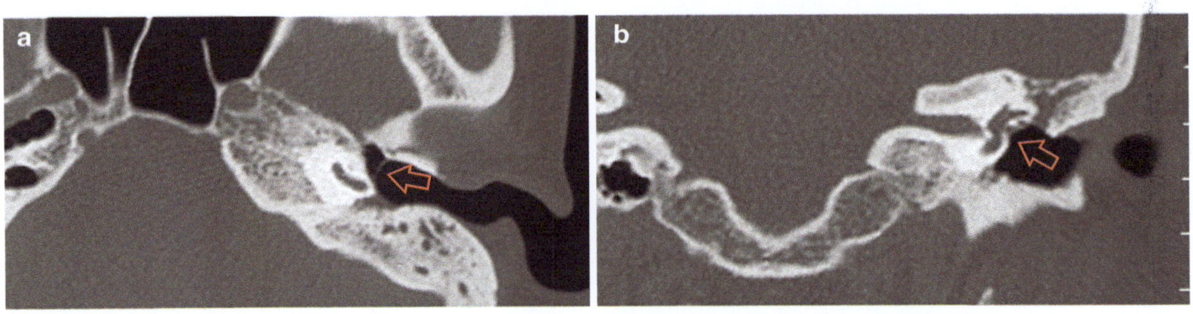

Fig. 5.6 Adhesive otitis media in left ear. (**a**) Axial CT; (**b**) Coronal CT. Tympanic membrane (⇧) was invaginated and adhered to promontory, eustachian tube contained air.

Note: Epithelialization and drying of the promontory mucosa could be seen before operation, and the ossicles (including manubrium, long foot of incus, and suprastapedial structure had been damaged and disappeared. This disease was easily misdiagnosed as large perforation of tympanic membrane, but large perforation of tympanic membrane was usually characterized by intact ossicular bone and residual edge of tympanic membrane and promontory mucosa was moist. Adhesive otitis media might be the sequela of secretory otitis media and could be complicated with cholesteatoma of the middle ear and mastoid process. Eustachian tube dysfunction may be the main cause

5.1.4 Chronic Suppurative Otitis Media and Sequelae

See Figs. 5.7, 5.8, 5.9, 5.10, 5.11, 5.12, 5.13, 5.14, 5.15, 5.16, 5.17, and 5.18.

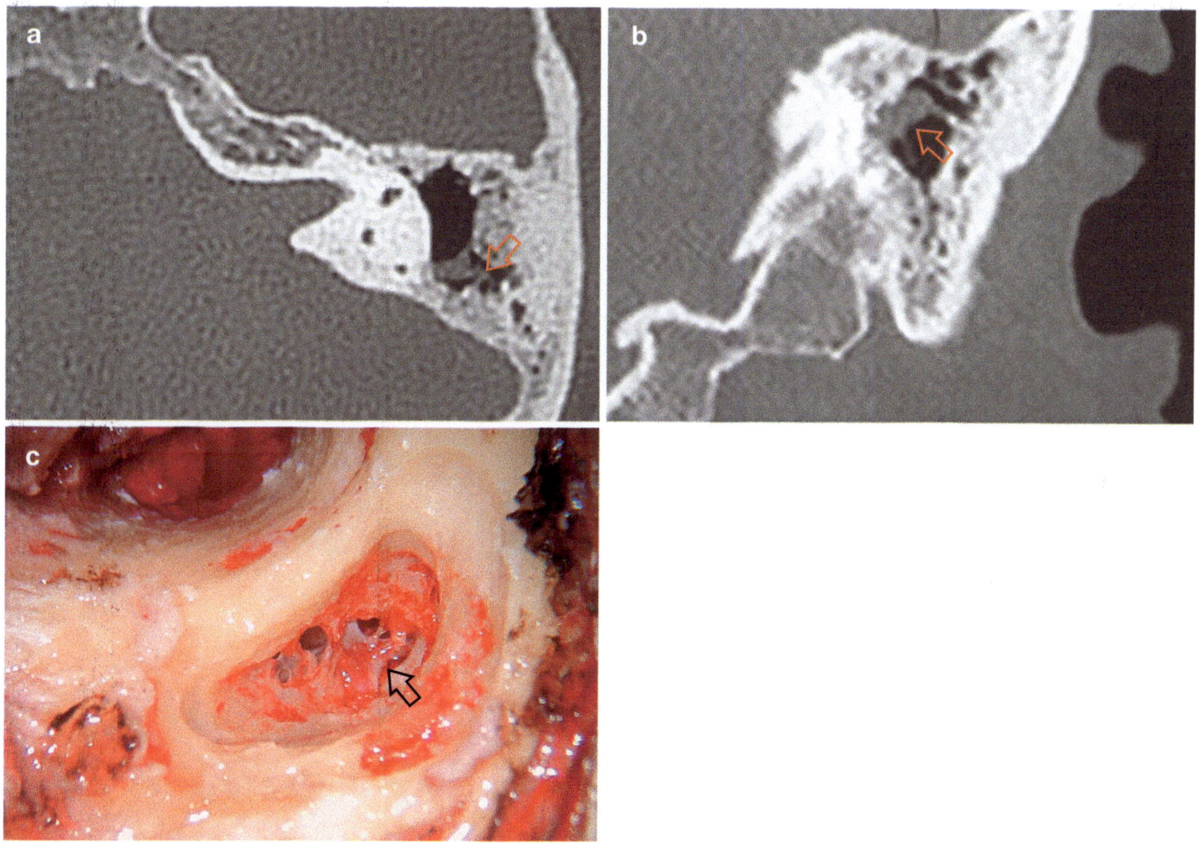

Fig. 5.7 Chronic suppurative otitis media and mastoiditis in left ear. (**a**) Axial CT; (**b**) Coronal CT; (**c**) Intraoperative finding. (**a**, **b**) Soft tissue shadows presented in the mastoid process (⇧) with clear boundary; (**c**) Mastoid exploration showed scar-like connective tissue in mastoid process (⇧)

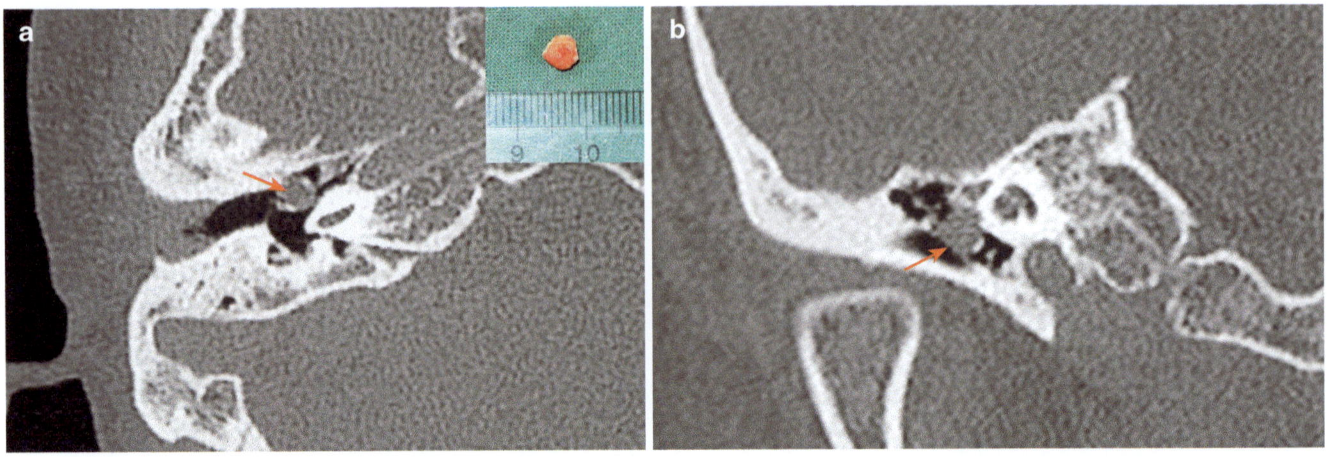

Fig. 5.8 Inflammatory calcification of right middle ear. (**a**) Axial CT and intraoperative finding; (**b**) Coronal CT. Calcification inflammatory tissue (↑) in tympanic cavity, illustration showed calcification tissue

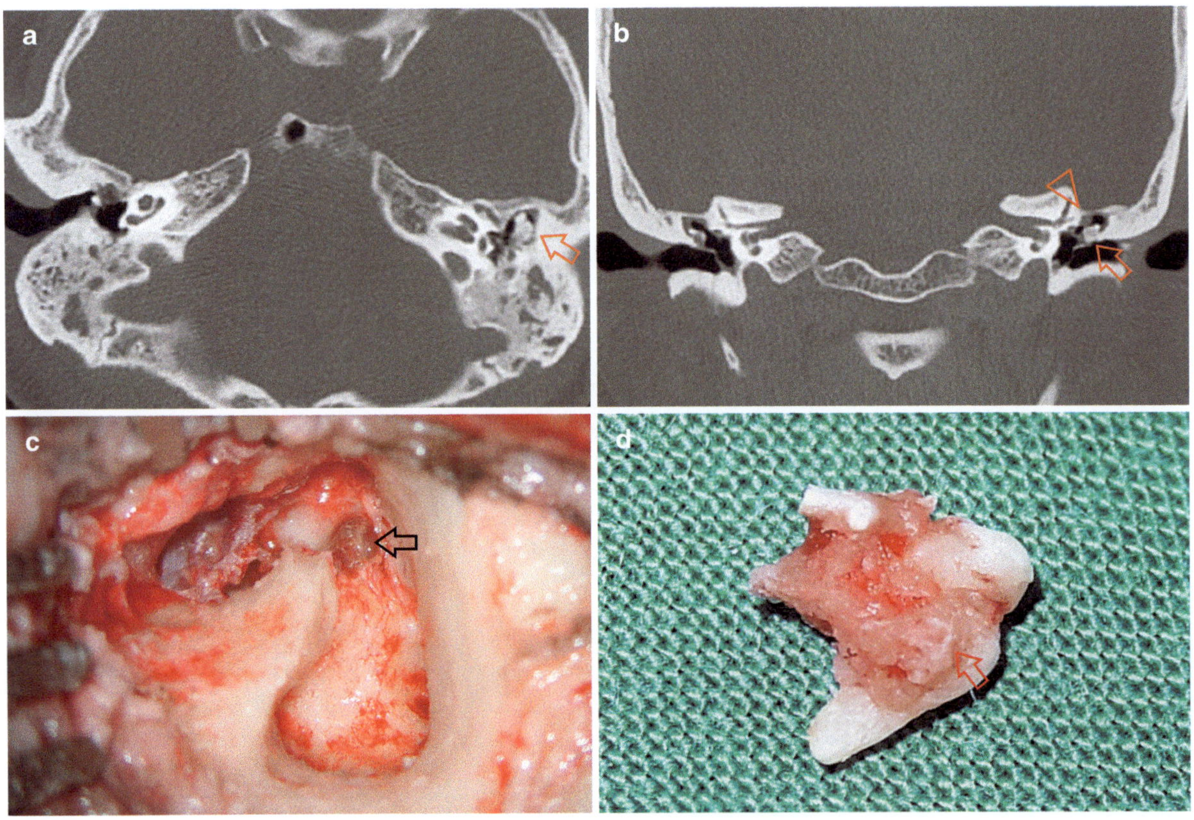

Fig. 5.9 Epitympanic type of tympanosclerosis (Incudomalleolar articulation fixation type). (**a**) Axial CT; (**b**) Coronal CT; (**c**, **d**) Intraoperative finding. (**a**, **b**) Incudomalleolar articulation fusion and adhesion to the tympanic scutum (⇧); (**b**) Soft tissue shadow (△) were found at the anterior crus of lateral semicircular canal; (**c**) Retention cyst (⇧) in epitympanum; (**d**) Fused incudomalleolar articulation (⇧) and its sclerosis focus

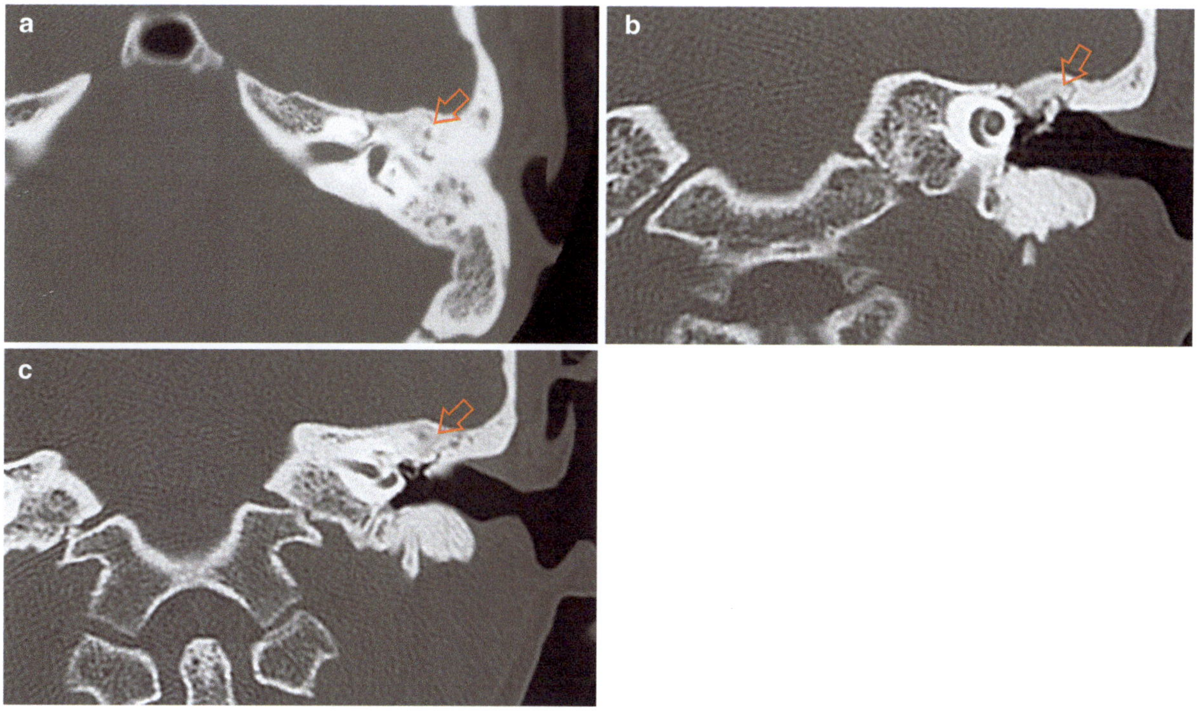

Fig. 5.10 Epitympanic type of tympanosclerosis in left ear. (**a**) Axial CT; (**b**, **c**). Coronal CT. Epitympanum and tympanic antrum were filled with sclerotic lesions (⇧), malleus and incus were deeply buried in it

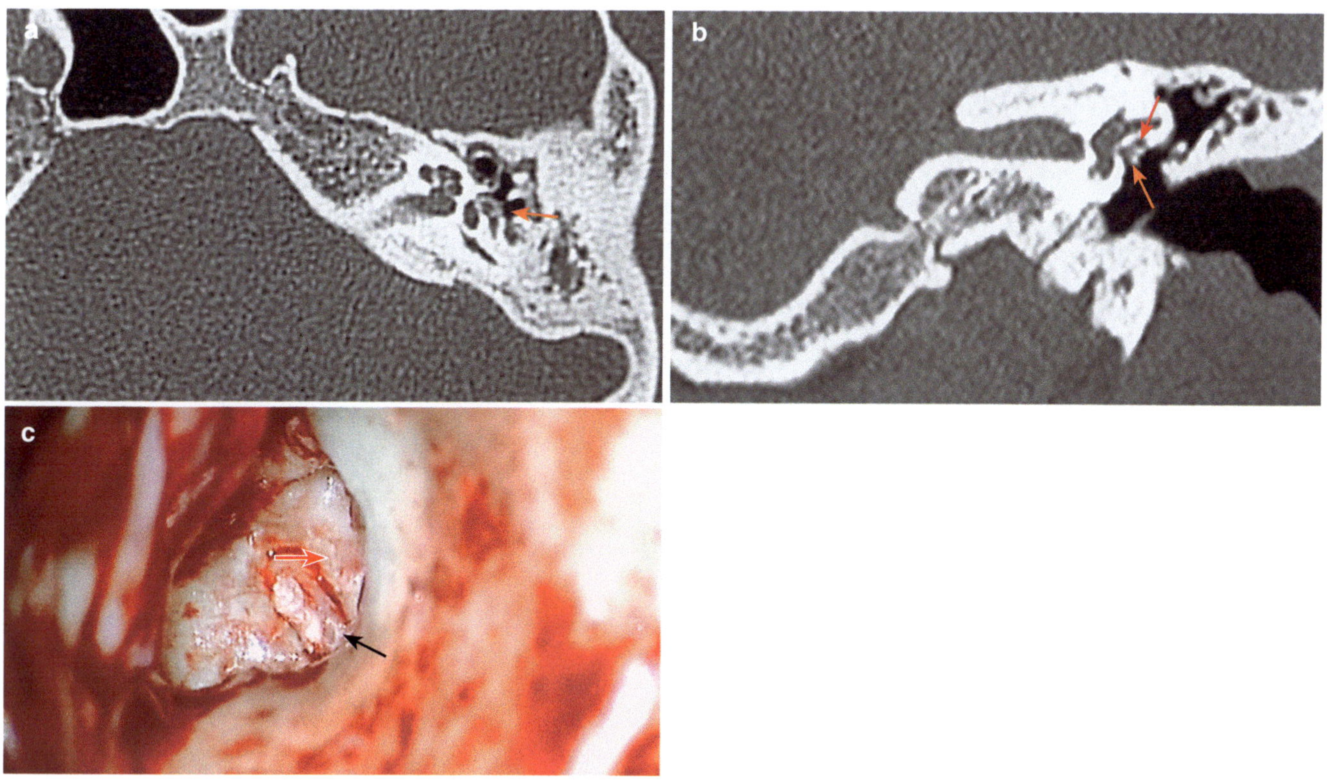

Fig. 5.11 Stapes fixation of tympanosclerosis in left ear. (**a**) Axial CT; (**b**) Coronal CT; (**c**) Intraoperative finding. (**a**) Thickened stapes (↑); (**b**) Thickened stapes (↑) was fused with facial nerve canal (↑); (**c**) There was no gap between thickened stapes (↑) and facial nerve canal (↑)

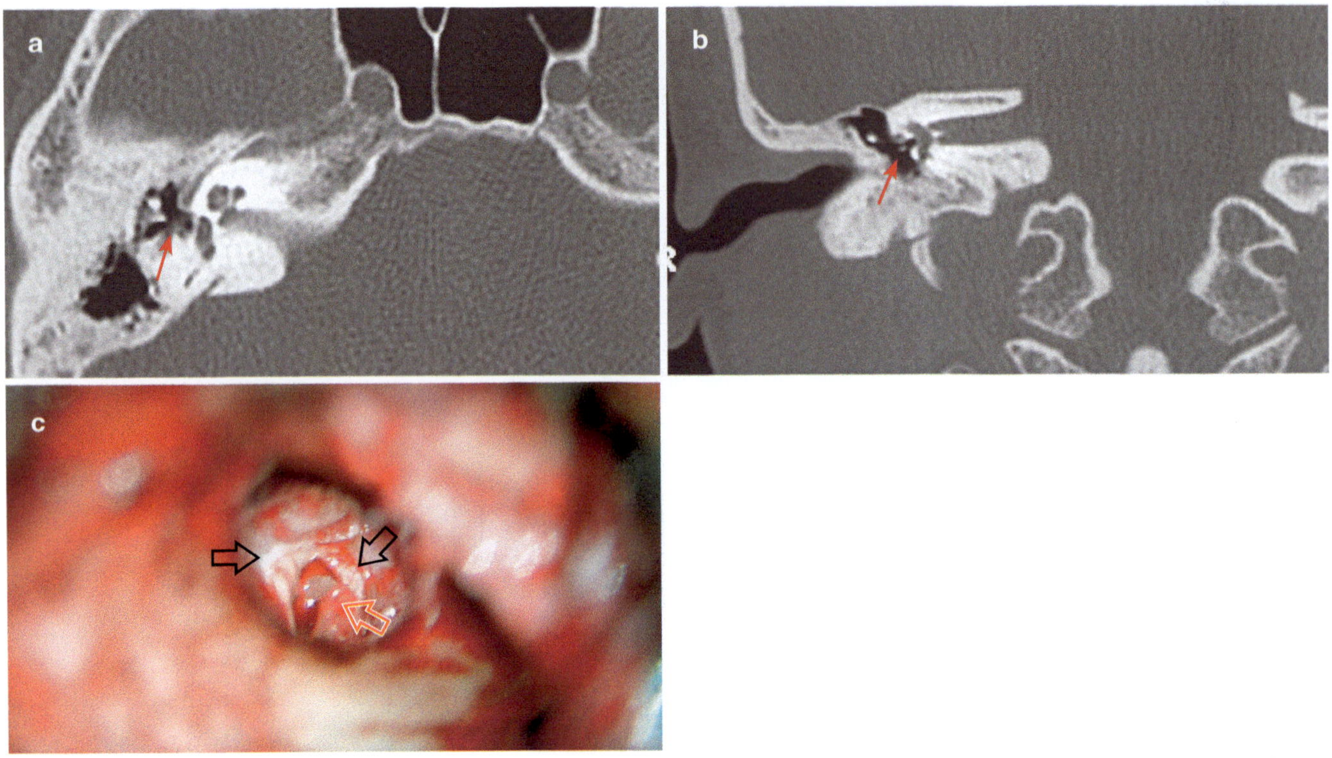

Fig. 5.12 Simple stapes fixed type of tympanosclerosis in right ear (vestibular window type of tympanosclerosis). (**a**) Axial CT; (**b**) Coronal CT; (**c**) Intraoperative finding. (**a**, **b**) No obvious sclerosis was showed around the ossicular chain and at the vestibular window, stapes (↑); (**c**) White sclerosis was located in vestibular window niche (⇧); stapes (⇧).

Note: CT scan has certain limitations in the diagnosis of this type of tympanosclerosis

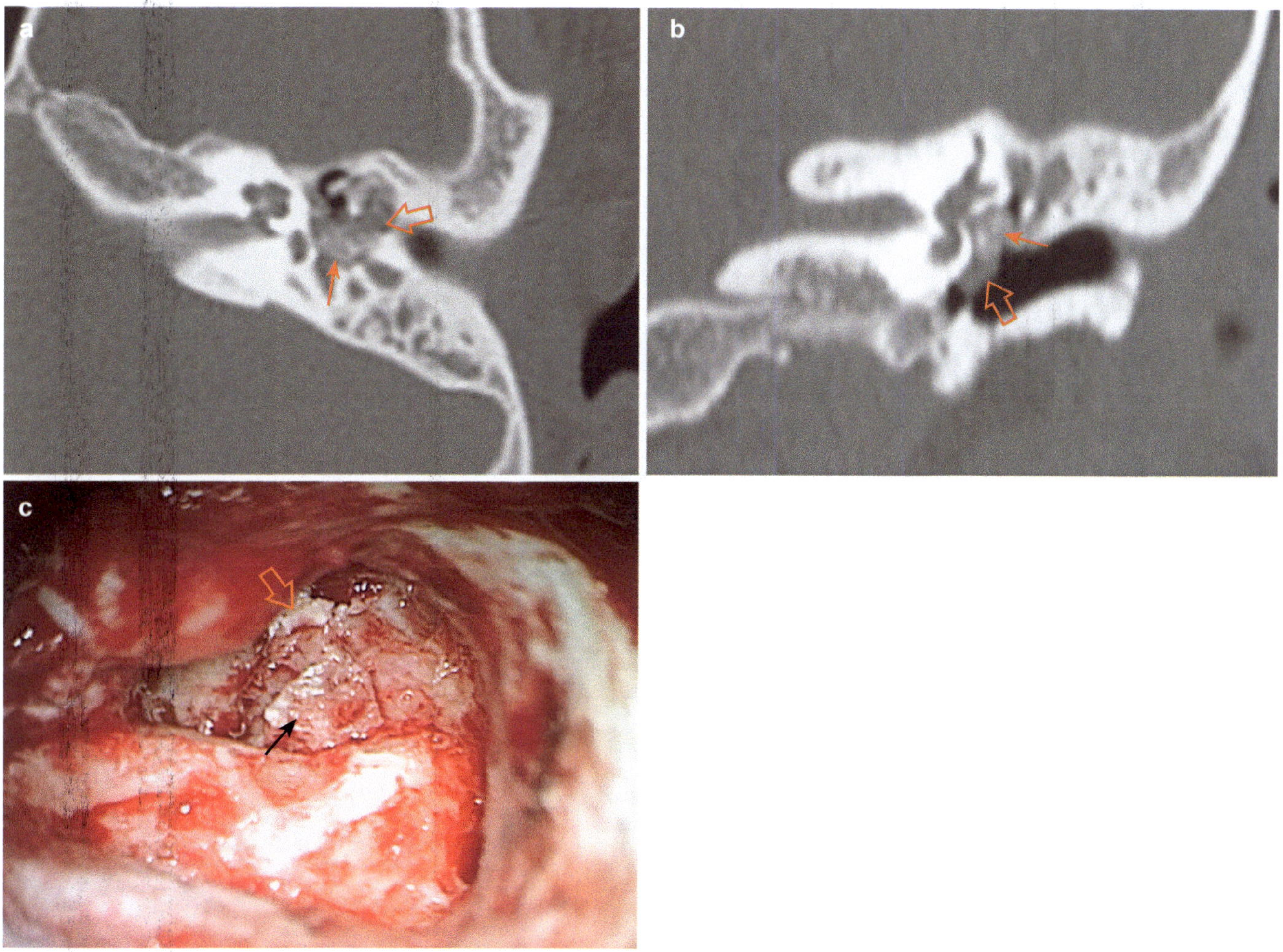

Fig. 5.13 Stapes fixed tympanosclerosis with cholesteatoma in left ear. (**a**) Axial CT; (**b**) Coronal CT; (**c**) Intraoperative finding. (**a**, **b**) Sclerotic focus located at vestibular window (↑), soft tissue shadow (⇧) in tympanum; (**c**) Sclerotic focus (↑) covering vestibular window niche, cholesteatoma epithelium (⇧) located in the gap between sclerotic focus and vestibular window niche

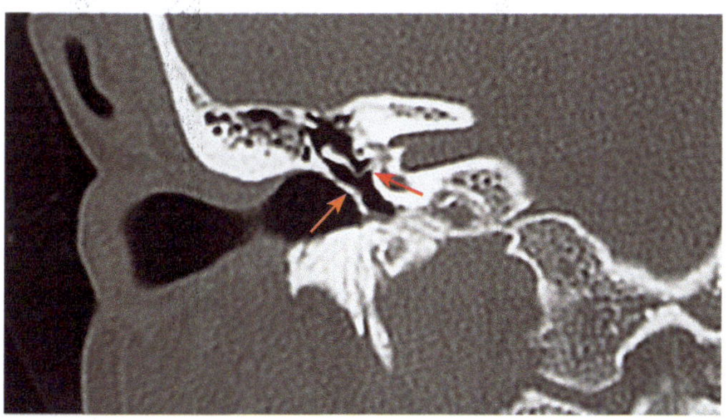

Fig. 5.14 Stapes fixation of tympanosclerosis in right ear on axial CT view. Tympanic membrane calcification (↑), stapes and promontory fusion (↑)

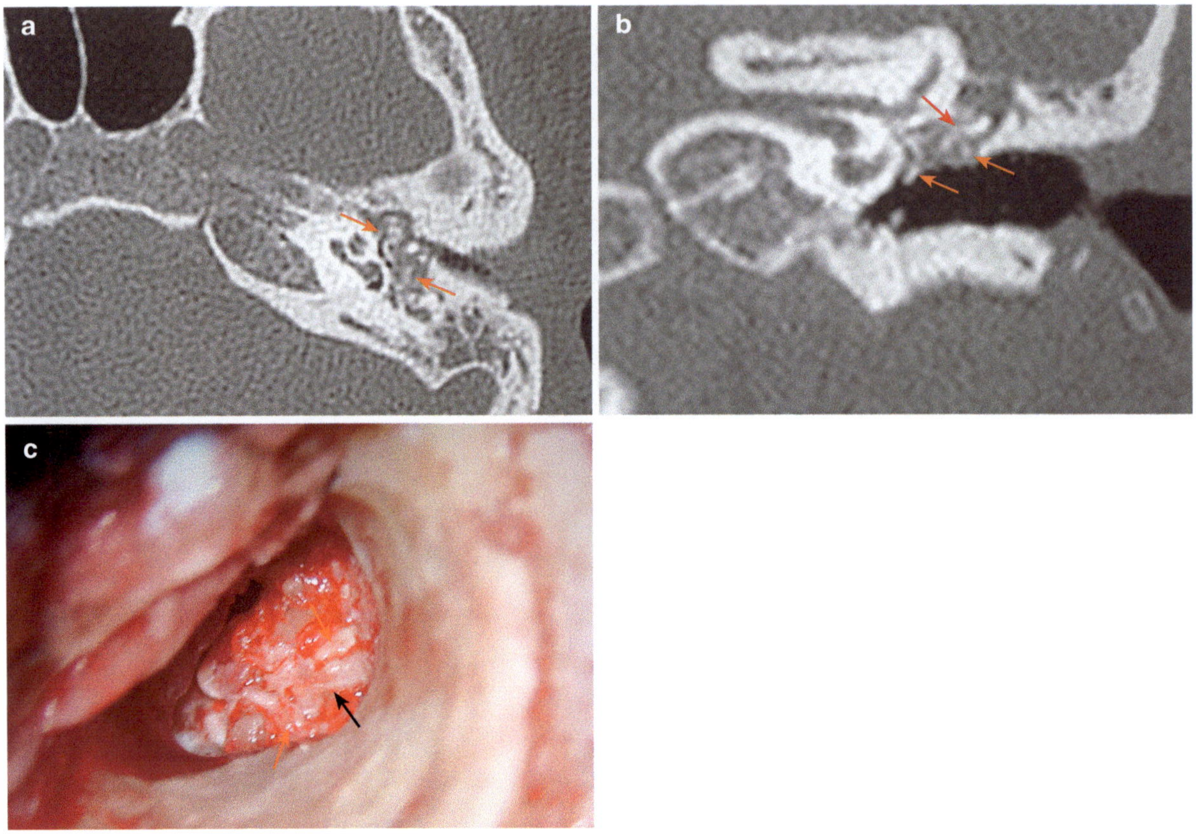

Fig. 5.15 Total tympanum type of tympanosclerosis in left ear. (**a**) Axial CT; (**b**) Coronal CT; (**c**) Intraoperative finding. (**a–c**) Scattered sclerotic foci (↑) were full of tympanum; (**b**) Ossicles (↑) were embedded in sclerotic foci; (**c**) Peeling off some sclerotic foci (↑), long crus of incus (↑) was exposed

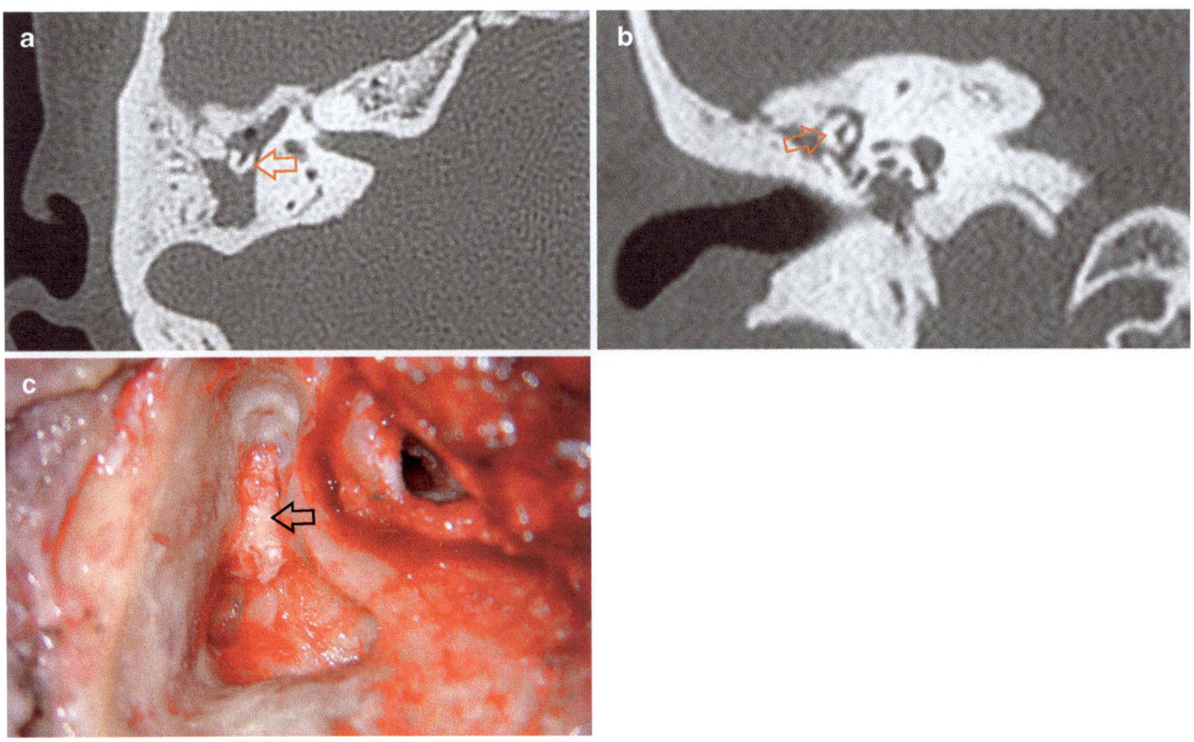

Fig. 5.16 Sclerotic lesions at aditus ad antrum in right ear. (**a**) Axial CT; (**b**) Coronal CT; (**c**) Intraoperative finding. (**a**, **b**) Aditus ad antrum was blocked by high-density shadow (⇧); (**c**) White sclerotic foci blocked aditus ad antrum (⇧)

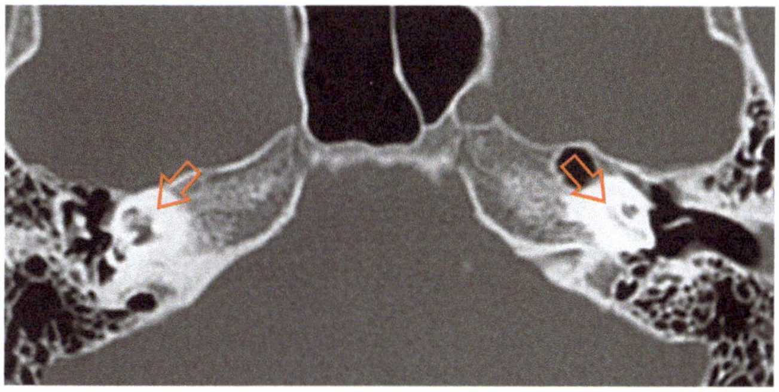

Fig. 5.17 Bilateral ossifying labyrinthitis on axial CT view. Cochlear duct had been ossified (⇧)

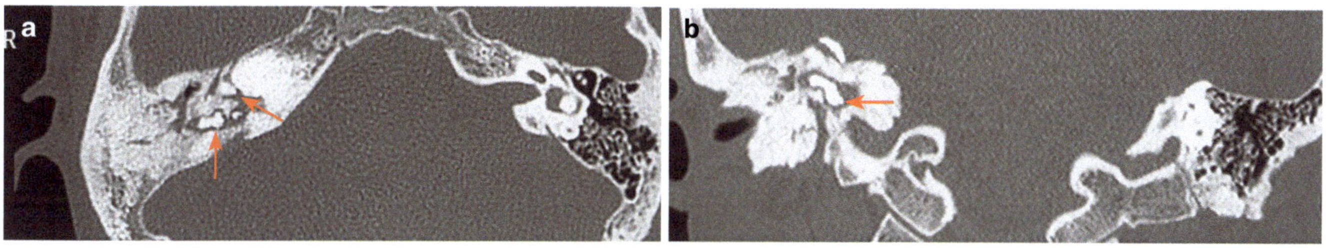

Fig. 5.18 Necrotic labyrinthitis in right ear. (**a**) Axial CT; (**b**) Coronal CT. Mastoid inflammatory changes and dead bone formed in labyrinthine area (↑) in right ear.

Note: Labyrinthitis ossificans is the late stage of labyrinthitis, where there is pathologic ossification of the normally fluid filled cavities in the cochlea, vestibule, and semicircular canals. Labyrinthitis occurs as a result of inner ear inflammation, which may be of post-traumatic (such as otic capsule fractures), autoimmune, or infectious etiologies (Aralasmak et al. 2009). The most extensive cases of labyrinthitis ossificans are seen in relation to meningitis, which are often with bilateral involvement (Juliano, 2018)

5.2 Cholesteatoma of Temporal Bone

This section includes cholesteatomas in external auditory canal, middle ear mastoid process, and petrous part of temporal bone. Cholesteatoma of petrous apex will be shown in petrous apex disease.

5.2.1 Cholesteatoma of External Auditory Canal

See Figs. 5.19, 5.20, 5.21, 5.22, 5.23, 5.24, and 5.25.

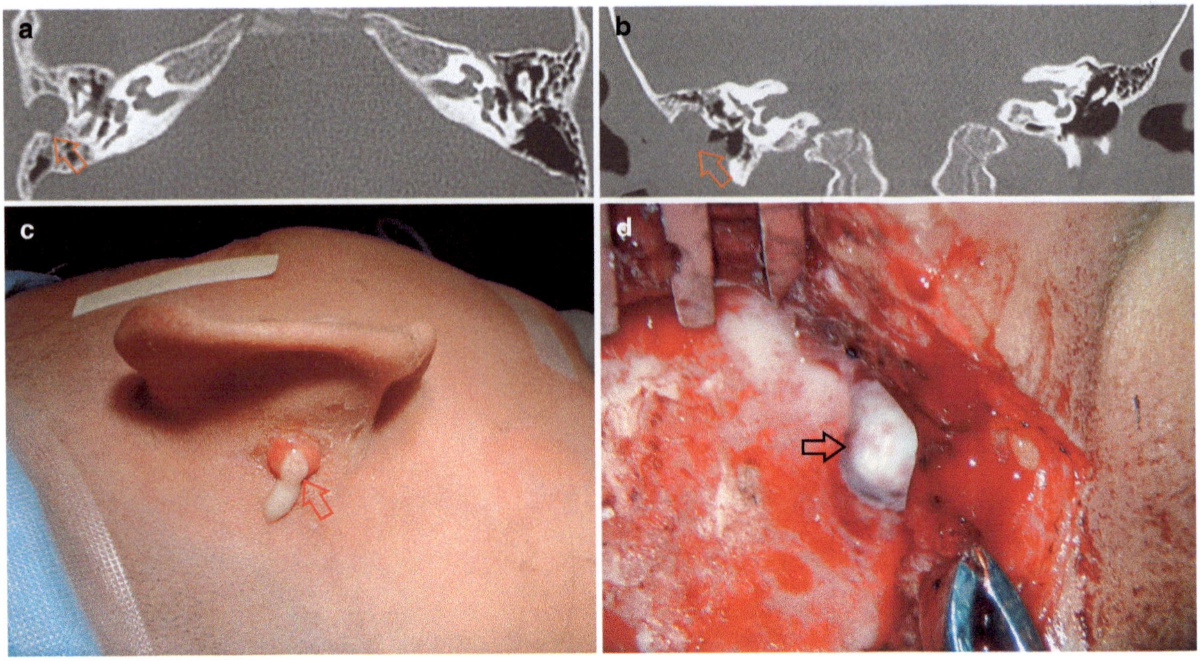

Fig. 5.19 Congenital stenosis of external auditory canal with cholesteatoma formation in right ear, (**a**). Axial CT; (**b**) Coronal CT; (**c**, **d**) Intraoperative finding. (**a**, **b**) Superior wall destruction (⇧) of right external auditory canal, where was instead by soft tissue; (**c**) Formation of postauricular fistula (⇧); (**d**) Enlargement of external auditory canal with epithelial mass (⇧).

Note: Six years old child showed stenosis of external auditory canal during examination

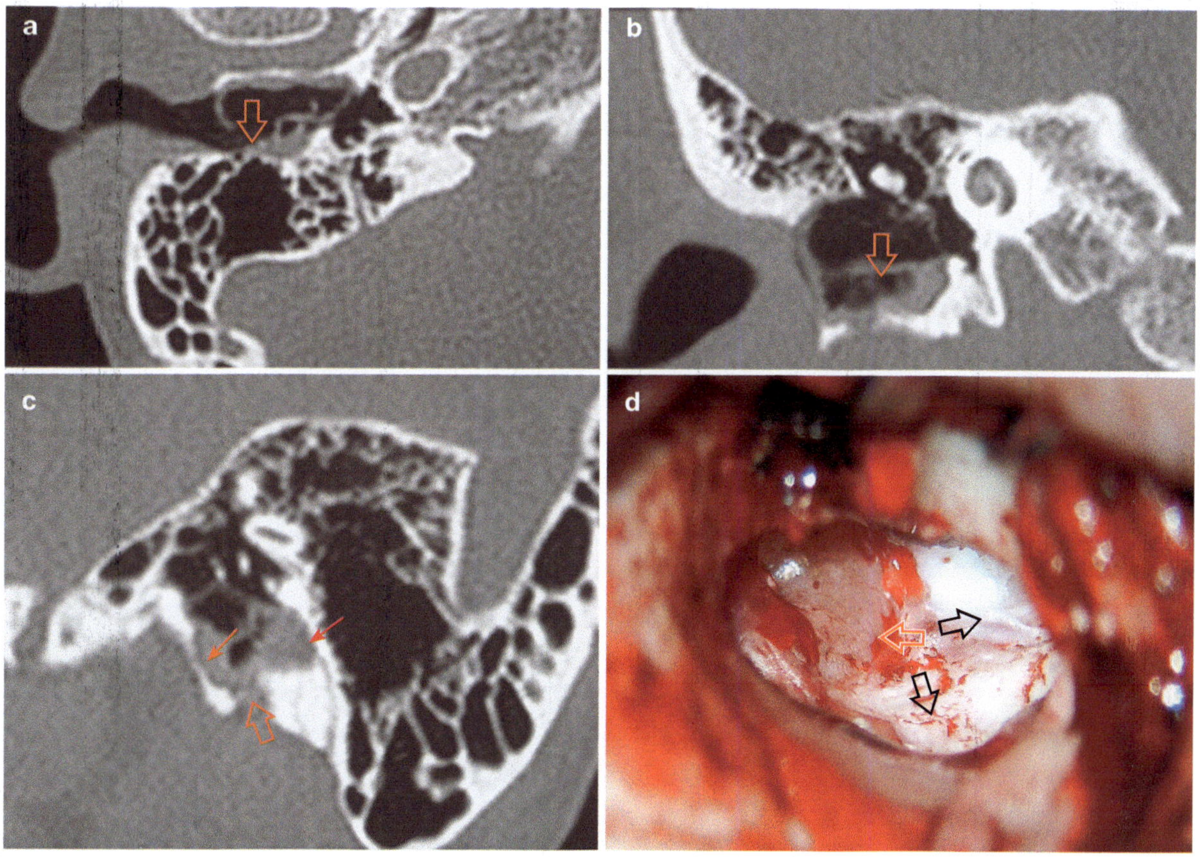

Fig. 5.20 Cholesteatoma of right external auditory canal. (**a**) Axial CT; (**b**) Coronal CT; (**c**) Sagittal CT; (**d**) Intraoperative finding. (**a**, **b**) Soft tissue shadow in external auditory canal, bone cortex destruction of posterior wall (⇧); (**c**) Bone destruction of anterior wall (↑), posterior wall (↑), and inferior wall (⇧); (**d**) External auditory canal expansion, inferior and posterior walls (⬆) were covered with white epithelial tissue, tympanic membrane was intact (⇧).

Note: The mastoid of acquired primary cholesteatoma of external auditory canal is mostly pneumatized or over-pneumatized. Bone cortex destruction of external auditory canal cholesteatoma was always accompanying the expansion of external auditory canal, and it could be communicated with mastoid cavity, but the cartilage segment of external auditory canal remained unchanged, therefore this segment is relatively narrow, resulting in a state of small outside and large inside. One of the purposes of surgical treatment is to repair the bony part of the external auditory canal and expand the cartilage part of the external auditory canal (including the plasty of the external auditory canal opening), so as to facilitate postoperative observation and cleaning. If the part of the bony external auditory canal cannot be repaired, it is recommended that the mastoid cavity be filled (including the transfer of pedicled temporal muscle) after the mastoidectomy with canal wall down to reduce or eliminate the mastoid cavity

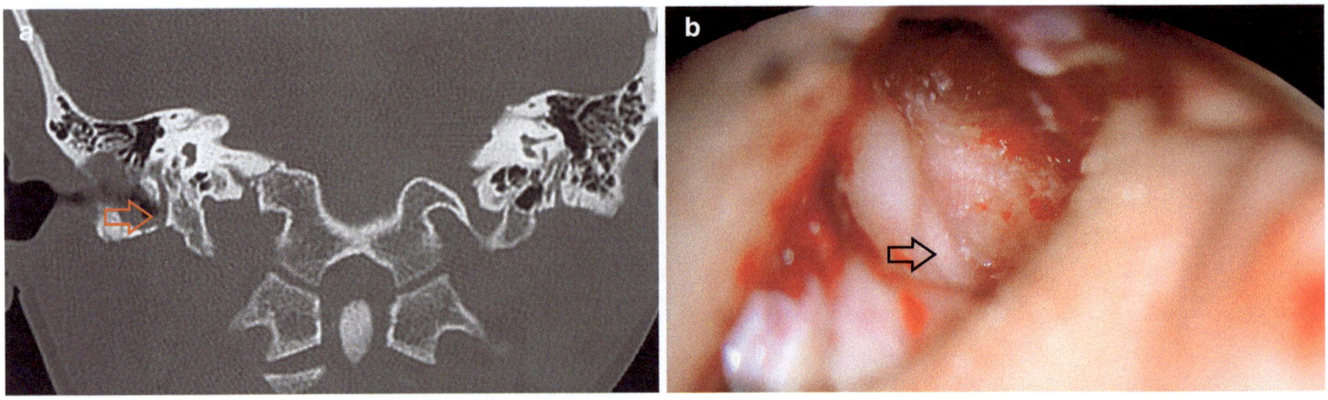

Fig. 5.21 Cholesteatoma of right external auditory canal causing vertical segment exposure of facial nerve. (**a**) Coronal CT; (**b**) Intraoperative finding. (**a**) Bone cortex destruction of mastoid and lateral walls (⇧) of vertical segment of facial nerve; (**b**) External auditory canal was enlarged, facial nerve was partially exposed (⇧).

As mentioned in Sect. 1.5 Intratemporal anatomy of facial nerve, Facial nerve at the level of the bottom wall of external auditory canal, is closed to posterior wall of external auditory canal, so facial nerve is vulnerable because of the erosion of external auditory canal cholesteatoma and other diseases. In order to understand the bone condition of external auditory canal and whether the facial nerve has been exposed, HRCT scanning is required before removal of cholesteatoma of external auditory canal

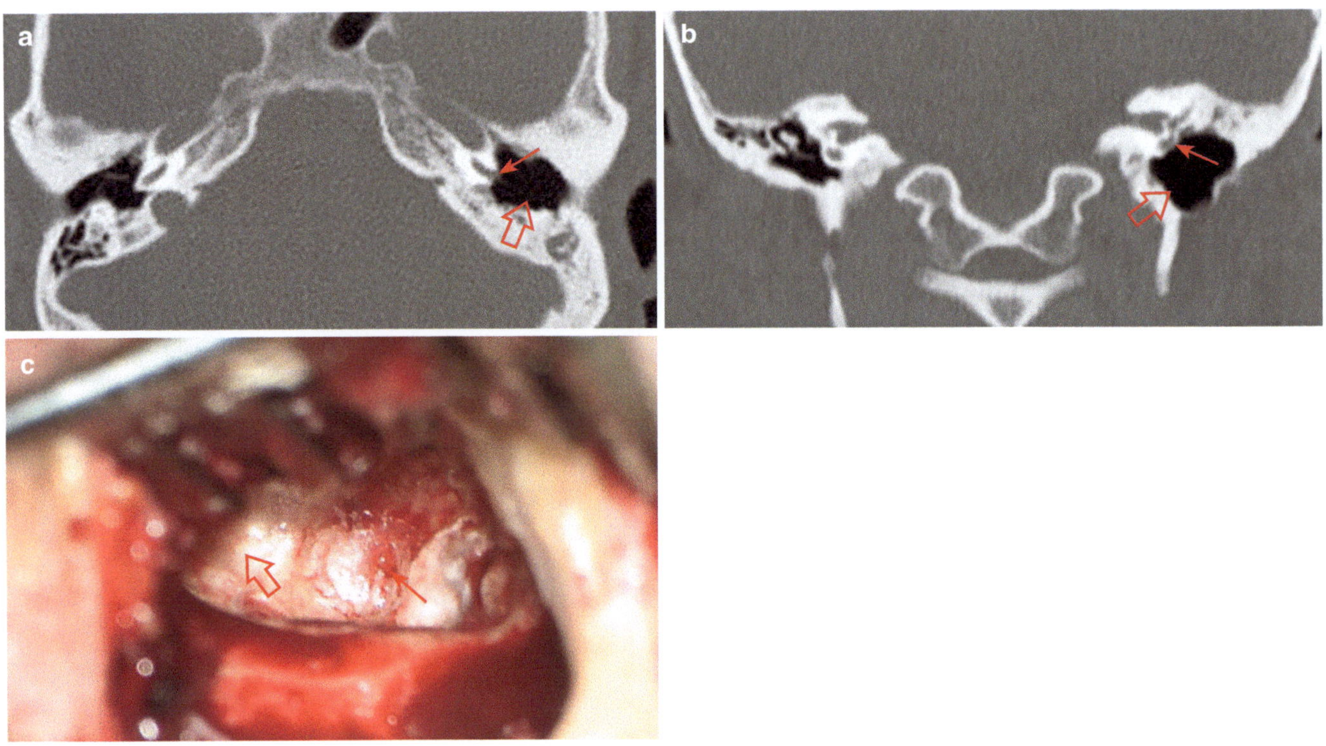

Fig. 5.22 Cholesteatoma of left external auditory canal invading cochlea. (**a**) Axial CT; (**b**) Coronal CT; (**c**) Intraoperative finding. (**a**, **b**) Expansion of left external auditory canal (⇧), and destruction of promontory (↑); (**c**) Expanded external auditory canal and epithelial tissue (⇧), bone absorption and granulation formation (↑) of promontory

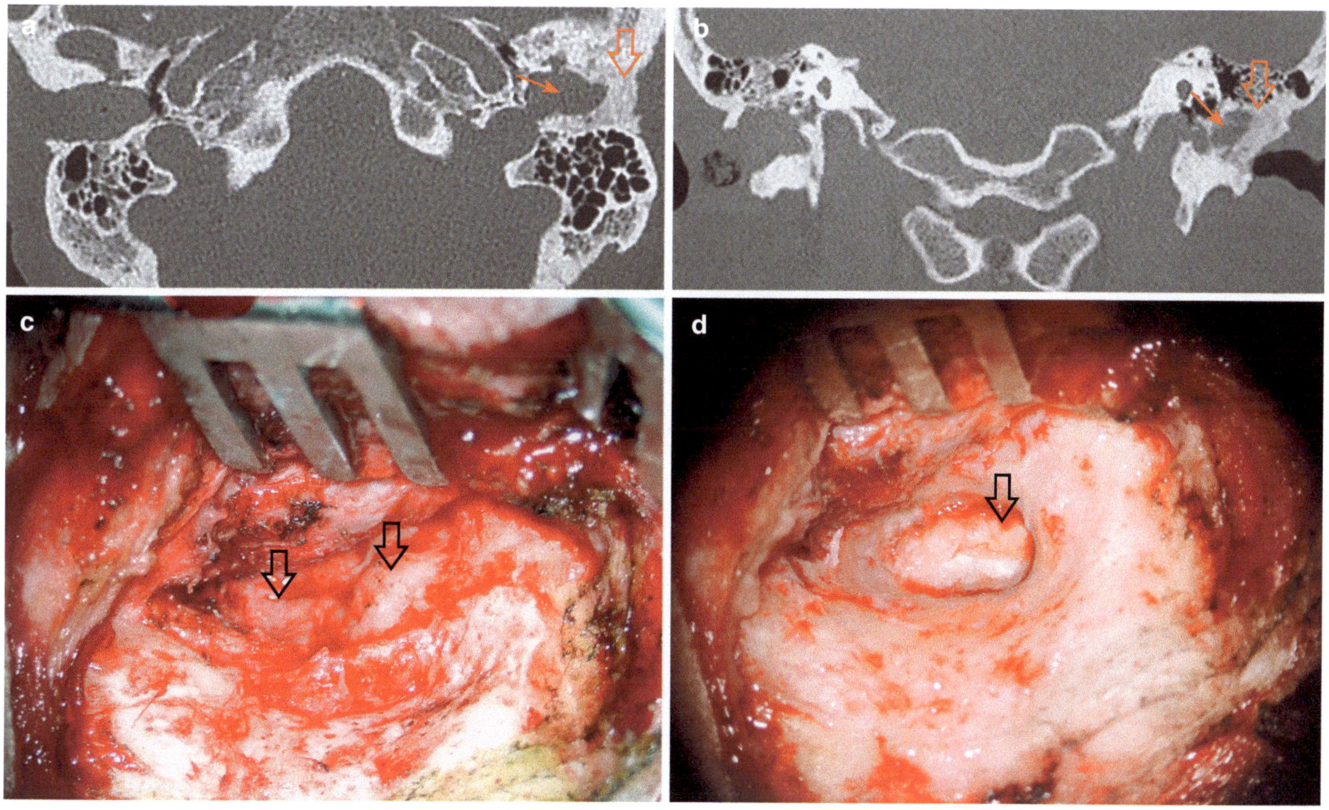

Fig. 5.23 Left external auditory canal atresia with acquired cholesteatoma. (**a**) Axial CT; (**b**) Coronal CT; (**c, d**). Intraoperative finding. (**a**, **b**) Hyperosteogeny (⇧) of lateral segment of external auditory canal resulted in atresia with deep soft tissue shadow (↑); (**c**) Hyperosteogeny and atresia (⇧) was found in opening of the external auditory canal; (**d**) When atretic plate was removed, cholesteatoma (⇧) could be seen in medial segment of external auditory canal

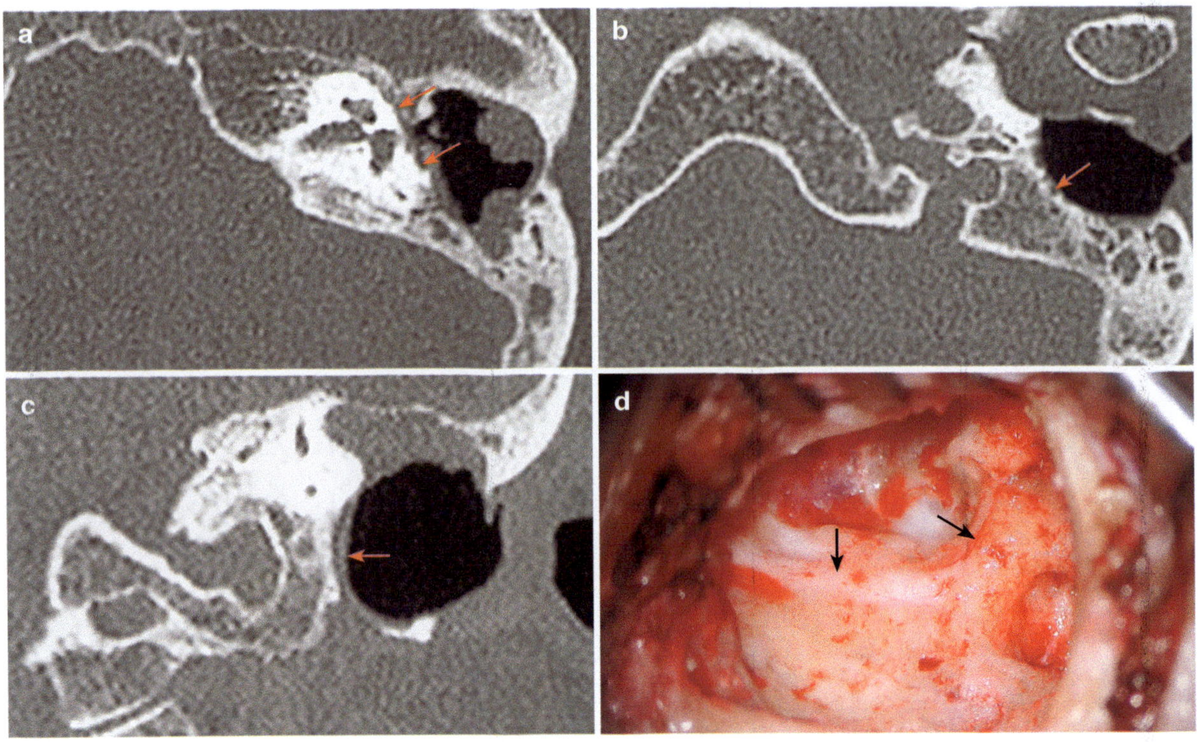

Fig. 5.24 Cholesteatoma of left external auditory canal invaded mastoid and tympanum. (**a**, **b**). Axial CT; (**c**) Coronal CT; (**d**) Intraoperative finding. (**a**) Destruction of horizontal segment (↑) of facial nerve canal; (**b**, **c**). Destruction of vertical segment (↑) of facial nerve canal; (**d**) Exposure of segment and vertical segment of facial nerve (↑)

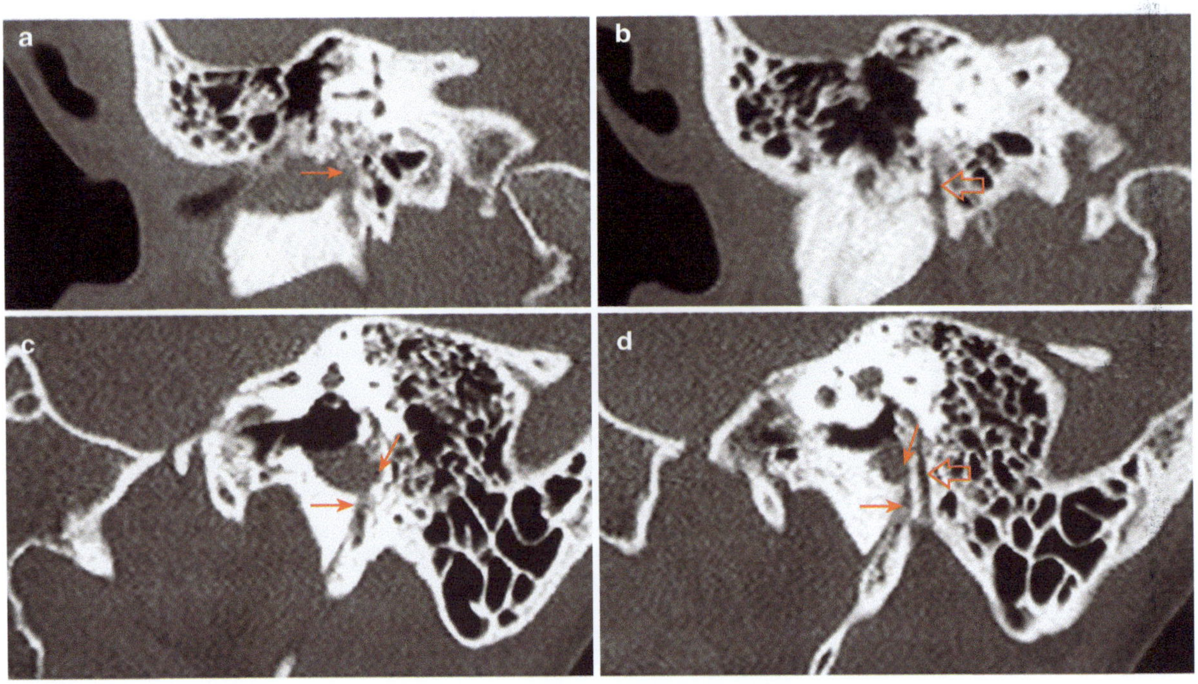

Fig. 5.25 Cholesteatoma of external auditory canal invaded styloid bone marrow (right). (**a**, **b**). Axial CT; (**c**, **d**). Sagittal CT. (**a**, **c**, **d**) Exposed marrow of styloid process (↑); (**b**, **d**) Intact canal of facial nerve canal (⇧)

5.2.2 Congenital Cholesteatoma of Tympanomastoid Cavity

See Figs. 5.26, 5.27, 5.28, 5.29, and 5.30.

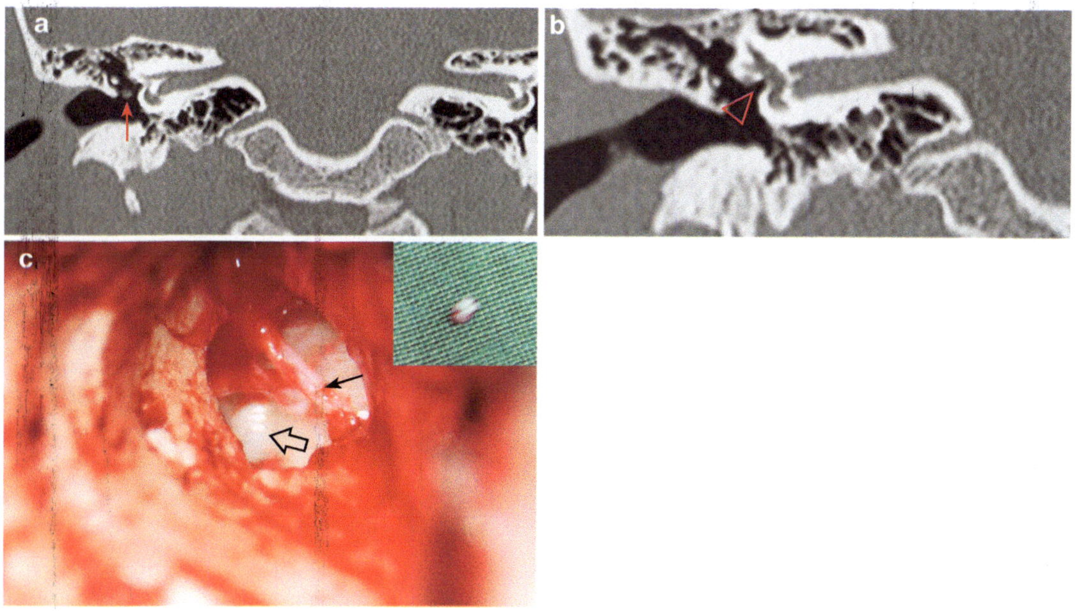

Fig. 5.26 Congenital cholesteatoma of right middle ear (**a**, **b**). Coronal CT; (**c**) Intraoperative finding. (**a**) Soft tissue shadow at lenticular process of incus (↑); (**b**) Disappearance of suprastapedial structure (△); (**c**) Disappearance of suprastapedial structure (⇧) after cholesteatoma (insert figure) cleaned up, chordal tympanic nerve (↑)

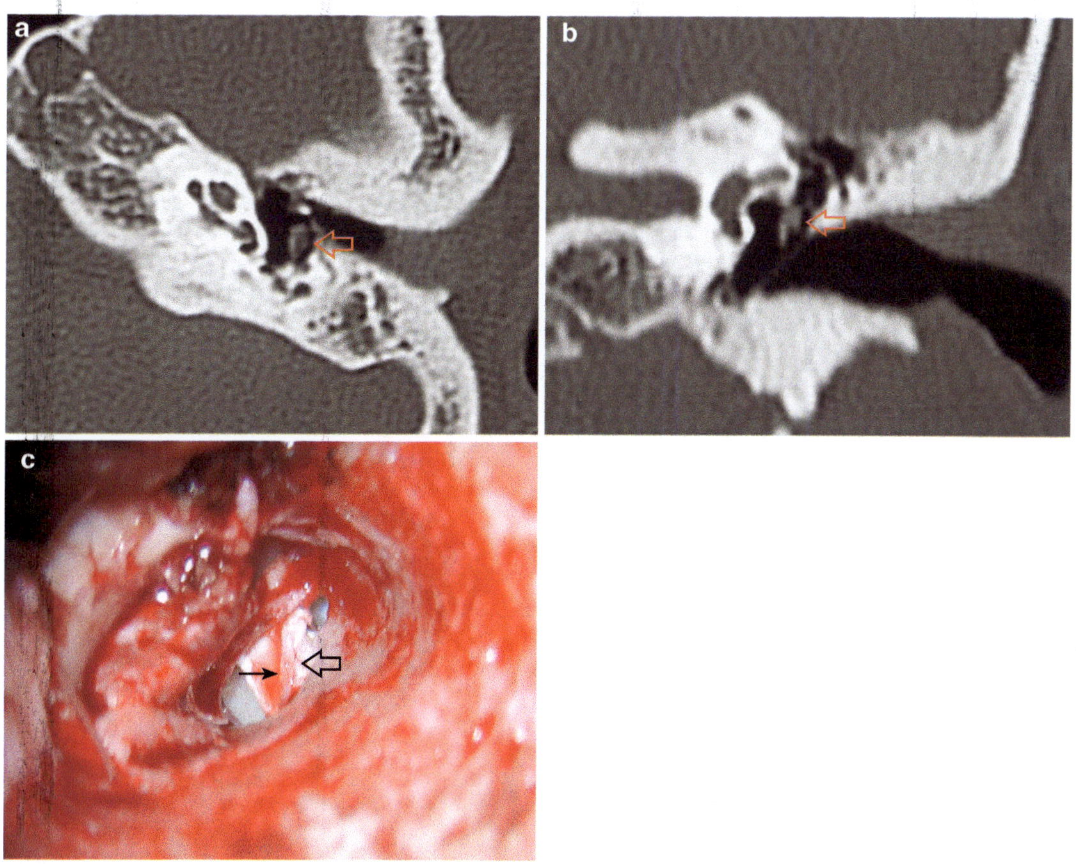

Fig. 5.27 Congenital cholesteatoma of left middle ear. (**a**) Axial CT; (**b**) Coronal CT; C. Intraoperative finding. (**a**, **b**). Long crus of incus was missing, and it was replaced by soft tissue shadow (⇧); (**c**) Tympanic membrane was intact, and exploration of retrotympanum showed epithelial mass (⇧) under chorda tympani nerve (↑)

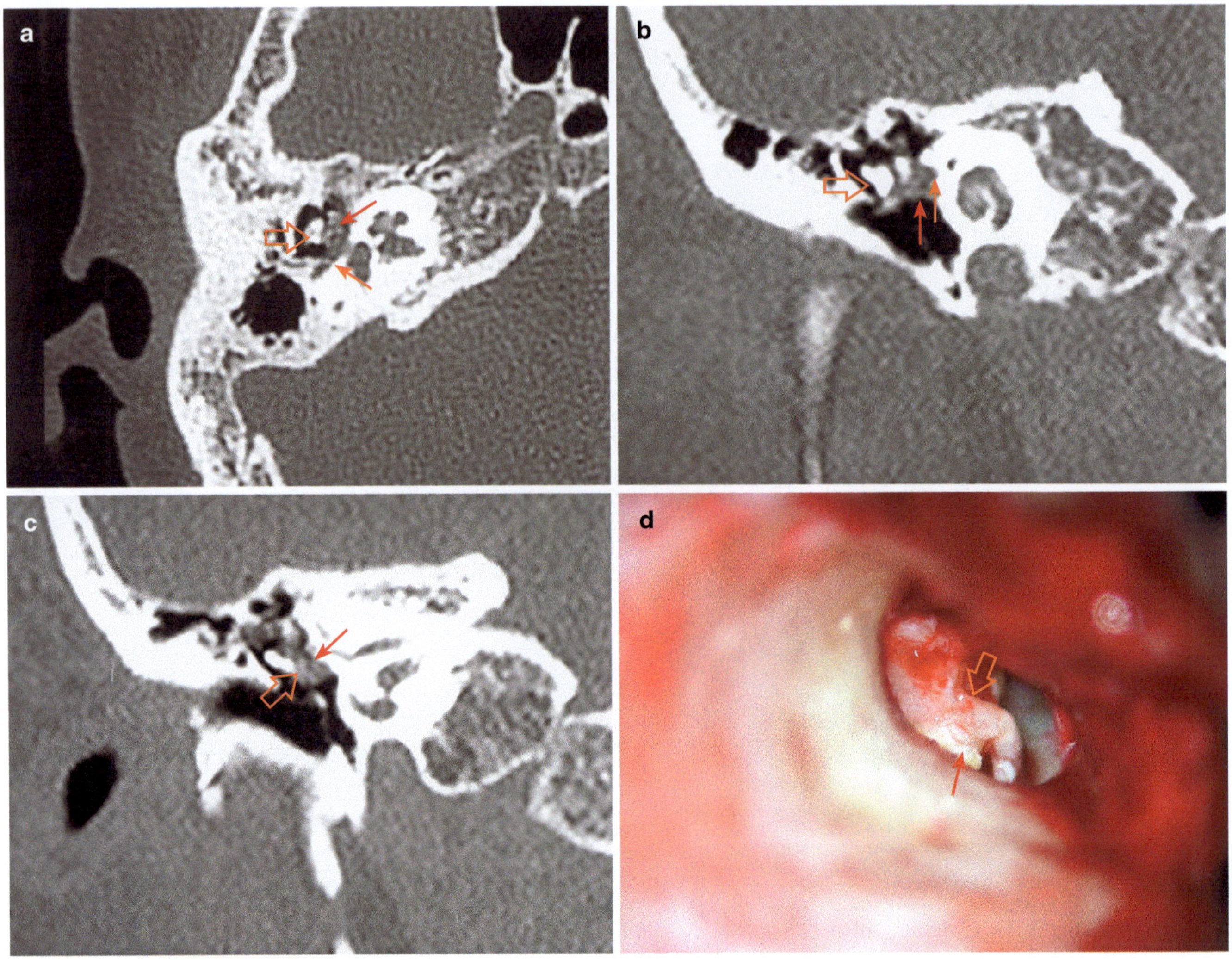

Fig. 5.28 Congenital cholesteatoma in right middle ear. (**a**) Axial CT; (**b**, **c**). Coronal CT; (**d**) Intraoperative finding. (**a**–**c**). Soft tissue shadow (↑) located between incudomalleolar articulation (⇧) and facial nerve (↑); (**d**) Exploration of retrotympanum showed intact tympanic membrane, white epithelium mass (↑) was under medial side of long crus of incus (⇧).

Main diagnostic points of congenital cholesteatoma of middle ear: (1) Without a history of otorrhea, infection, perforation or previous otologic surgery (Gilberto et al. 2020); (2) Progressive conductive deafness, complete tympanic membrane without invagination; (3) There is no connection between (solitary) soft tissue shadow (CT) and tympanic membrane.

Congenital cholesteatoma of middle ear, as a kind of white pearl-like lesion behind a normal tympanic membrane, is usually located at the anterior or posterior region of tympanum

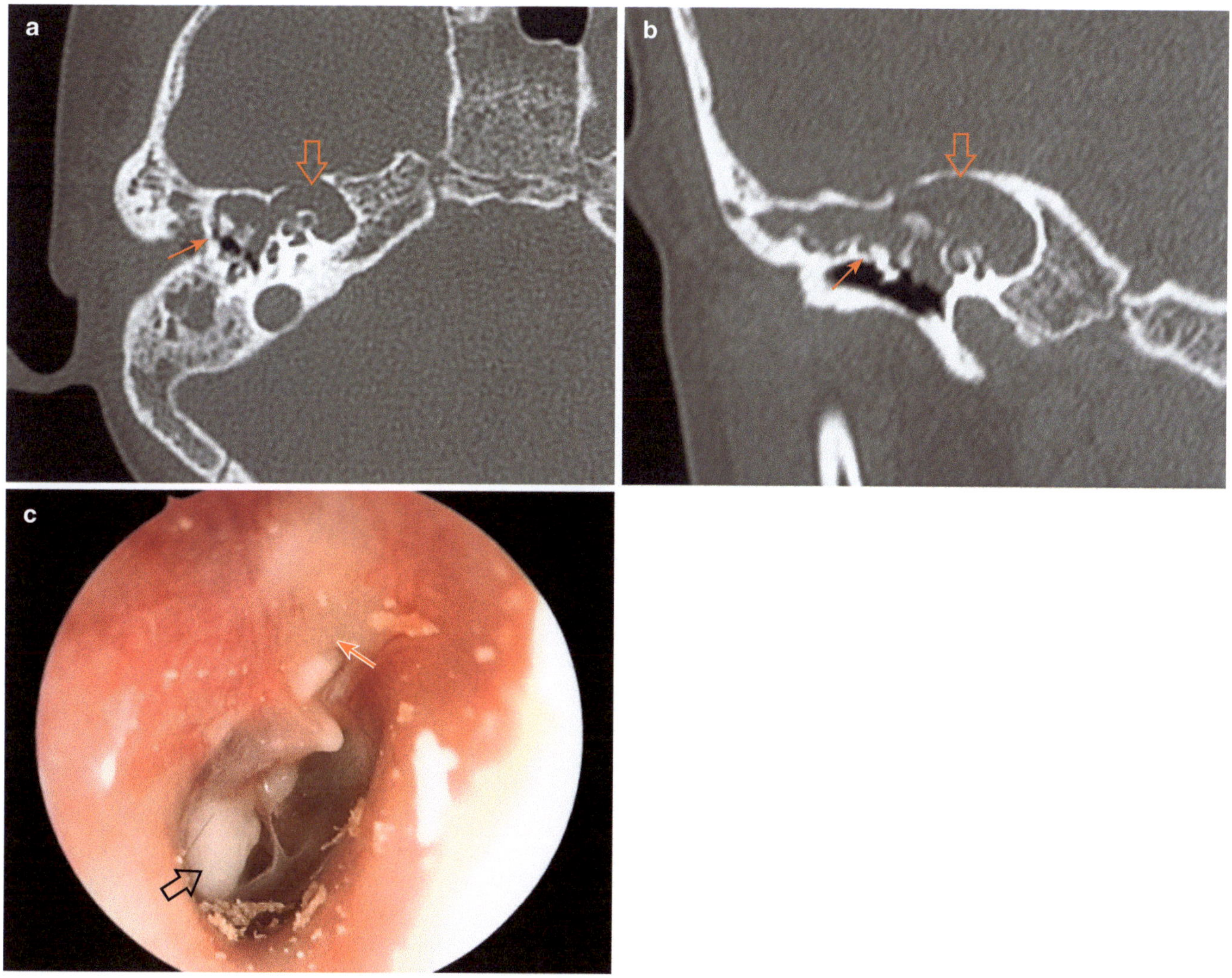

Fig. 5.29 Congenital cholesteatoma of petrous portion of temporal bone in right ear. (**a**) Axial CT; (**b**) Coronal CT; (**c**) Endoscopy of tympanic membrane. (**a**, **b**) Soft tissue shadow (⇧) located at anterosuperior area of labyrinth. Osseous cochlea had been destroyed partially, facial nerve canal also involved, but with intact tympanic membrane and tympanic scutum (↑); (**c**) White epithelial mass (⇧) could be seen through transparent tympanic membrane (↑)

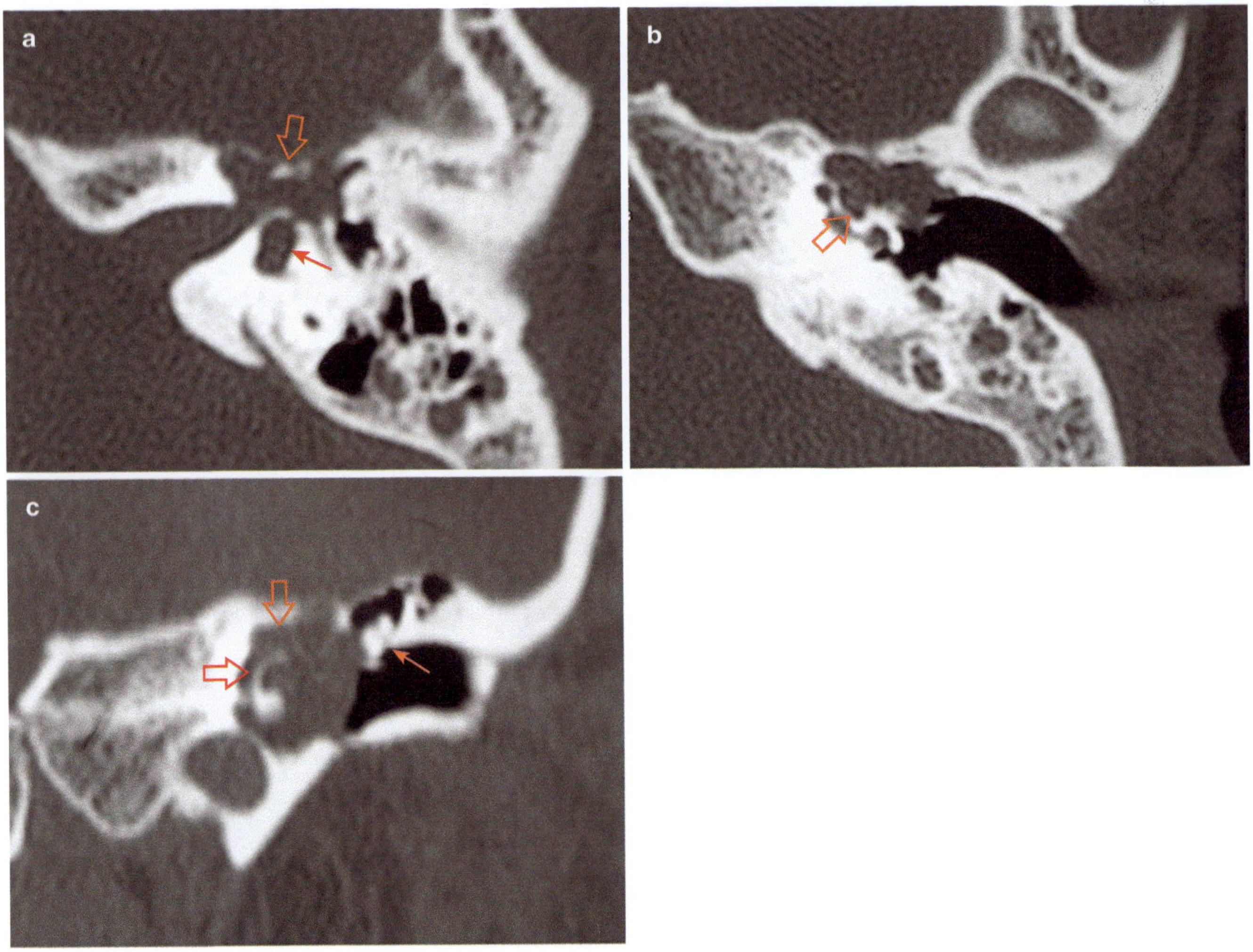

Fig. 5.30 Congenital cholesteatoma in anterosuperior area of labyrinth in left ear and ipsilateral facial paralysis. (**a**, **b**). Axial CT; (**c**) Coronal CT. (**a**) Soft tissue shadow and bone destruction could be seen between labyrinthine segment, geniculate ganglion, beginning of horizontal segment of facial nerve (⇧), vestibule (↑); (**b**) Destruction of cochlea (⇧); (**c**) Destruction of labyrinthine segment, beginning of horizontal segment of facial nerve canal (⇧), cochlear duct (⇧) was destroyed and surrounded by soft tissue (⇧), malleus and incus fused with intact tympanic scutum (↑)

5.2.3 Acquired Cholesteatoma of Middle Ear and Mastoid Process

See Figs. 5.31, 5.32, 5.33, 5.34, 5.35, 5.36, 5.37, 5.38, 5.39, 5.40, 5.41, 5.42, 5.43, 5.44, 5.45, 5.46, 5.47, 5.48, 5.49, 5.50, 5.51, 5.52, and 5.53.

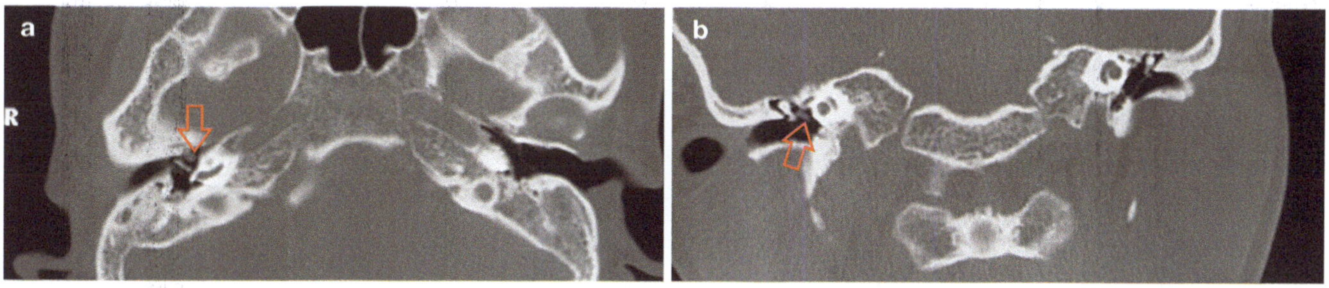

Fig. 5.31 Pars tensa perforation of tympanic membrane with formation of cholesteatoma in right ear. (**a**) Axial CT; (**b**) Coronal CT. Isolated soft tissue shadow could be seen on the anteromedial side of malleus handle (⇧)

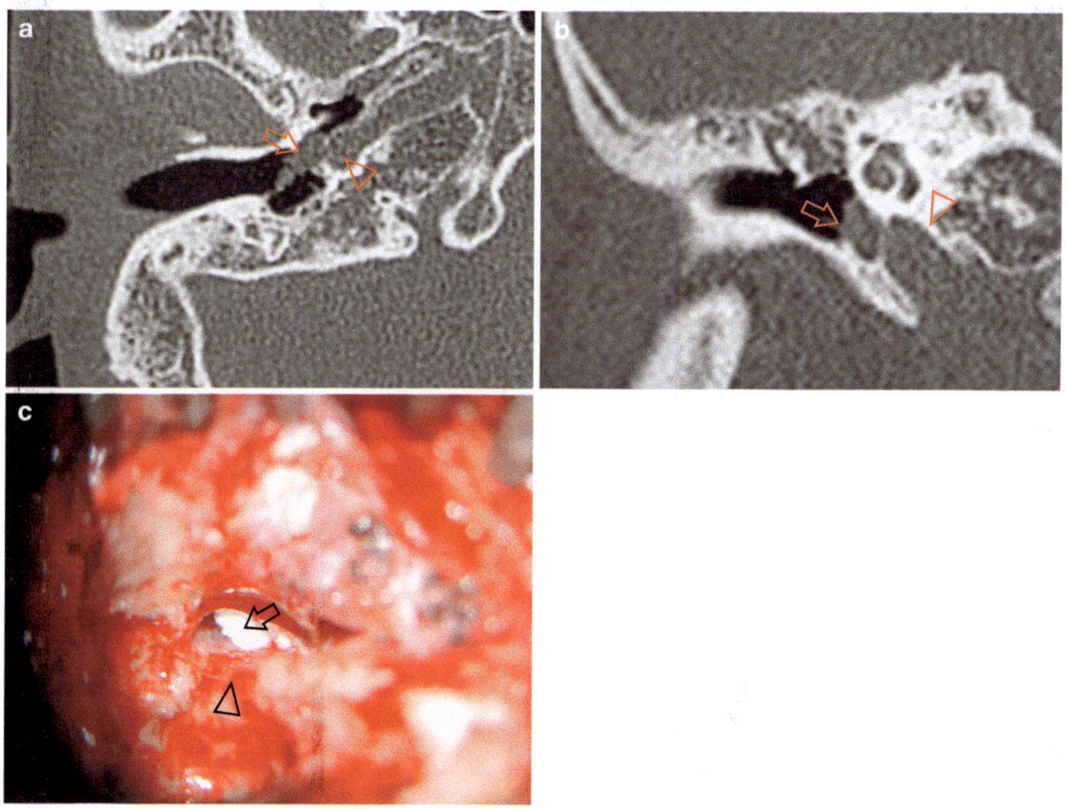

Fig. 5.32 Pars tensa perforation of tympanic membrane with formation of cholesteatoma in hypotympanic cavity of right ear. (**a**) Axial CT; (**b**) Coronal CT; (**c**) Intraoperative finding. (**a**, **b**) Soft tissue shadow (⇧) was located at outside of carotid artery canal (△) and anteroinferior area of tympanic cavity; (**c**) White epithelial mass (⇧) was found in tympanic orifice of eustachian tube, posterior wall of external auditory canal (△)

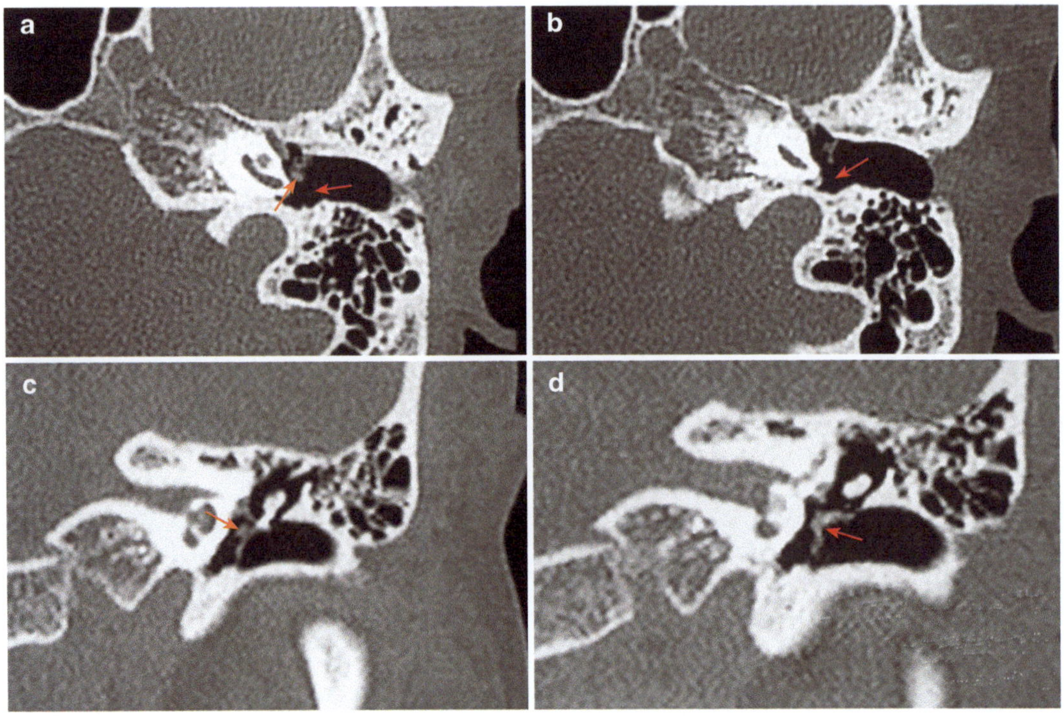

Fig. 5.33 Marginal perforation of tympanic membrane with cholesteatoma formation in left ear. (**a**) Axial CT; (**b**) Coronal CT. (**a**, **c**). Soft tissue (↑) attached on mucosa side of tympanic membrane (↑); (**b**) Marginal perforation (↑) of tympanic membrane; (**d**) Obvious thickening tympanic membrane (↑).

The soft tissue shadow on mucosa side of tympanic membrane was confirmed to be epithelial tissue during operation

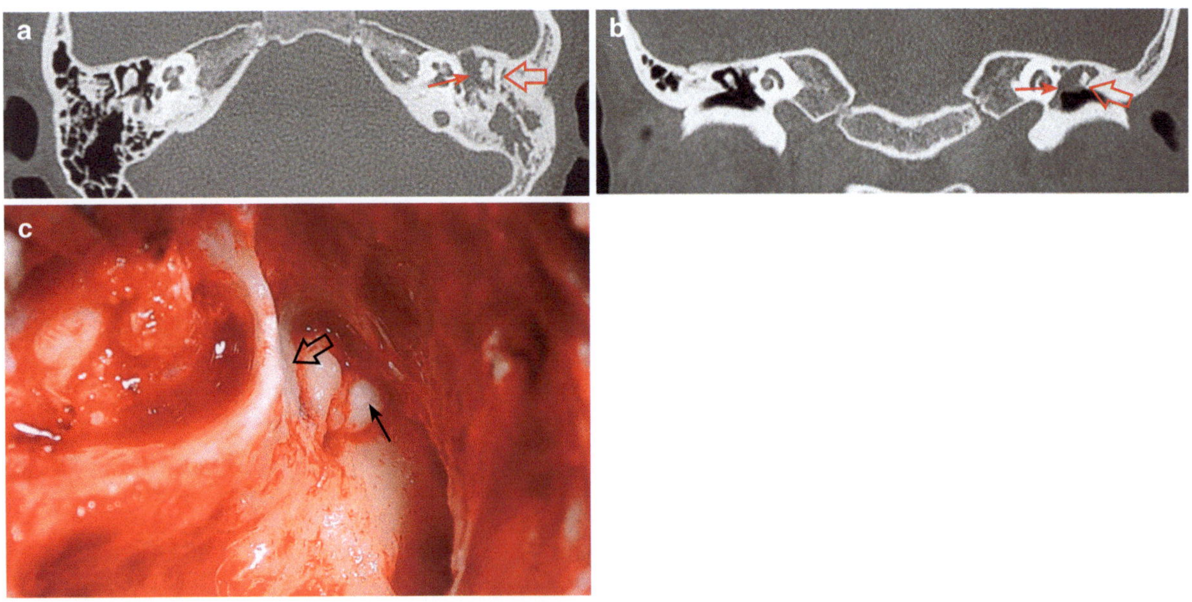

Fig. 5.34 Adhesive otitis media with cholesteatoma formation in left ear. (**a**) Axial CT; (**b**) Coronal CT; (**c**) Intraoperative finding. (**a**, **b**) Epitympanic shadow (↑), intact tympanic scutum (⇧); (**c**) Epithelial mass (↑) was located under medial side of incudomalleolar articulation, tympanic scutum (⇧) was intact

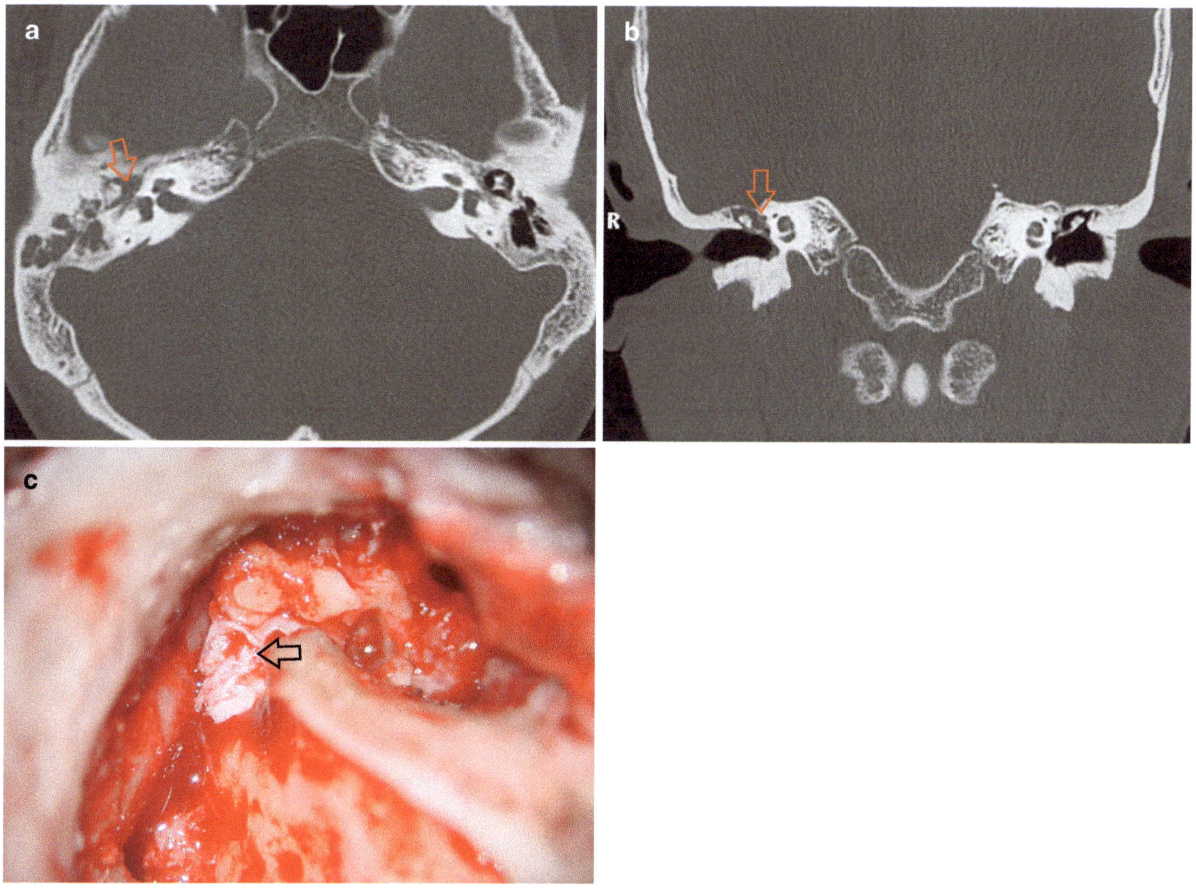

Fig. 5.35 Right adhesive otitis media with cholesteatoma formation in right ear. (**a**) Axial CT; (**b**) Coronal CT; (**c**) Intraoperative finding. (**a**, **b**). Soft tissue shadow (⇧) was mainly located in medial side of incudomalleolar articulation; tympanic membrane was invaginated and adhered to promontory, there is no obvious destroy of tympanic scutum; (**c**) Epithelial tissue (⇧) was seen after removal of incus, which was located at the medial to the incudomalleolar articulation.

Summary: Invaginated sag behind pars tensa of tympanic membrane can develop towards the epitympanum and tympanic antrum, which can cause destruction of incus and suprastapedial structure, and the gap between incudomalleolar articulation and medial wall of epitympanum will increases, but the tympanic scutum remains intact (Yu et al. 2010).

As characteristic changes of cholesteatoma in epitympanum (prussak space), the erosion of tympanic scutum plays an important role in diagnosis of **epitympanic cholesteatoma**, but the tympanic scutum intact cannot be exclude the possibility of temporal bone cholesteatoma (Yu et al. 2010).

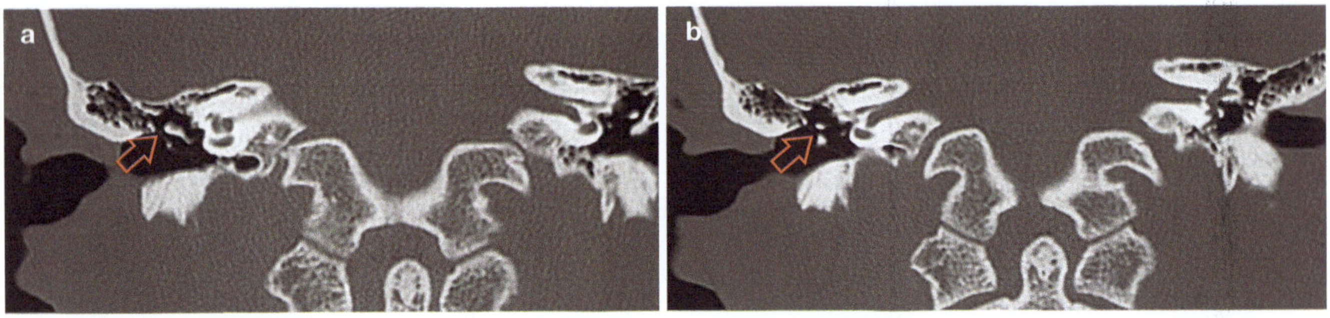

Fig. 5.36 Right tympanum scutum erosion in right ear. (**a**) Axial CT; (**b**) Coronal CT. Tympanic scutum (⇧) was destroyed, and it was partially replaced by membranous tissue

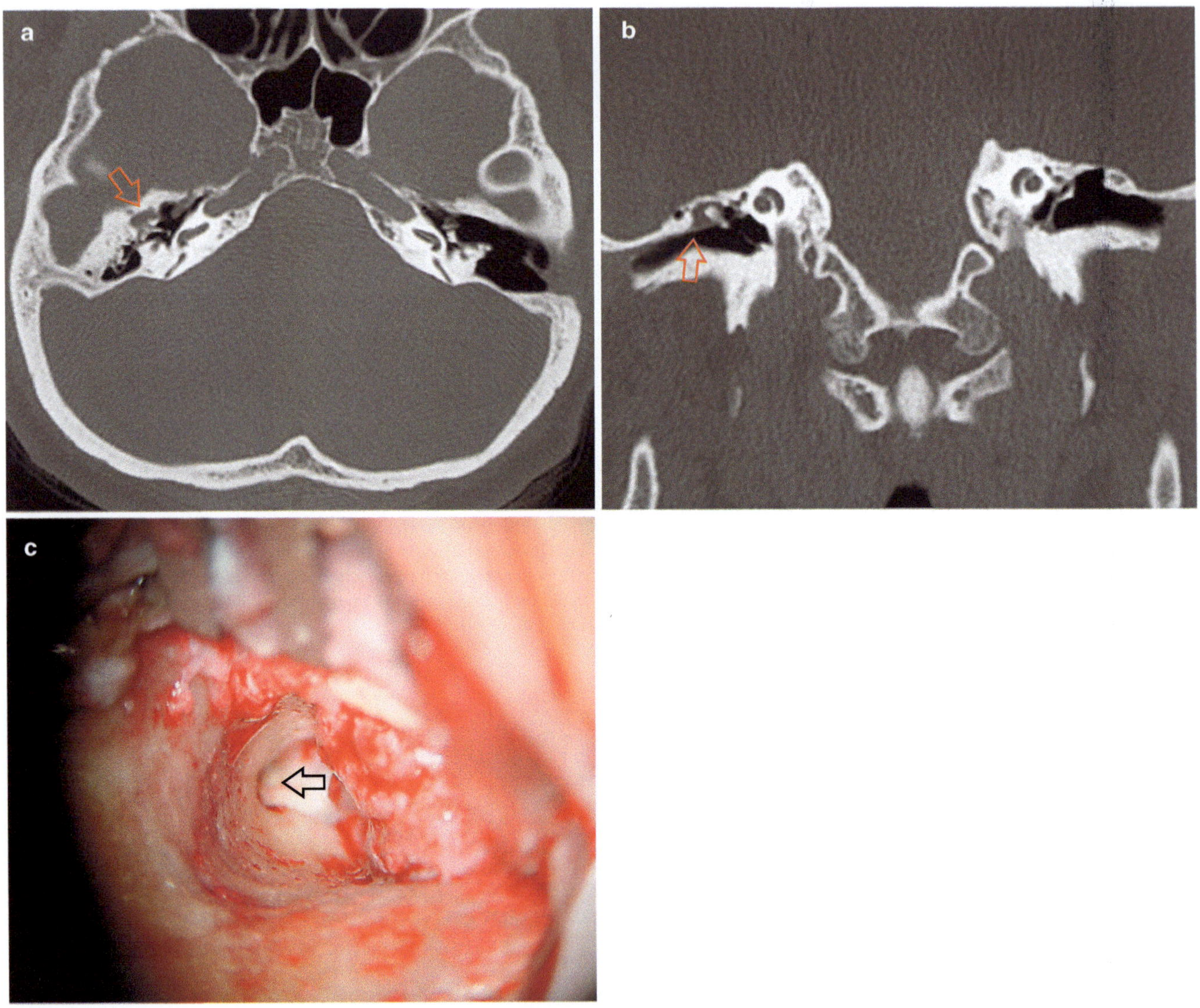

Fig. 5.37 Epitympanic cholesteatoma with erosion of tympanic scutum in right ear. (**a**) Axial CT; (**b**) Coronal CT; (**c**) Intraoperative finding. (**a**, **b**). Space between ossicles and tympanic scutum was enlarged and filled with soft tissue (⇧); (**c**) Tympanic scutum was partially absent (⇧), and epitympanum contained epithelial tissue

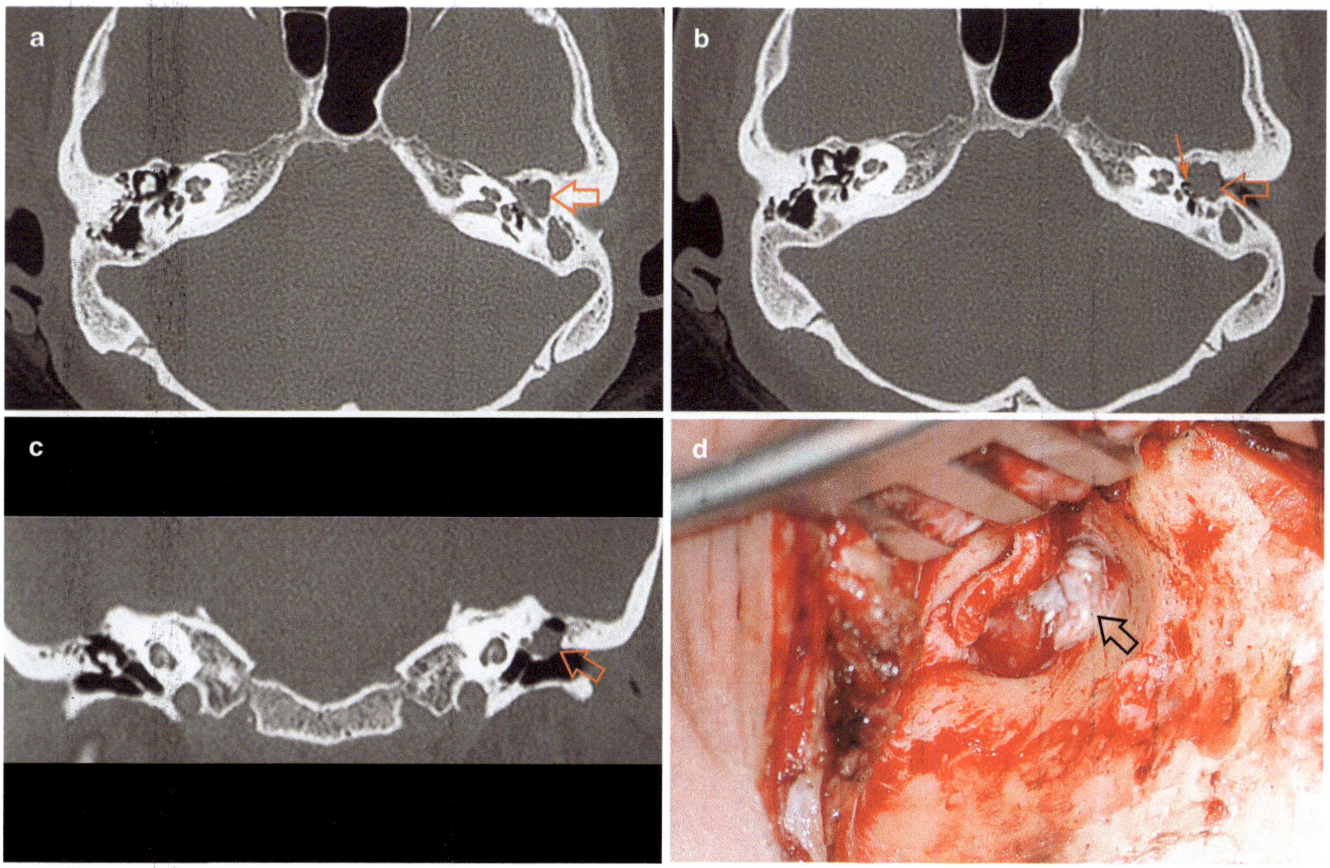

Fig. 5.38 Tympanomastoid cholesteatoma with ossicle erosion in left ear. (**a**, **b**) Axial CT; (**c**) Coronal CT; (**d**) Intraoperative finding. (**a**–**c**). Soft tissue shadow in left epitympanum and tympanic antrum, malleus and incus disappear (⇧), stapes still exist (↑); (**c**) Malleus and incus disappeared, white epithelial tissue (⇧) could be found in epitympanum

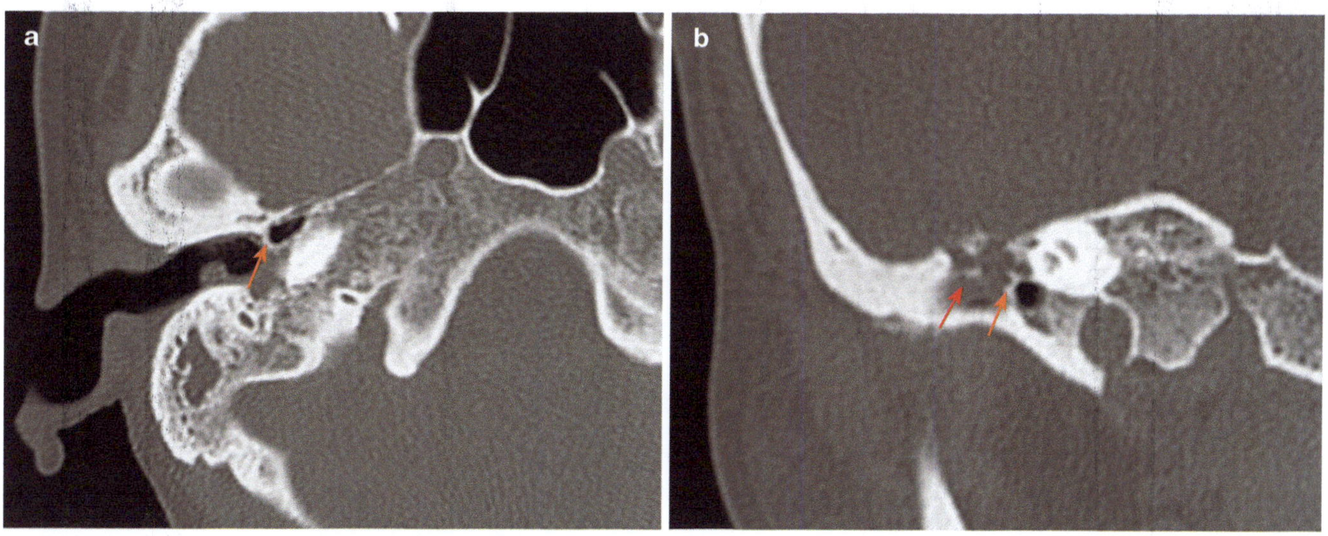

Fig. 5.39 Osseous block of eustachian tube tympanic orifice with cholesteatoma in epitympanum. (**a**) Axial CT; (**b**) Coronal CT . (**a**, **b**) Arc-shaped bone closure (↑) of eustachian tube tympanic orifice, erosion of tympanic scutum, soft tissue shadow (↑) in epitympanum

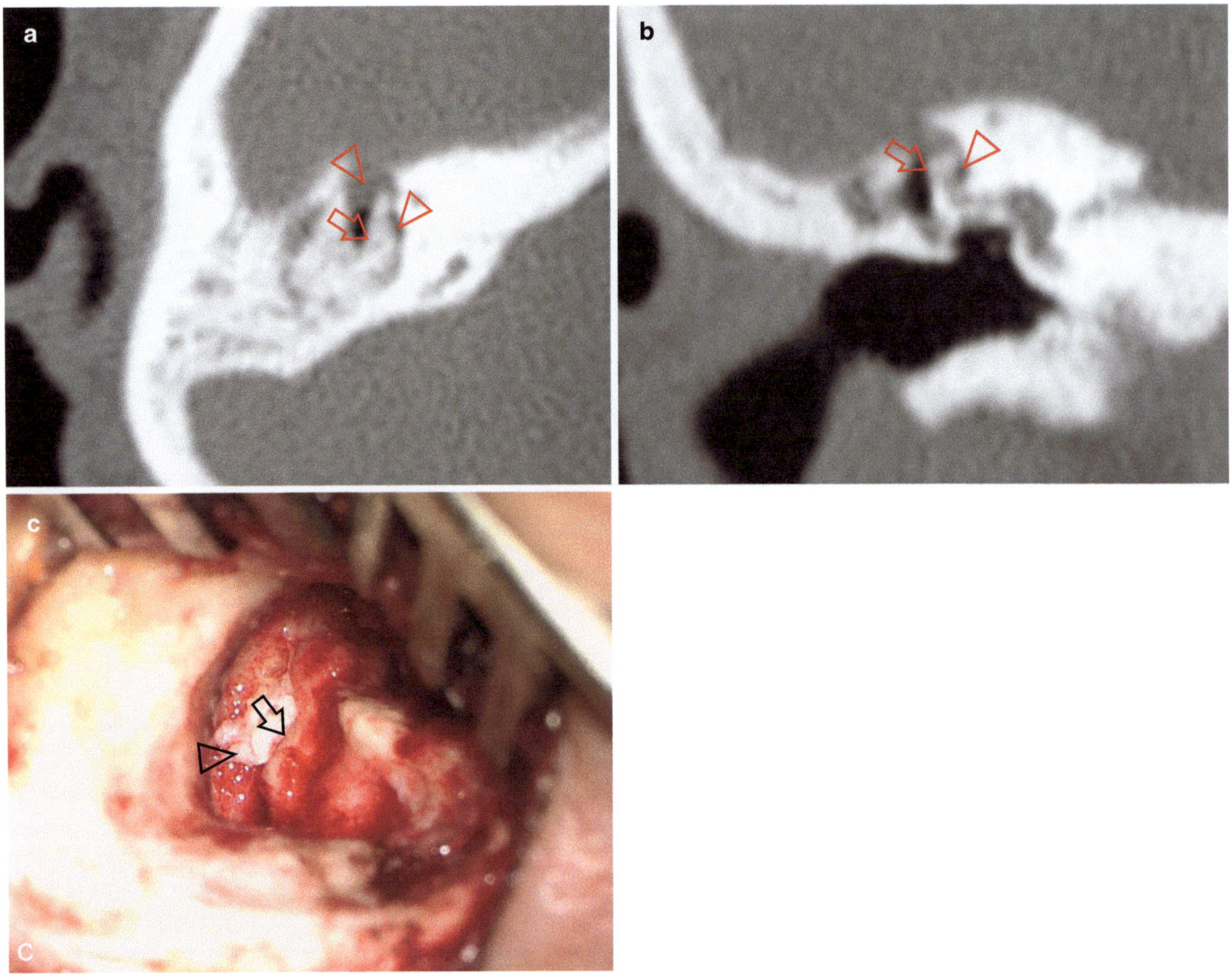

Fig. 5.40 Tympanosclerosis with cholesteatoma. (**a**). Axial CT; (**b**) Coronal CT; C. Intraoperative finding. (**a**, **b**). Soft tissue shadow (Δ) with bone destruction of anterior semicircular canal convex, hyperosteogeny (⇧); (**c**) Cholesteatoma epithelium (Δ) existed in the slit between sclerotic lesions (⇧)

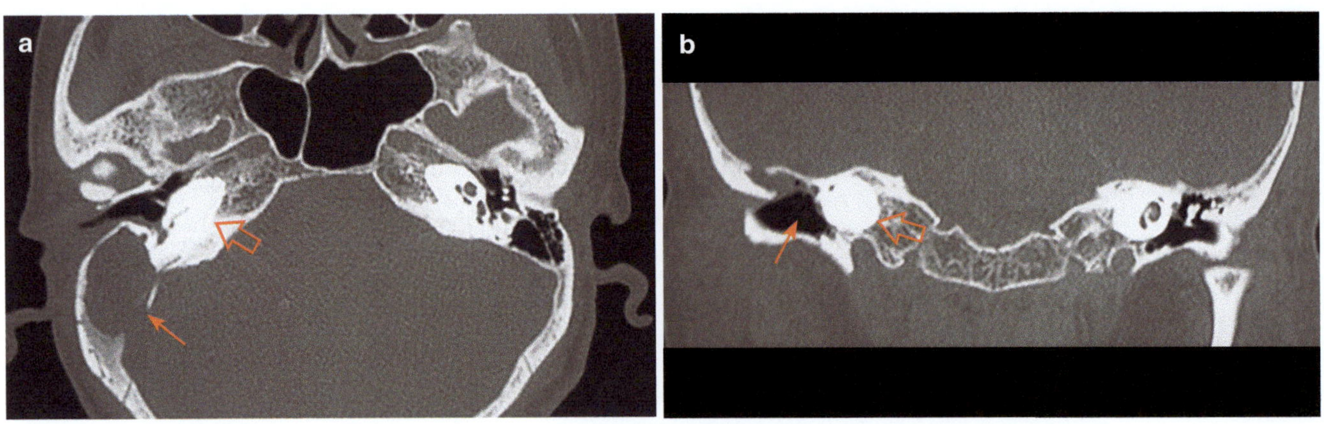

Fig. 5.41 Mastoid cholesteatoma with ossification of cochlea in right ear. (**a**) Axial CT; (**b**) Coronal CT. (**a**, **b**) Ossification of right ear cochlea, disappearance of cochlear duct (⇧), soft tissue occupancy of tympano-mastoid cavity (↑)

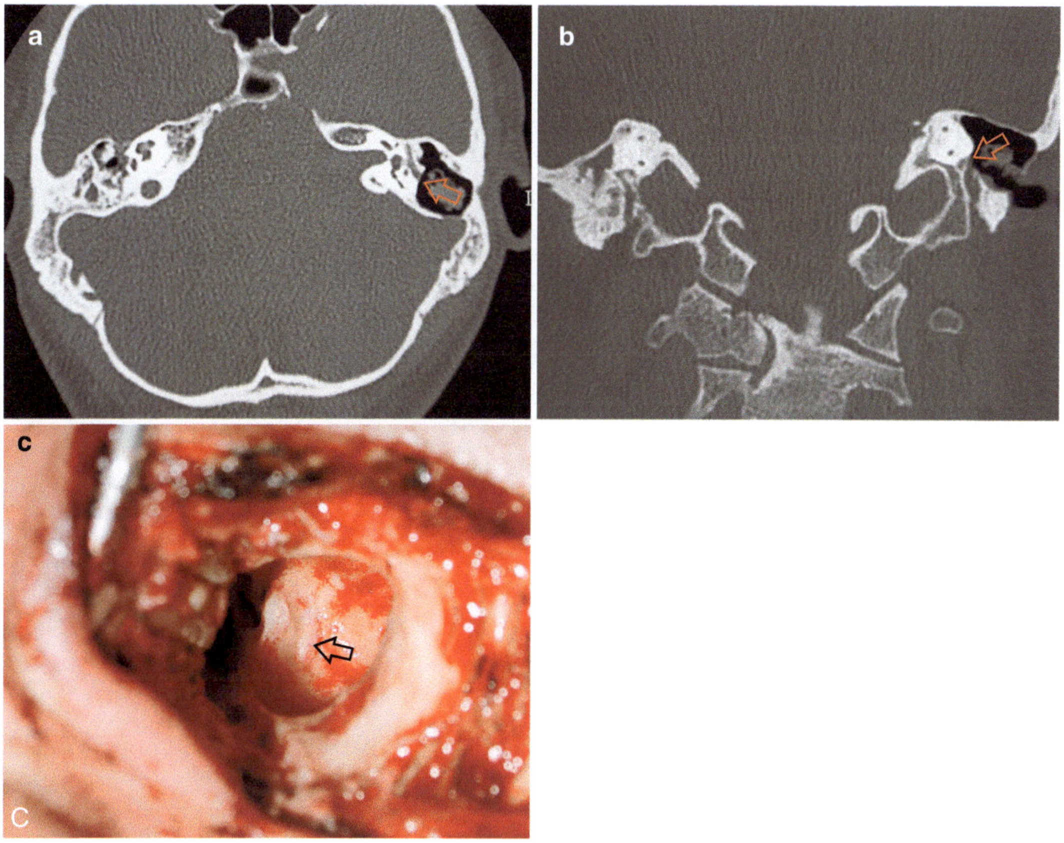

Fig. 5.42 Exposure of second genu of facial nerve caused by cholesteatoma in left ear. (**a**) Axial CT; (**b**) Coronal CT; (**c**) Intraoperative finding. Erosion of second genu (⇧ ⇧) of facial nerve canal

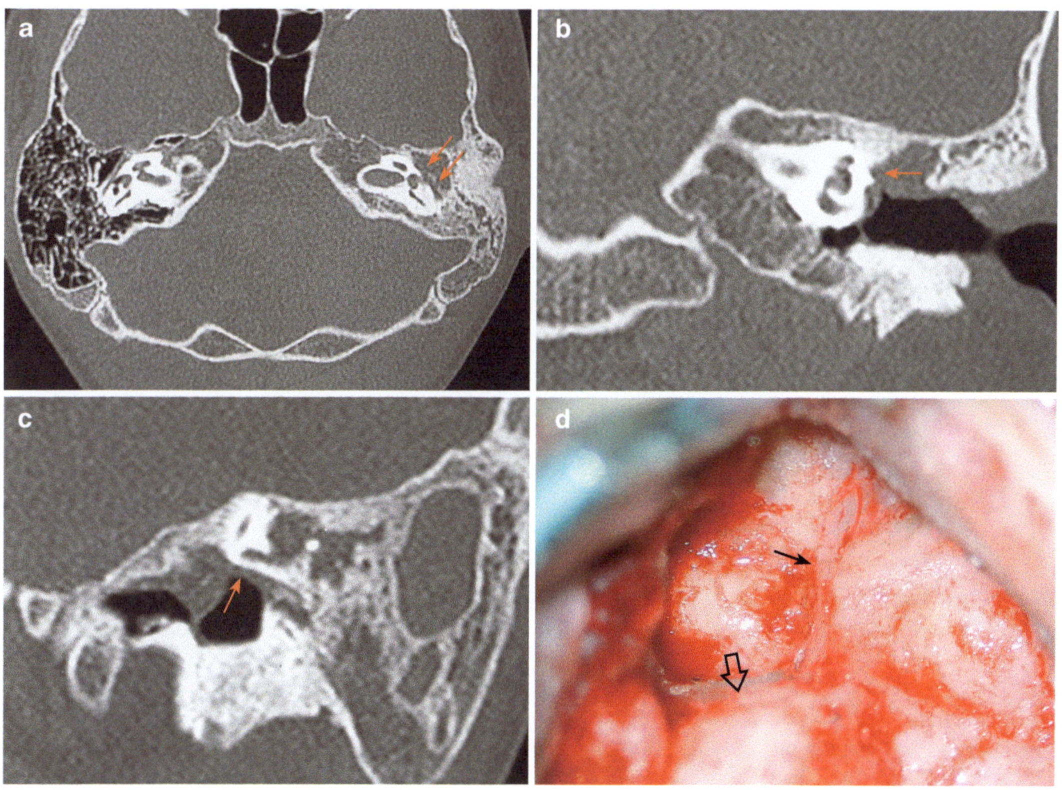

Fig. 5.43 Horizontal segment exposure of facial nerve accompanying cholesteatoma. (**a**) Axial CT; (**b**) Coronal CT; (**c**) Sagittal CT; (**d**) Intraoperative finding. (**a**–**c**) Horizontal segment exposure (↑) of facial nerve; (**d**) Exposed horizontal segment (↑) and vertical segment (⇧) of facial nerve

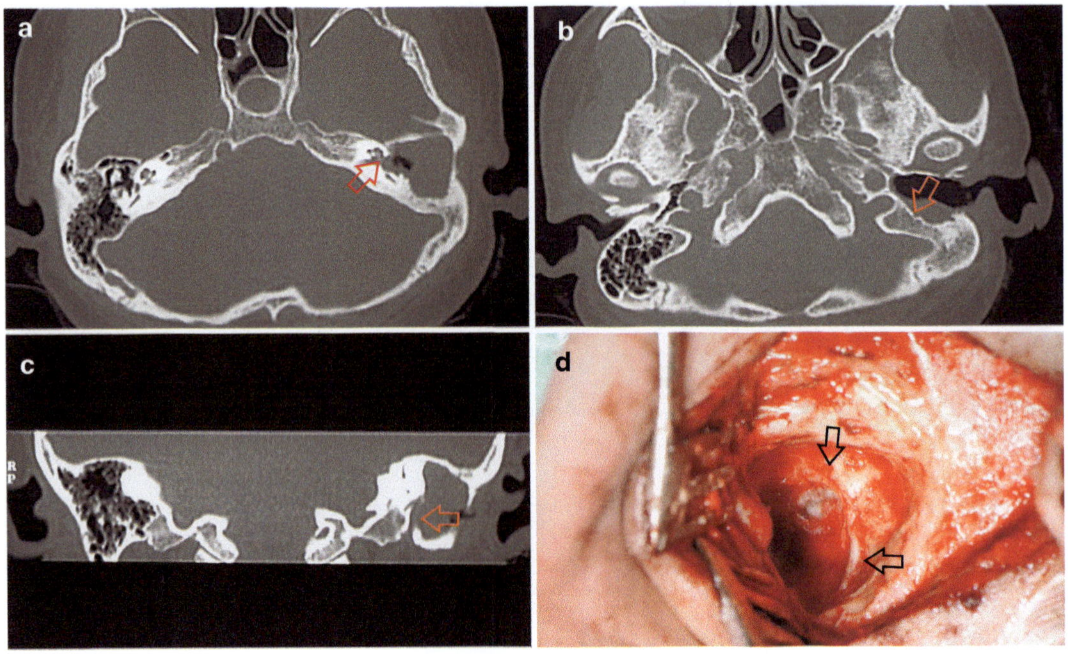

Fig. 5.44 Cholesteatoma invaded horizontal segment and second genu and vertical segment of facial nerve canal in left ear. (**a**, **b**). Axial CT; (**c**) Coronal CT; (**d**) Intraoperative finding. (**a**) Horizontal segment of facial nerve canal and cochlea was destroyed (⇧); (**b**, **c**) Vertical segment (⇧) of facial nerve canal was also destroyed; (**d**) Horizontal–vertical segment of facial nerve (⇧) were exposed.

Note: The patient had a history of suppurative meningitis 45 days ago and ipsilateral ear was total hearing loss

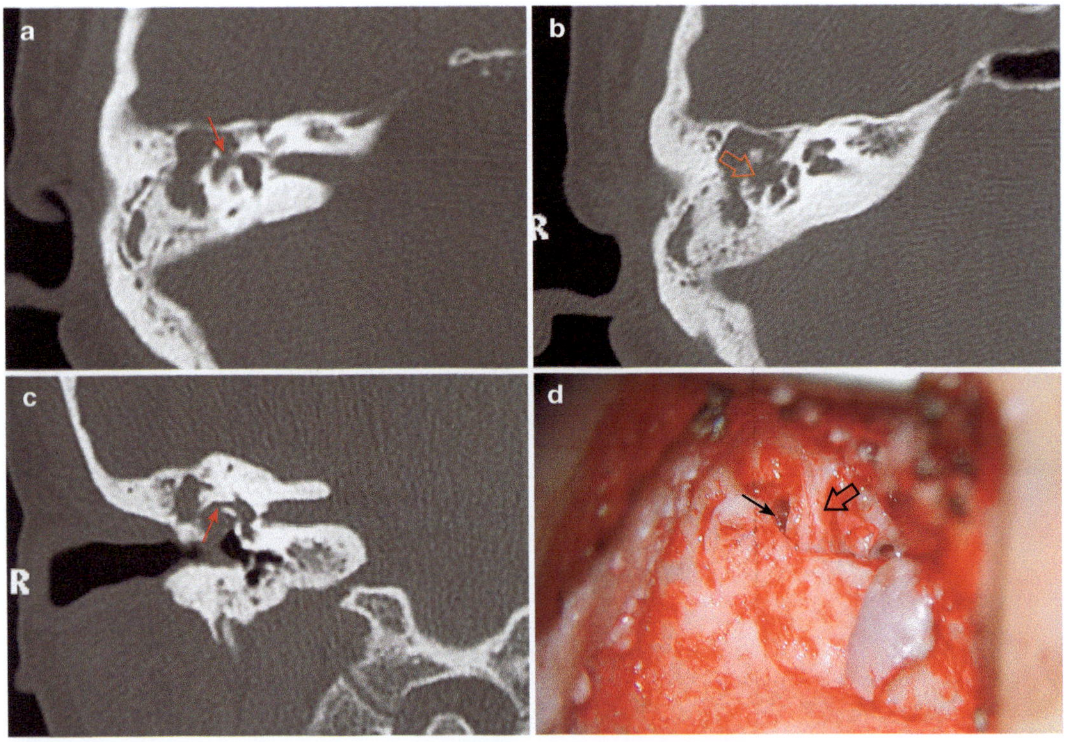

Fig. 5.45 Tympanomastoid cholesteatoma with erosion of lateral semicircular canal and exposure of facial nerve. (**a**, **b**). Axial CT; C. Coronal CT; (**d**) Intraoperative finding. (**a**, **b**) Erosion of horizontal segment of facial nerve canal (↑ , ⇧); (**c**) Erosion of lateral semicircular canal (↑); (**d**) Anteroinferior osseous defect (↑) of lateral semicircular canal and exposure of horizontal segment of facial nerve (⇧)

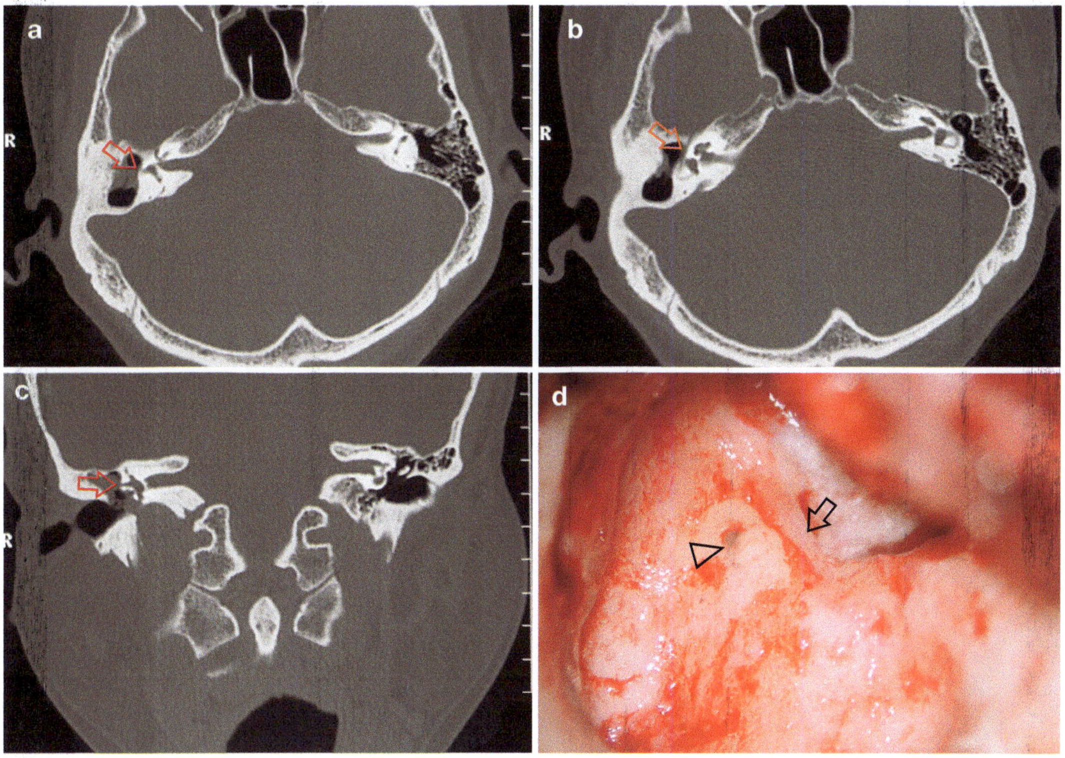

Fig. 5.46 Tympanomastoid cholesteatoma with exposure of facial nerve and erosion of lateral semicircular canal in right ear. (**a**, **b**) Axial CT; (**c**) Coronal CT; (**d**) Intraoperative finding. (**a**–**c**) Enlargement of aditus ad antrum, erosion of lateral semicircular canal (⇧) and horizontal segment of facial nerve canal (⇧); (**d**) Exposure of horizontal segment of the facial nerve (▲) and membranous lateral semicircular canal (⇧)

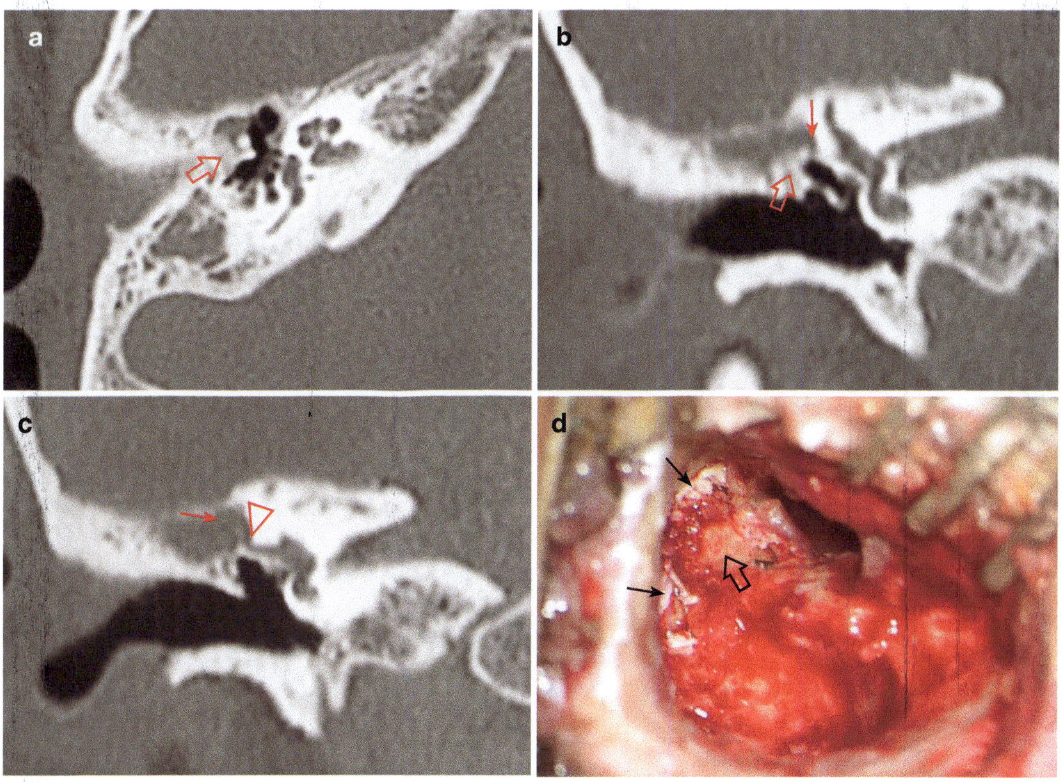

Fig. 5.47 Tympanosclerosis with cholesteatoma and destruction of lateral semicircular canal in right ear. (**a**) Axial CT; (**b**, **c**) Coronal CT; (**d**) Intraoperative finding. (**a**–**c**) Osteogeny (⇧) at incus, incus fixation, epitympanic soft tissue (↑), destruction of lateral semicircular canal bone (△); (**d**) Epithelial tissue in epitympanum(↑), Osteogeny (⇧)

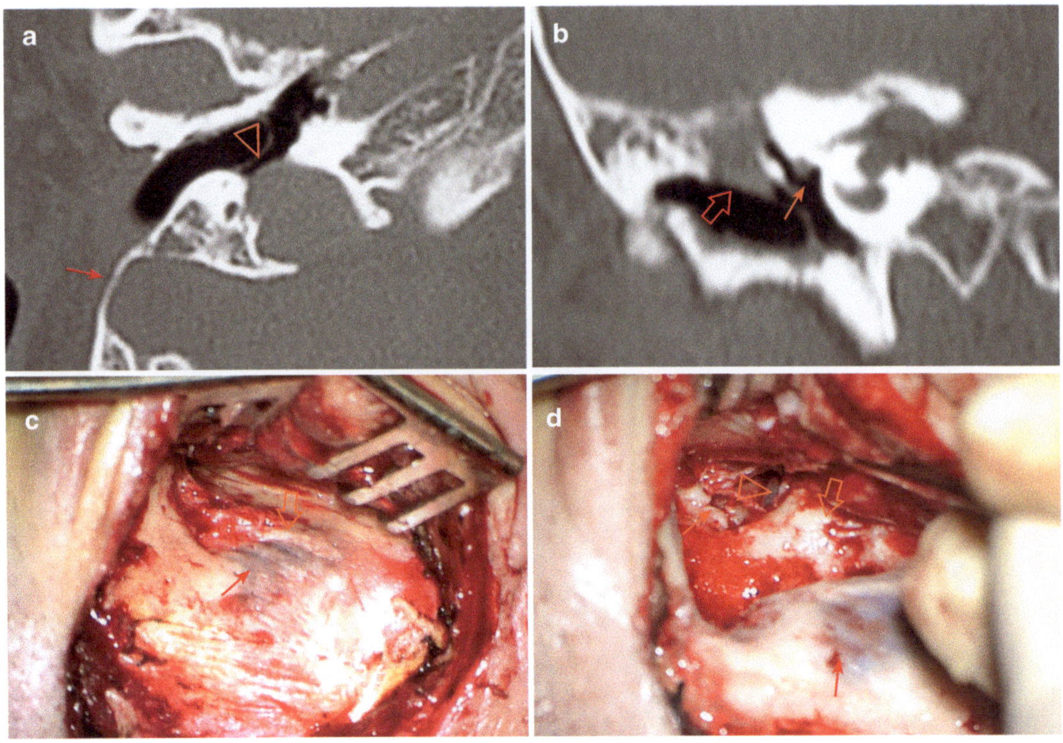

Fig. 5.48 Anterolateral position of sigmoid sinus-exposure of jugular glomus with tympanomastoid cholesteatoma in right ear. (**a**) Axial CT; (**b**) Coronal CT; (**c, d**) Intraoperative finding. (**a**) High position and exposure of jugular glomus (△); (**b**) Epitympanic soft tissue shadow with destruction of tympanic scutum (⇧), facial nerve (↑); (**c, d**) Anterolateral position of sigmoid sinus (↑), thin posterior wall (⇧) of external auditory canal, exposure of facial nerve (↑) and jugular glomus (△)

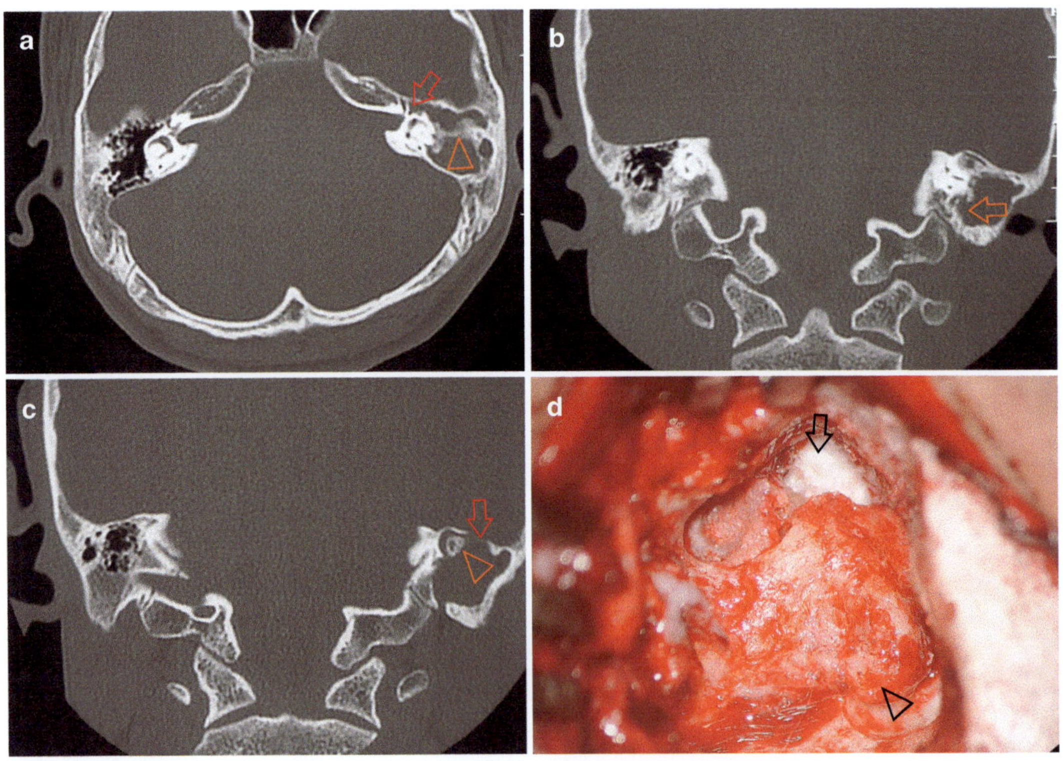

Fig. 5.49 Cholesteatoma of anterior-superior tympanum in left ear. (**a**) Axial CT; (**b, c**) Coronal CT; (**d**) Intraoperative finding. (**a**) Anteromedial cholesteatoma (⇧) of anterior semicircular canal, osteogeny (△) of mastoid cavity; (**b**) Erosion of vertical segment of facial nerve canal (⇧); (**c**) Osteogeny (△) in mastoid cavity, soft tissue and erosion of tegmen of tympanic antrum (⇧); (**d**) Anteromedial cholesteatoma (⇧) of anterior semicircular canal, osteogeny (△) in mastoid cavity

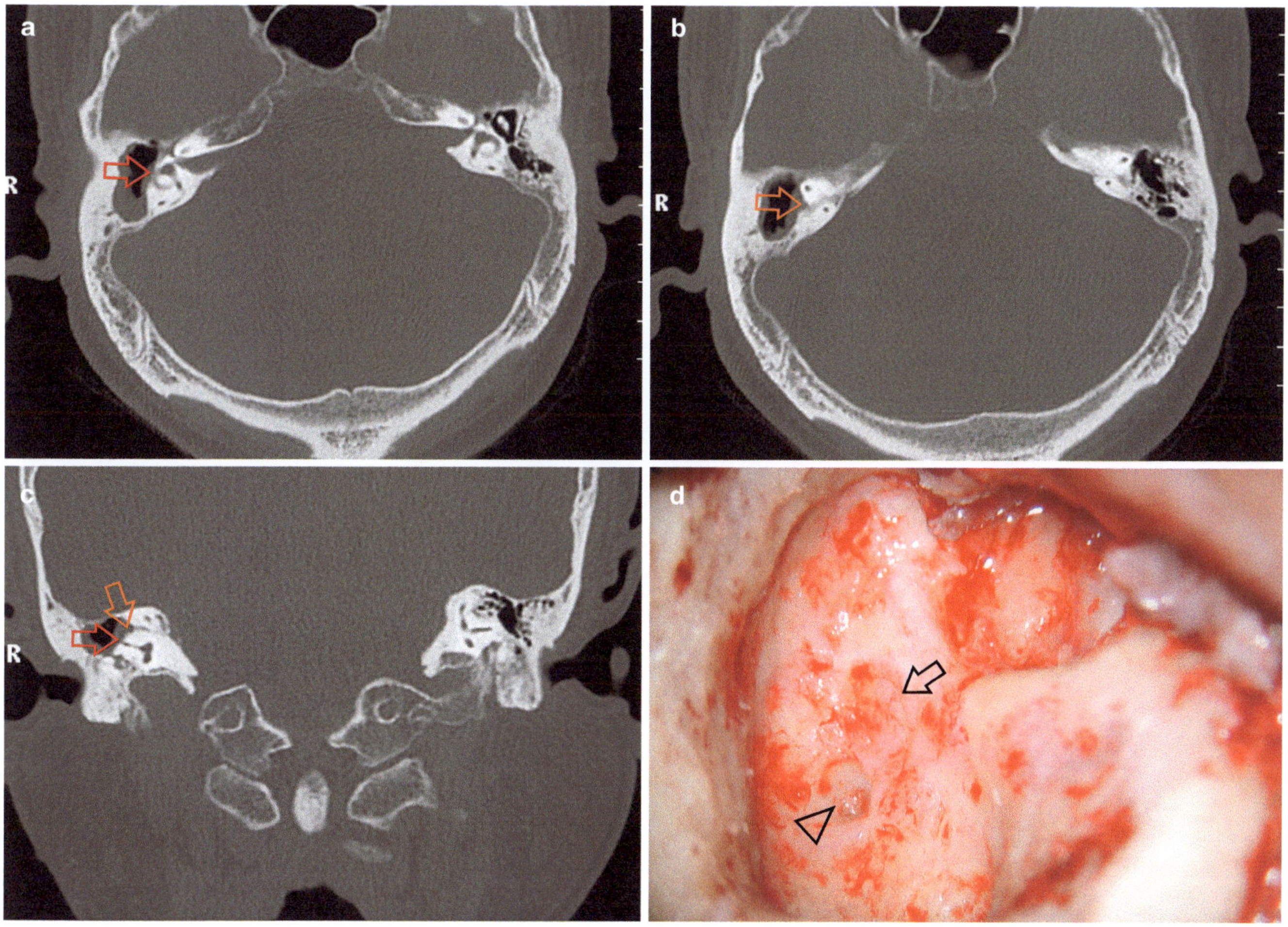

Fig. 5.50 Destruction of lateral semicircular canal and enlargement of petromastoid canal caused by tympanomastoid cholesteatoma in right ear. (**a**, **b**) Axial CT; (**c**) Coronal CT; (**d**) Intraoperative finding. Destruction of lateral semicircular canal convex (⇧, ⇧), enlarged mastoid end of petromastoid canal (⇧, △) and aditus ad antrum

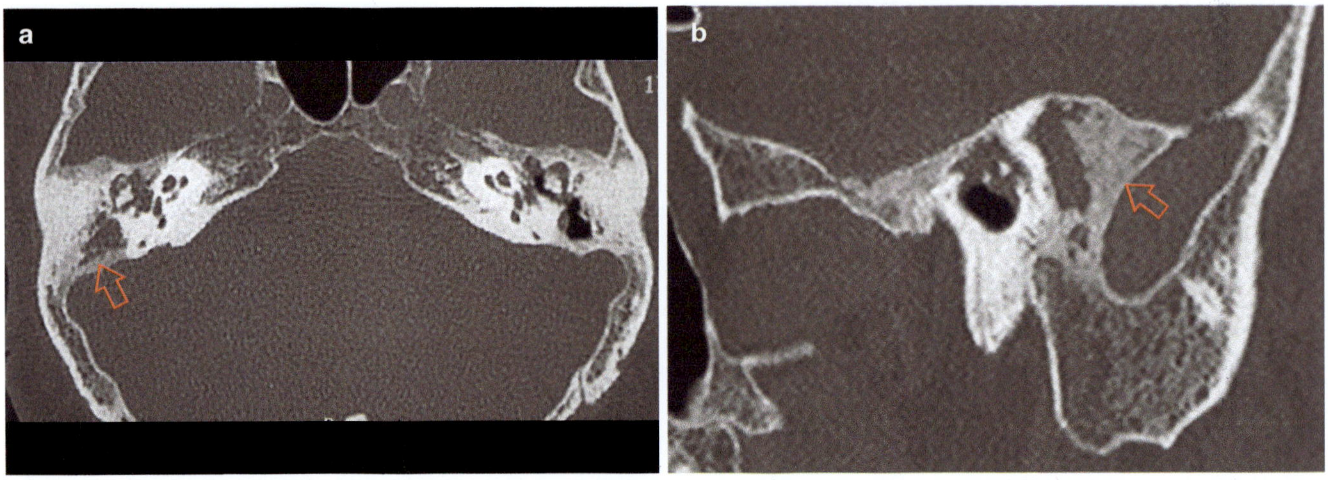

Fig. 5.51 Bilateral tympanomastoid cholesteatoma with osteomyelitis in right sigmoid sulus. (**a**) Axial CT; (**b**) Sagittal CT. Osteomyelitis of right sigmoid sulcus (⇧) and ipsilateral tympano-mastoiditis

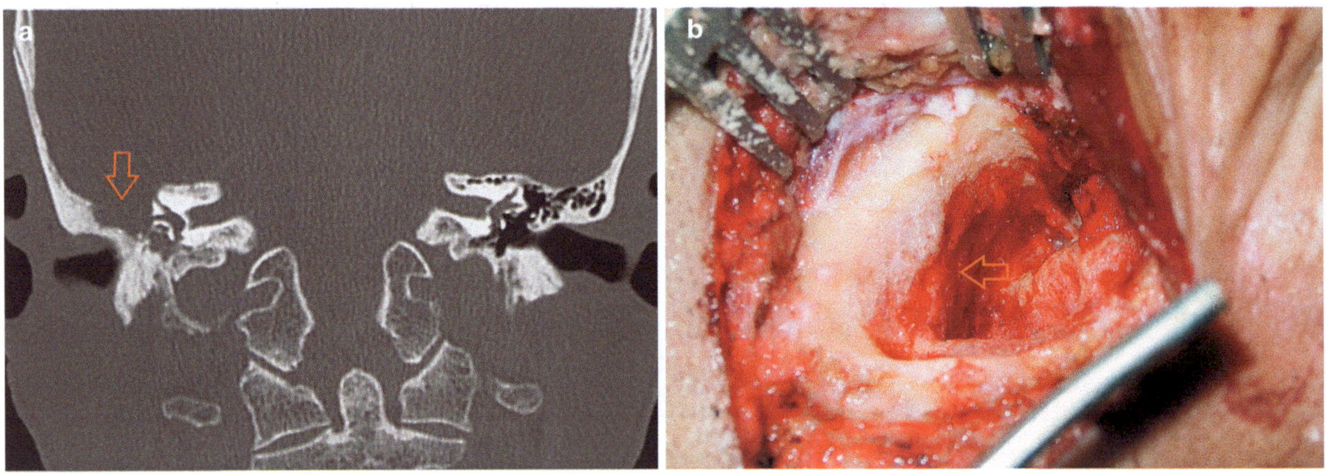

Fig. 5.52 Tympanomastoid cholesteatoma with dural exposure in right ear. (**a**) Coronal CT; (**b**) Intraoperative finding. (**a**) Bony destruction of tegmen of tympanic antrum (⇧); (**b**) Dural exposure (⇧)

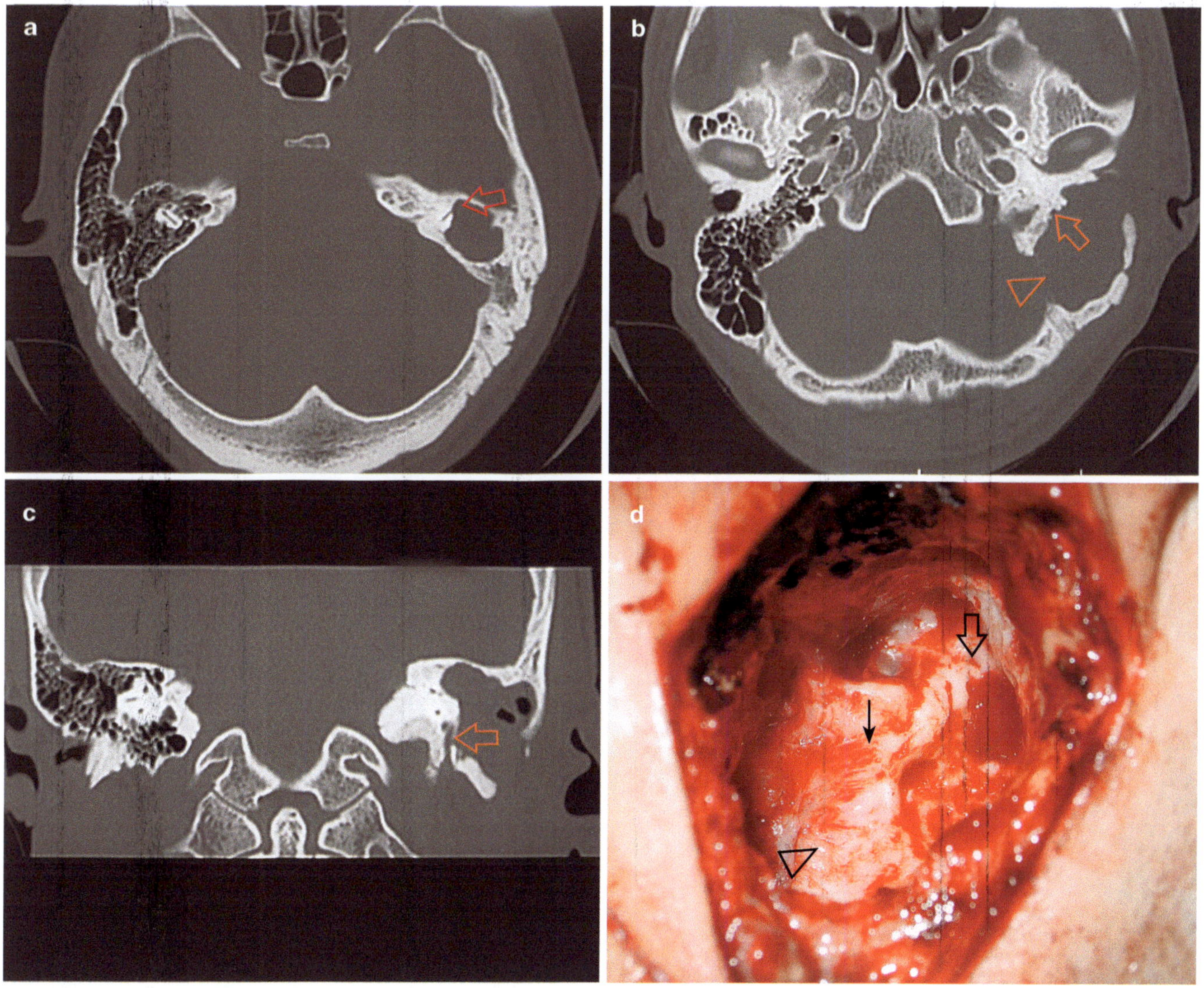

Fig. 5.53 Tympanomastoid cholesteatoma with erosion of facial nerve canal and anterior semicircular canal & sigmoid sulcus. (**a**, **b**) Axial CT; (**c**) Coronal CT; (**d**) Intraoperative finding. (**a–c**) Cholesteatoma resulted in erosion of anterior semicircular canal (⇧), posterolateral wall of facial nerve vertical segment (⇧) and sigmoid sulcus (△); (**d**) Surface of vertical segment of facial nerve(↑), sigmoid sinus (**▲**) and anterior semicircular canal (**⇧**) were covered with connective tissue.

Note: In otitis media with cholesteatoma, pathological exposure of the facial nerve is very common. Preoperative CT imaging diagnosis is helpful for intraoperative management and protection (Yu et al. 2007; Yu et al. 2011). This Facial nerve has produced a certain tolerance for the pathological exposure. If we are careful enough, addition injure usually does not occur, the routine supply of glucocorticoids are not required to prevent facial paralysis after surgery

5.3 Post-operative Changes of Tympanomastoid Surgery

See Figs. 5.54, 5.55, 5.56, 5.57, 5.58, and 5.59.

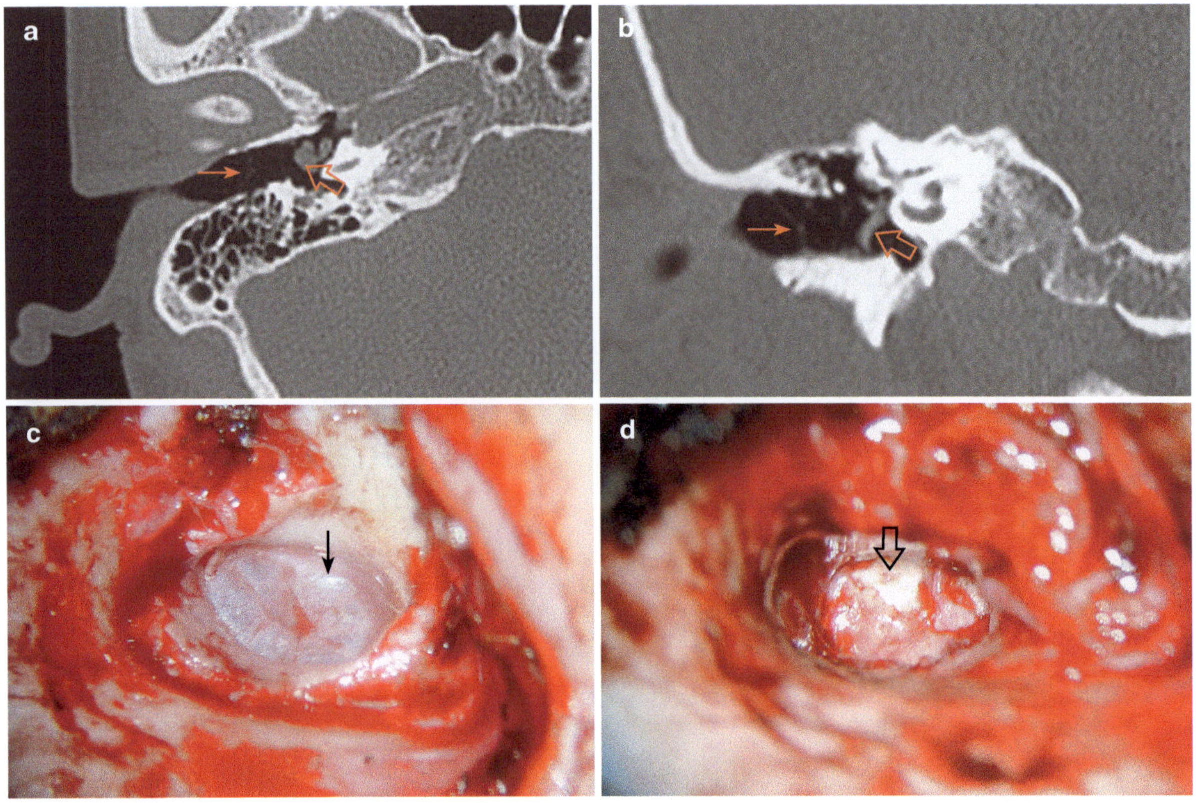

Fig. 5.54 Membranous atresia of external auditory canal and cholesteatoma formation in tympanic cavity after tympanoplasty in right ear. (**a**) Axial CT; (**b**) Coronal CT; (**c**, **d**) Intraoperative finding. (**a**, **b**) Soft tissue shallow of membranous sealing (↑) could be seen in the middle segment of external auditory canal, strip shadow could also be seen in the tympanum (⇧); (**c**) Membranous tissue (↑) in middle segment of external auditory canal; (**d**) When membranous sealing tissue removed, white epithelial mass was found in tympanum (⇧)

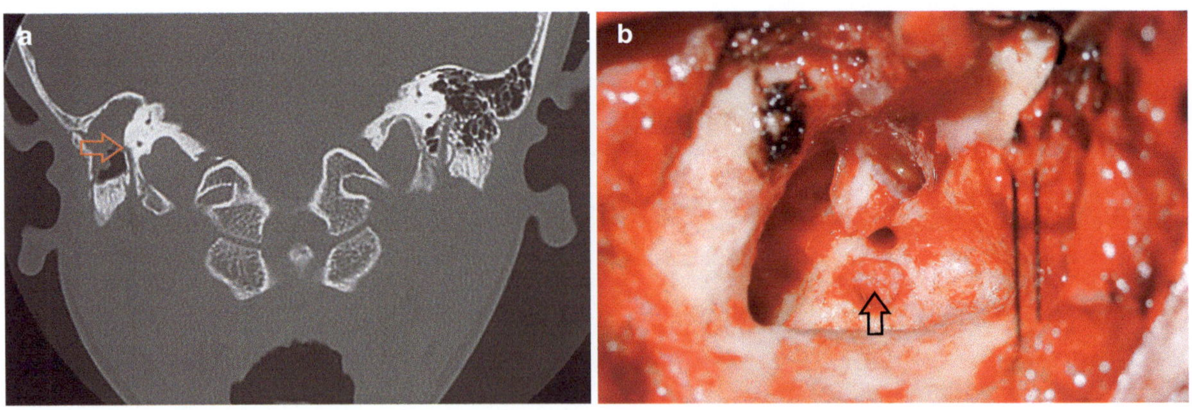

Fig. 5.55 Postoperative recurrence of cholesteatoma in right ear. (**a**) Coronal CT; (**b**) Intraoperative finding. (**a**) Bony absence of second genu (⇧) of facial nerve canal; (**b**) Granulation tissue formation at exposure site of facial nerve canal (⇧)

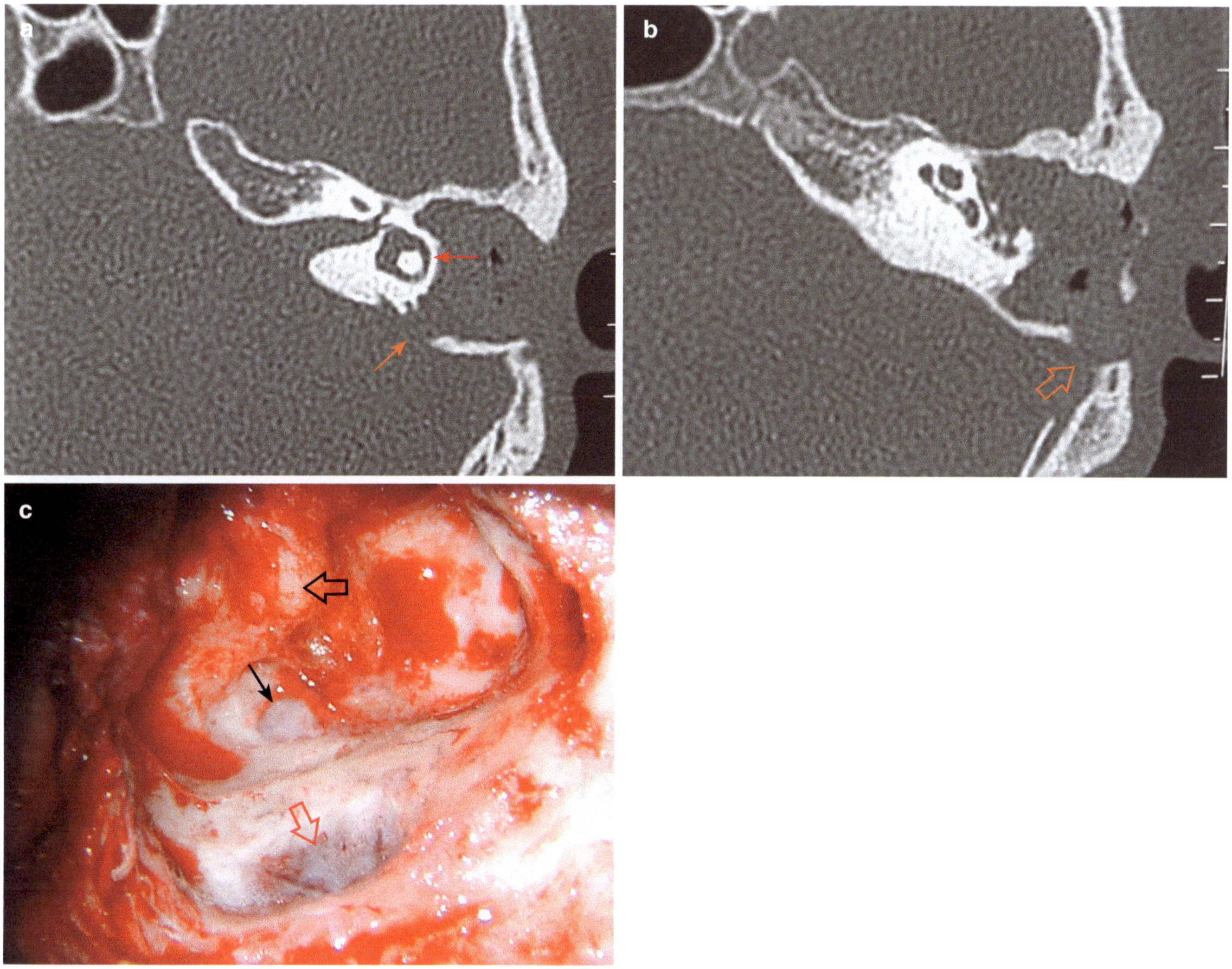

Fig. 5.56 Postoperative recurrence of cholesteatoma and exposure of sigmoid sinus and endolymphatic sac in left ear. (**a**, **b**) Axial CT; (**c**) Intraoperative finding. (**a**) Exposure of endolymphatic sac (↑), external semicircular canal (↑); (**b**) Exposure of sigmoid sinus (⇧); (**c**) Exposure of endolymphatic sac (↑) and sigmoid sinus (⇧), lateral semicircular canal (⇧)

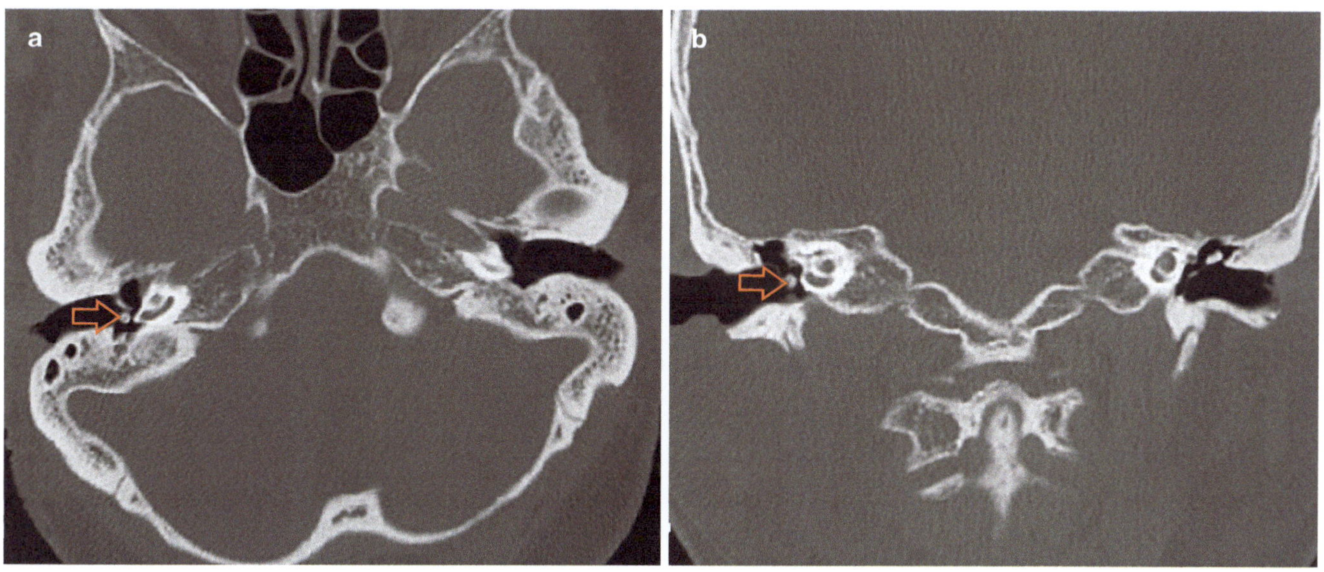

Fig. 5.57 Postoperative imaging of tympanoplasty in right ear. (**a**) Axial CT; (**b**) Coronal CT. Trimmed malleus head was used as artificial ossicles (⇧)

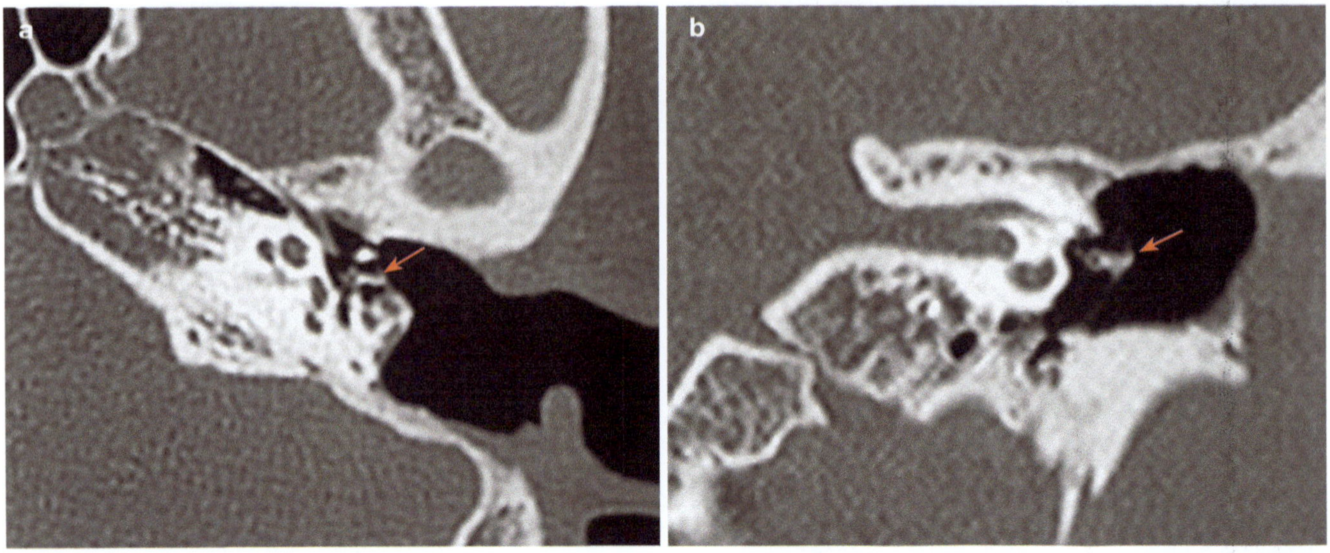

Fig. 5.58 Tympanoplasty and mastoidectomy with canal wall down in left ear. Artificial ossicles (↑) scanned showed by CT showed no displacement and no absorption 6 years after operation.

Note: Autogenous mastoid bone cortex was used to make partial ossicles replacement of prothesis, which remains one of the best available materials for ossiculoplasty (Yu et al. 2014)

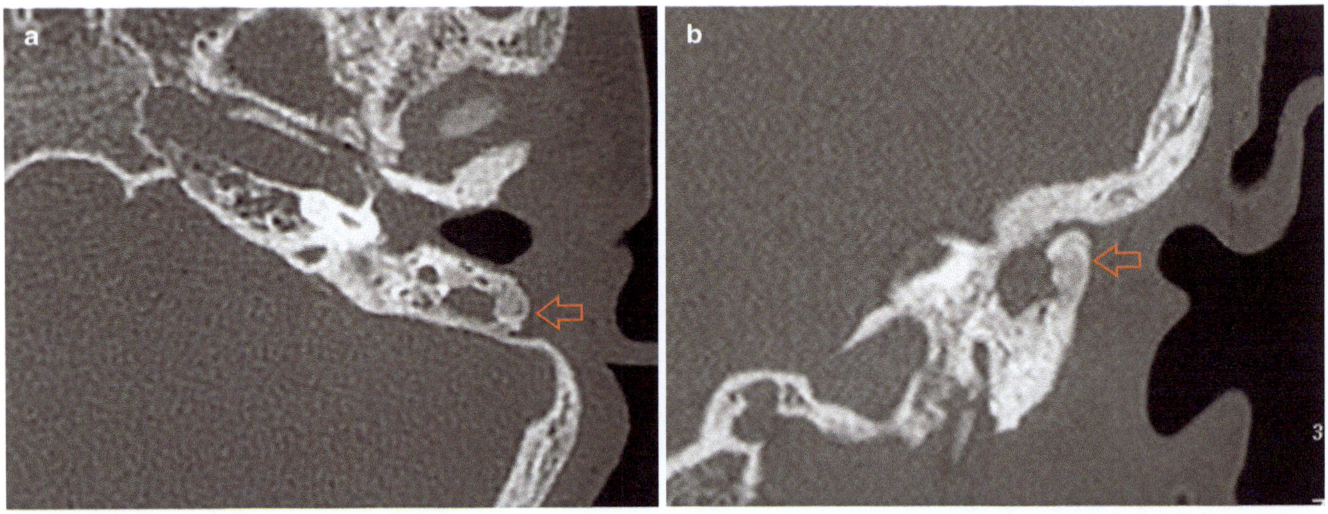

Fig. 5.59 Hyperosteogeny after mastoidectomy with canal wall down in left ear. (**a**) Axial CT; (**b**) Coronal CT. Hyperosteogeny could be seen in mastoid cavity (⇧)

5.4 Otogenic Complications

The inflammation of the middle ear and mastoid can spread to extra- and intra-crania through the natural channels or fissure of temporal bone or through destructive bone, occasionally can reach the distant organs through blood circulation, causing infection. When intra-cranial infection occurs, mild cases have local dural thickening, severe cases include meningitis, brain abscess, thrombophlebitis of sigmoid sinus and peripheral abscess, even threatening life. Extra-cranial infection includes the labyrinthitis, facial paralysis, sensorineural hearing loss, vertigo, lateral abscess of temporal bone, osteomyelitis of temporal bone, postauricular subperiosteal abscess, deep neck abscess, even distant organs complications such as lung abscess and mediastinal abscess. In case of existing or suspected intracranial and extracranial complications, enhanced temporal bone MRI (or soft tissue window brain CT) should be performed in time to make a clear diagnosis and understand the scope of the lesion. The bony cortex destruction of the sigmoid sulcus, tegmen of tympanum or tympanic antrum and so on, can provide an important reminder in the diagnosis of otogenic intracranial and extracranial complications.

Bony anatomy and structures surrounded by air are best evaluated by CT, but MR is preferred for soft tissue assessment.

5.4.1 Otogenic Extracranial Complications

See Figs. 5.60, 5.61, and 5.62.

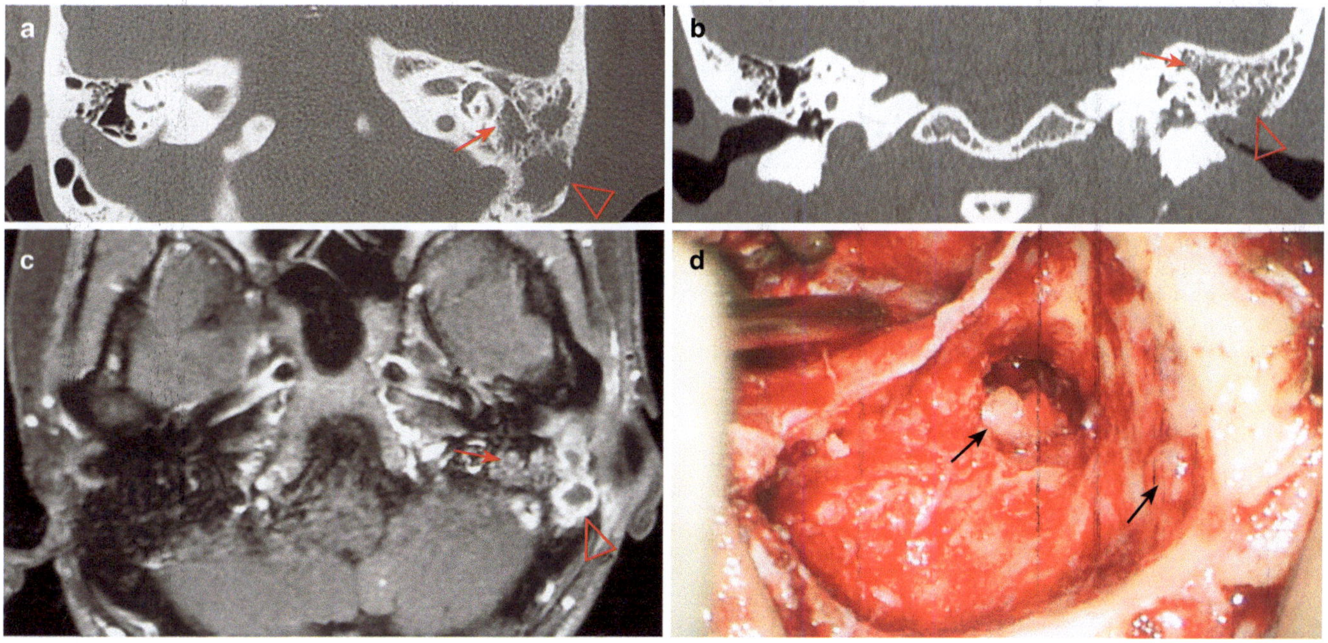

Fig. 5.60 Masked mastoiditis with postauricular periostitis in left ear. (**a**) Axial CT; (**b**) Coronal CT; (**c**) Axial MRI T_1WI postgadolinium; (**d**) Intraoperative finding. (**a, b**) Pneumatic mastoid in left ear, inflammatory obstructive change of mastoid cavity (↑), destruction of mastoid bone cortex (Δ); (**c**) Enhanced soft tissue shadow with hyperintense signal at the margin and hypointense signal at the center of mastoid cavity empyema (Δ), and slightly hyperintense signal at the mastoid cavity(inflammation) (↑). After anti-inflammatory treatment, the postauricular swelling was reduced (compared with CT), (**d**) Granulation (↑), mucosa edema of mastoid cavity

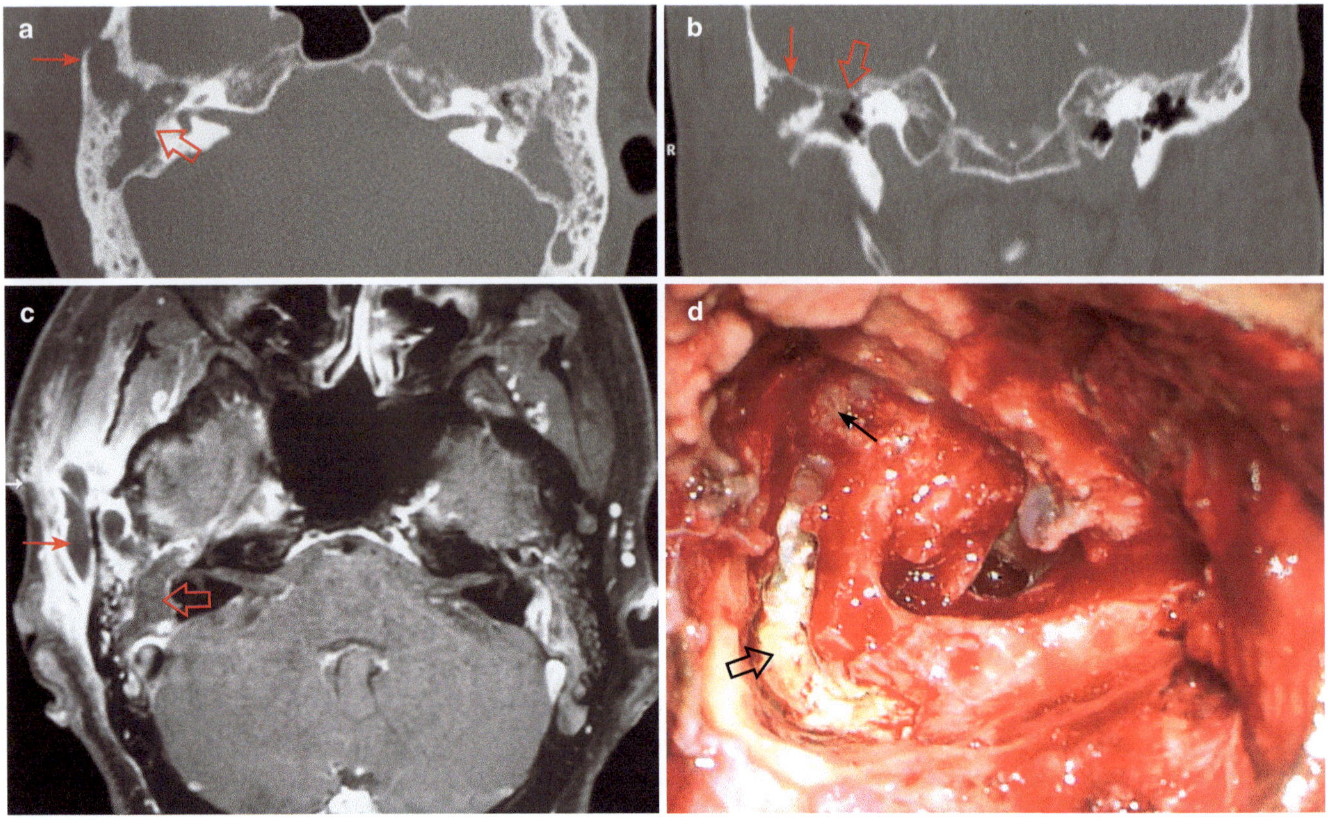

Fig. 5.61 Right tympanomastoid cholesteatoma with abscess of squamous portion of temporal bone. (**a**) Axial CT; (**b**) Coronal CT; (**c**) Axial MRI T_1WI postgadolinium; (**d**) Intraoperative finding. (**a, b**). Diploetic mastoid of right ear, soft tissue shadow (⇧) in tympanomastoid with bone erosion (↑) in squamous portion of temporal bone; (**c**) MRI T_1 WI enhancement showed hyperintense signal shadow in squamous portion of temporal bone and central hypointense signal shadow indicated local abscess formation (↑), and mastoid cavity (⇧) showed hyperintense signal shadow in the periphery and hypointense signal shadow in the center indicated cholesteatoma forms (⇧); (**d**) Granulation (↑) and abscess on squamous portion of temporal bone scale, and cholesteatoma (⇧) in mastoid cavity

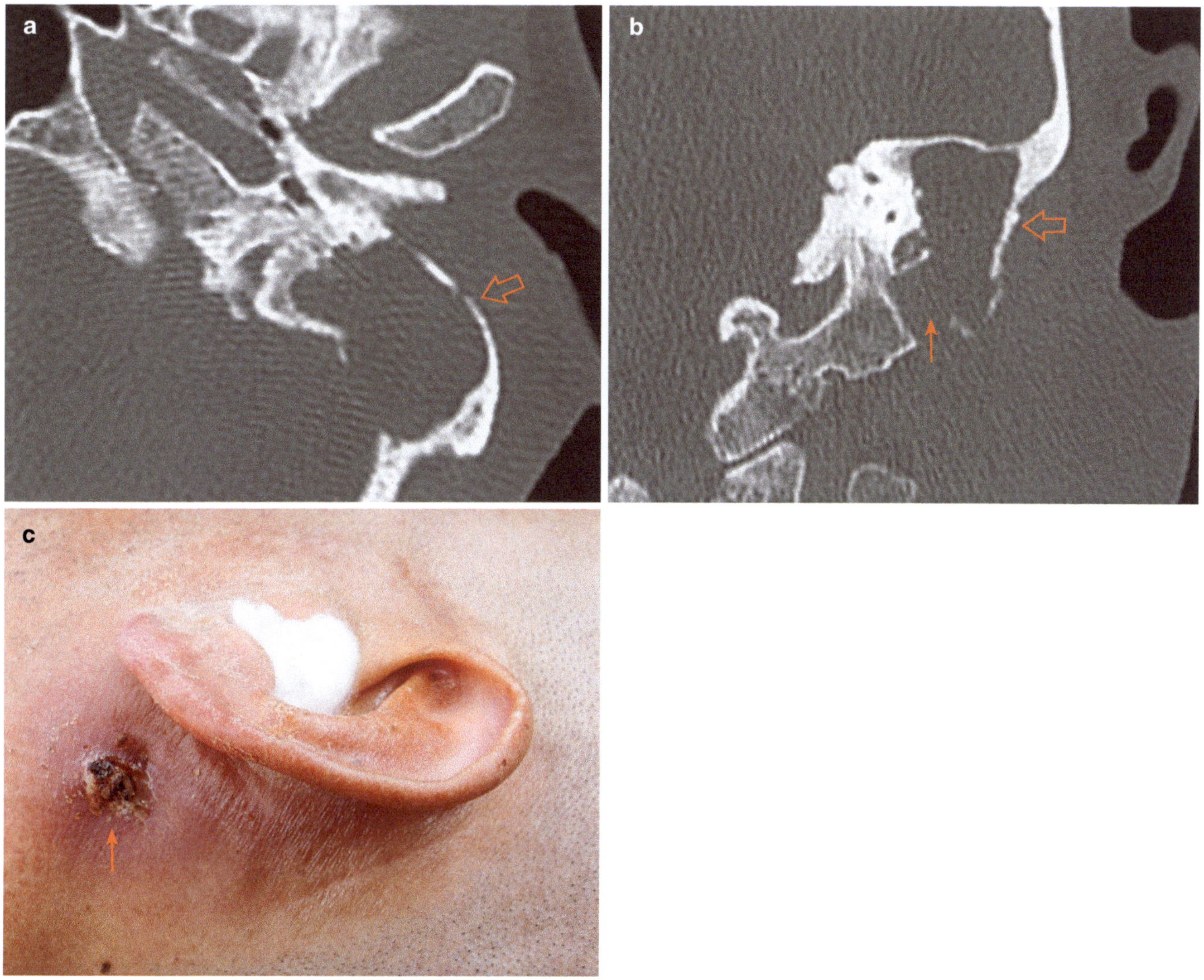

Fig. 5.62 Tympanomastoid cholesteatoma in left ear with Bezold abscess. (**a**) Axial CT; (**b**) Coronal CT; (**c**) Intraoperative finding. (**a**, **b**). Left sclerotic mastoid, soft tissue shadow in mastoid process, lateral bone cortex still intact (⇧), bone destruction in digastric groove (↑); (**c**) Skin rupture under mastoid tip of left ear, fistula formation (↑), no obvious postauricular swelling

5.4.2 Intracranial and Neck Complications

See Figs. 5.63, 5.64, 5.65, 5.66, 5.67, 5.68, and 5.69.

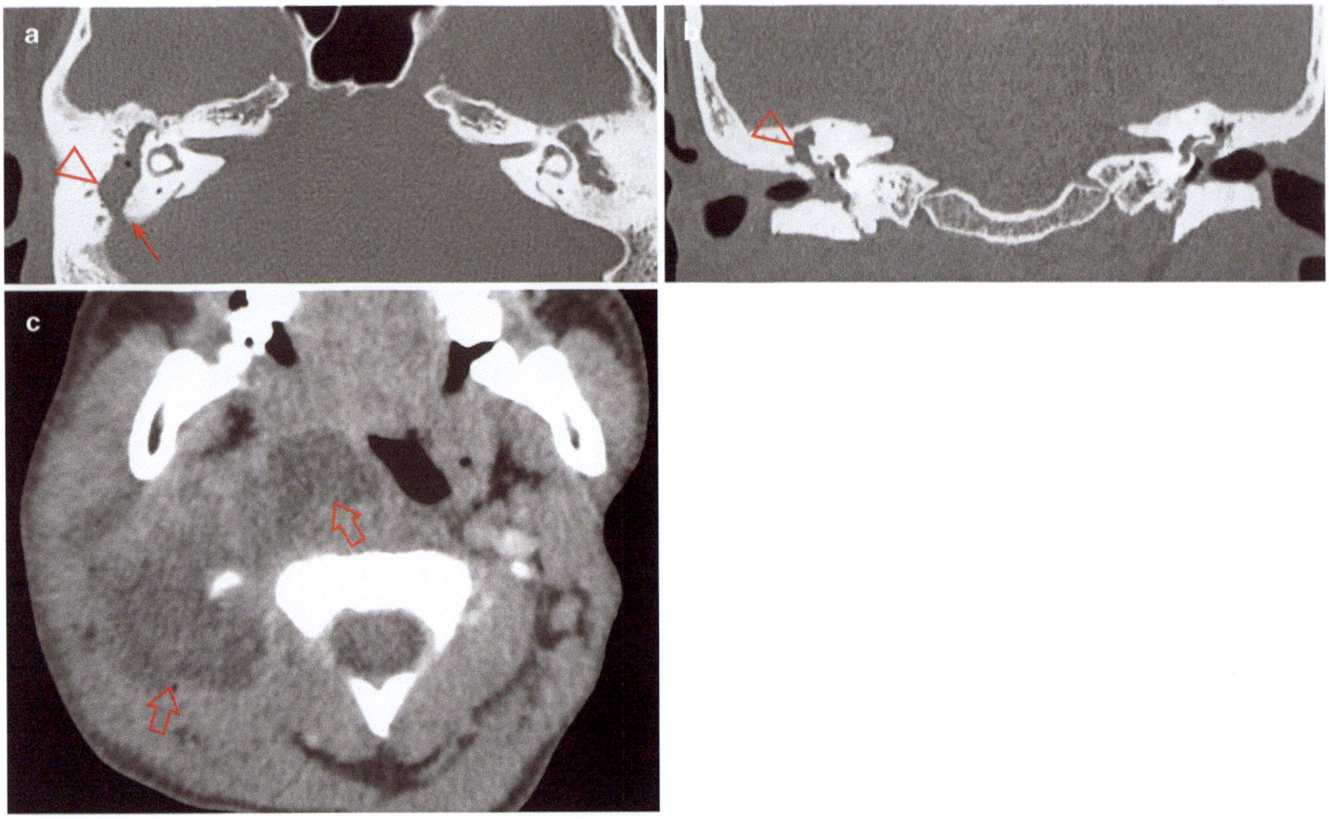

Fig. 5.63 Tympanomastoid cholesteatoma with sigmoid sinus thrombophlebitis accompanying deep neck abscess in left ear. (**a**) Axial CT; (**b**) Coronal CT; (**c**). Neck CT. Right sclerotic mastoid, tympanomastoid soft tissue shadow (▲), and ossicular erosion, bone loss of sigmoid sulcus (↑), low density shadow on neck CT (⇧)

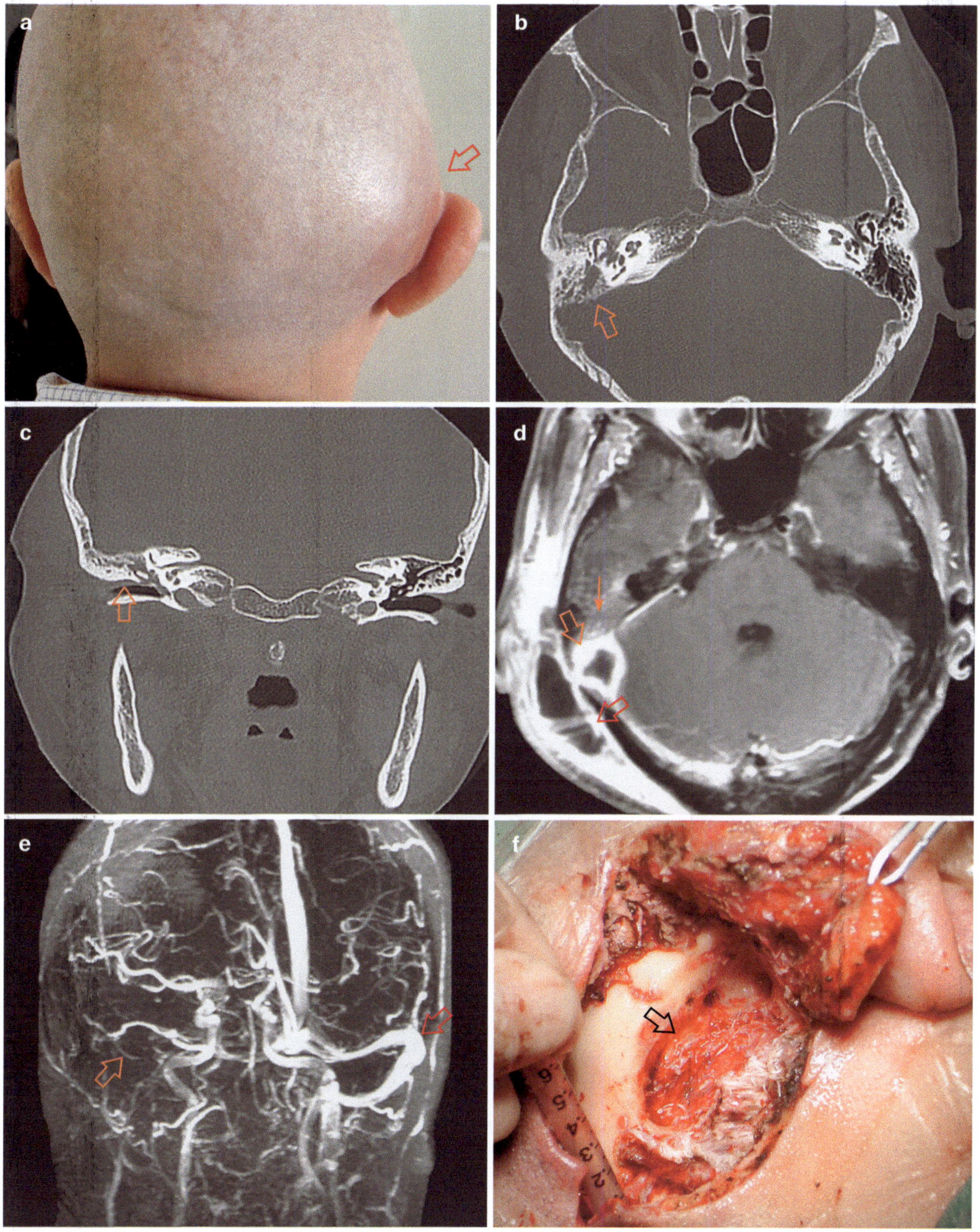

Fig. 5.64 Masked otitis media and mastoiditis in right ear with sigmoid sinus thrombophlebitis and postauricular subperiosteal abscess. (**a**) Axial CT; (**b**) Coronal CT; (**c**) Neck CT; (**d**) Axial MRI T1WI postgadolinium; (**e**) Coronal MRV. (**a**) Right pneumatic mastoid, there was obvious inflammatory swelling at posterosuperior area (⇧) of right ear before operation; (**b**, **c**). Right Mastoid process presented acute inflammatory changes and sigmoid sinus osteoporotic (⇧), soft tissue swelling of upper wall (⇧) of external auditory canal; (**d**) MRI T_1 WI enhancement scan: middle ear mastoid process (↑) showed slightly hyperintense signal shadow, abnormal hyperintense signal edge of ipsilateral sigmoid sinus, hypointense signal shadow in center of sigmoid sinus(pus cavity) (⇧), postauricular soft tissue (⇧) swelling and hypointense signal shadow in center and peripheral enhanced signal shadow (pus cavity); (**e**) MRV showed the filling absence of right sigmoid sinus (⇧), left sigmoid sinus was clearly displayed (⇧); (**f**) Wall of sigmoid sinus (⇧) was thickened and showed inflammatory granulomatous changes.

Note: This female patient had been ipsilateral headache and repeated fever for more than 1 month, without history of ear discharge, right tympanic membrane was congested, thickened and intact during physical examination

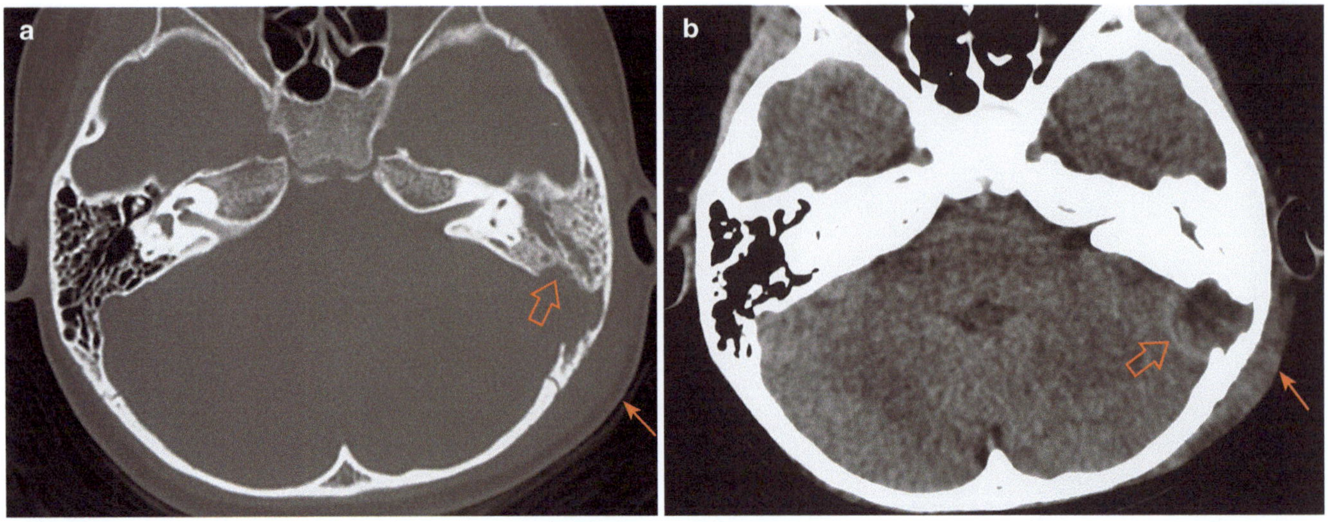

Fig. 5.65 Left chronic suppurative otitis media with peri-sigmoid abscess and postauricular subperiosteal abscess. (**a**) Axial CT; (**b**) Brain CT. (**a**) Diploetic mastoid of left ear, mastoid cavity presented inflammatory obstructive change, bone erosion of sigmoid sulcus (⇧), postauricular soft tissue swelling (↑); (**b**) Low density shadow with clear boundary of sigmoid sinus area (⇧), postauricular soft tissue swelling (↑)

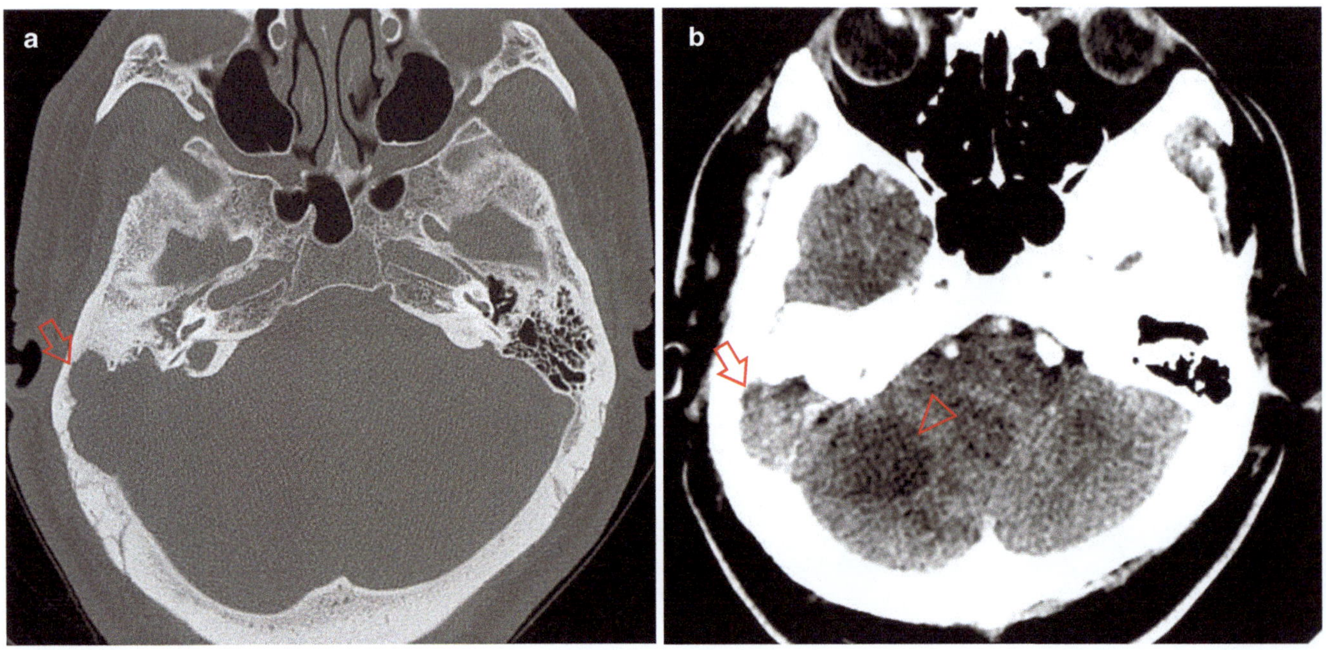

Fig. 5.66 Right mastoid cholesteatoma with brain abscess. (**a**) Axial CT; (**b**) Brain CT. Sclerotic mastoid of right ear, erosion of the bone cortex of sigmoid groove (⇧), low density shadow of cerebellum (abscess formation) (△)

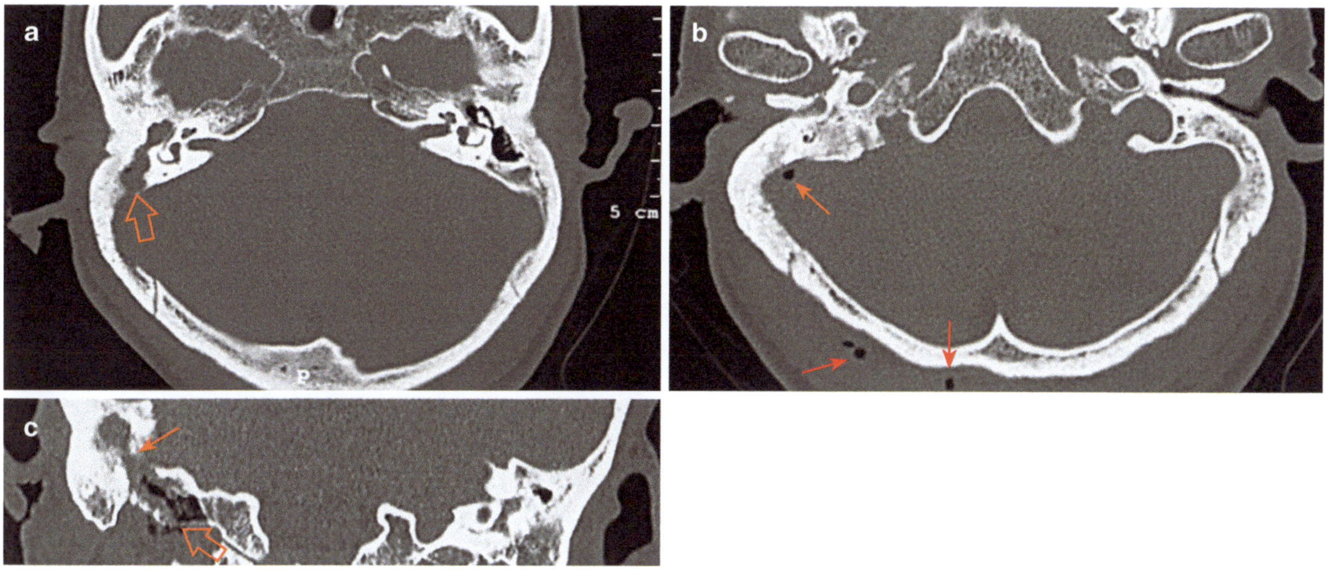

Fig. 5.67 Right middle ear and mastoid cholesteatoma with perisigmoiditis and occipital abscess. (**a**, **b**). Axial CT; (**c**) Coronal CT. (**a**) Sclerotic mastoid of right ear, middle ear and mastoid were full of soft tissue shadow, ossicles disappeared, bone wall of sigmoid sinus groove was destroyed (⇧); (**b**) Right sigmoid sinus contained air (↑), extracranial occipital and nuchal soft tissue has multiple air-containing cavities (↑), local swelling; (**c**) Right mastoid medial wall (↑), occipital bone erosion (⇧), local air-containing cavity communicating with extracranial tissue

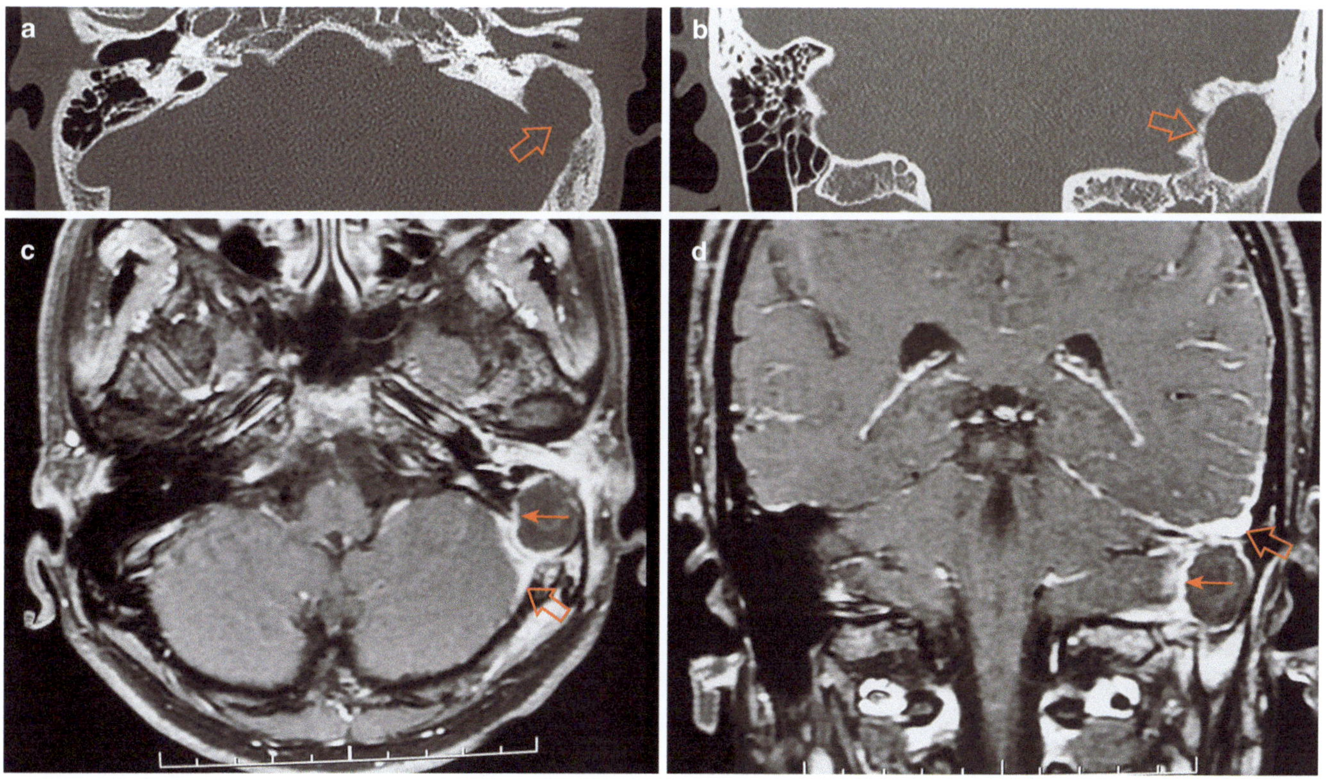

Fig. 5.68 Cholesteatoma in middle ear and mastoid process of left ear with localized meningitis. (**a**) Axial CT; (**b**) Coronal CT; (**c**) Axial MRI T1WI postgadolinium; (**d**) Coronal MRI T1WI postgadolinium. (**a**) and (**b**) Sclerotic mastoid of left ear, low density shadow (⇧) with smooth edge in mastoid process, bone erosion in sigmoid sinus groove; (**c**, **d**) Enhancement MRI T1 WI, edge hyperintense signal shadow in mastoid cavity of left ear (↑), adjacent meninges enhancement (⇧)

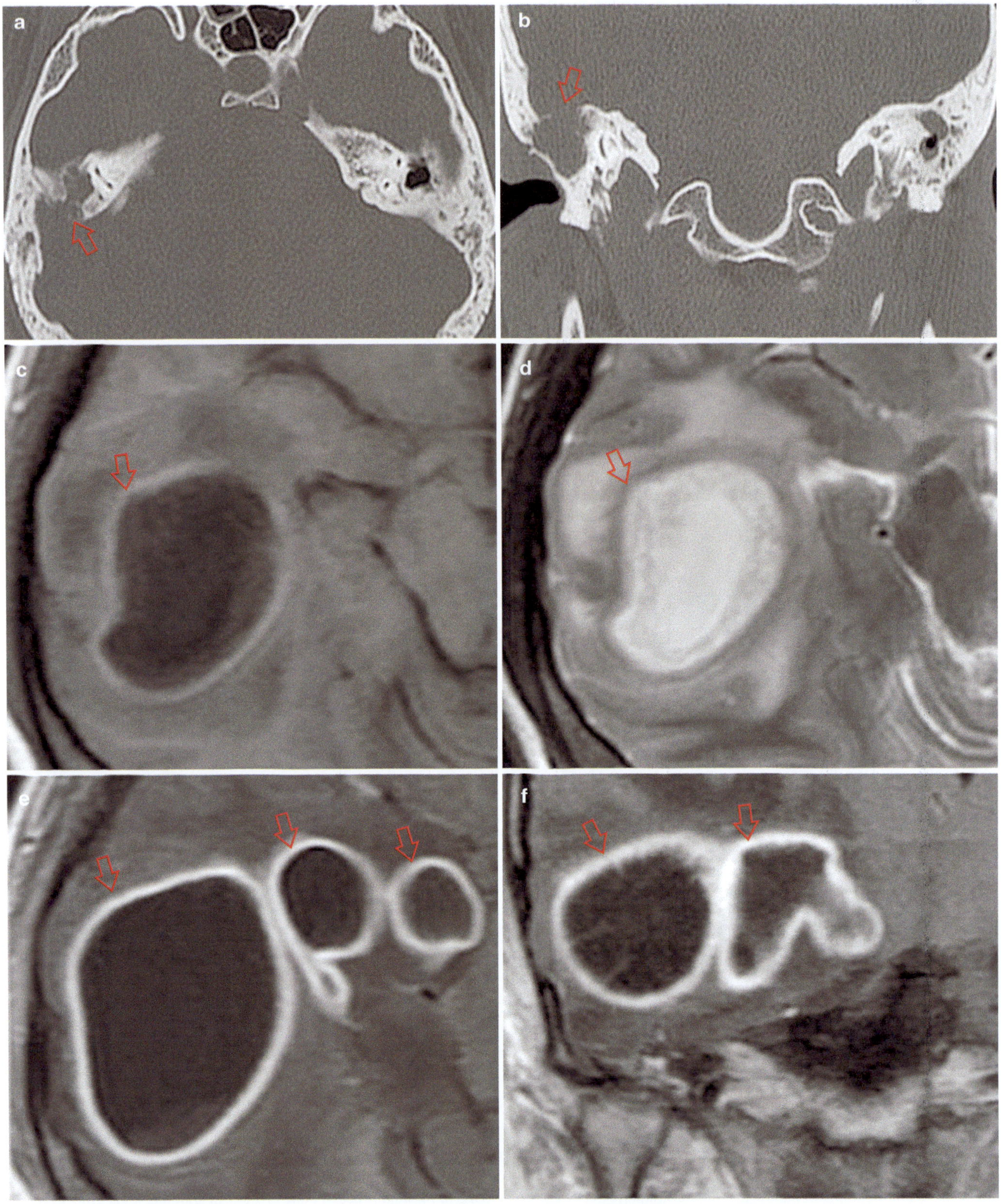

Fig. 5.69 Right middle ear mastoid cholesteatoma with brain abscess. (**a**) Axial CT; (**b**) Coronal CT; (**c**) Axial MRI T1WI; (**d**) Axial MRI T2 WI; (**e**) Axial MRI T1WI postgadolinium; (**f**) Coronal MRI T1WI postgadolinium. (**a, b**). Diploid mastoid of right ear with soft tissue shadow of upper tympanum and mastoid, and bone erosion of middle cranial fossa (⇧); (**c**) Pebble-shaped peripheral slightly hyperintense signal, central hypointense signal shadow (⇧); (**d**) Pebble-shaped hyperintense signal shadow (⇧); (**e, f**). Multiple (or lobulated) pebble-shaped peripheral strong signal and central hypointense signal shadows (⇧) in ipsilateral temporal lobe of brain tissue.

Note: A 45-year-old male with intermittent ear discharge in his right ear for many years, fever and headache for 1 week.

Note: Bone erosion or osteoporosis (osteomyelitis) in sigmoid groove and middle cranial fossa from Fig. 5.69 suggest the possibility of intracranial complications, and further examinations (including brain CT, temporal bone MRI, etc.) are needed to clarify the diagnosis

5.5 Specific Inflammation of Ear

Temporal bone specific inflammation is relatively rare, it is often accompanied by similar diseases in other parts of the human body or the manifestations of similar diseases in the ear (Fig. 5.70).

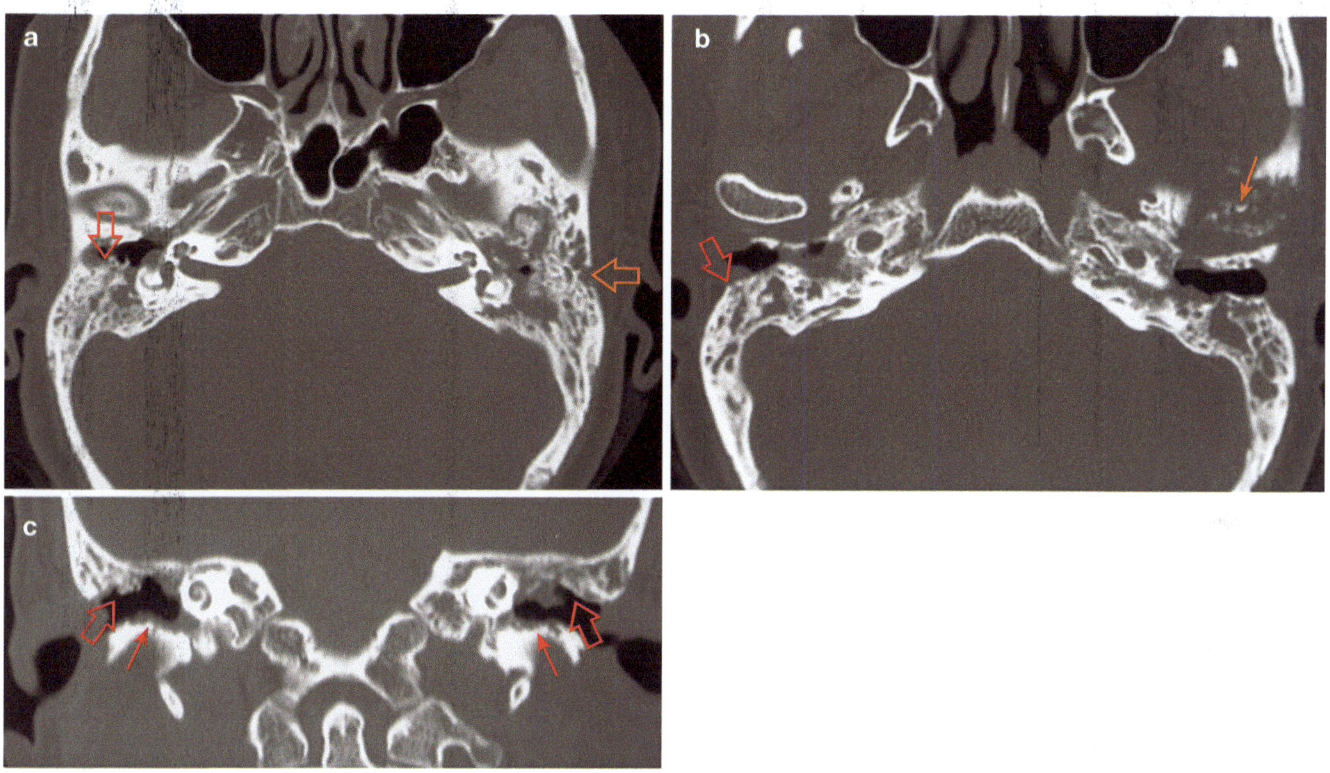

Fig. 5.70 Bilateral tuberculous otitis media. (**a**, **b**) Axial CT; (**c**) Coronal CT. Bilateral pneumatic mastoid showed soft tissue shadow in tympanic cavity and mastoid process, erosion of squamous portion of temporal bone (⇧), worm-bitten change of posterior (⇧), superior (⇧), and inferior (↑) wall of external auditory canal; condyle was also destroyed and absorbed (↑). Ossicle had disappeared

6 Tumor-Like Lesions and Tumors of Ear

Zilong Yu, Shubin Chen, Jie Wang, Shusheng Gong, and Bentao Yang

Although temporal bone tumors only account for a small part of the tumors in the whole body, imaging examination is one of the important means for their diagnosis because of their concealment location. This section will describe the imaging features of the tumors occurring in the temporal bone and some of them affiliated intraoperative findings.

6.1 Ear Granuloma

See Figs. 6.1, 6.2, 6.3, and 6.4.

Z. Yu (✉) · S. Chen · J. Wang
Department of Otolaryngology Head and Neck Surgery, Beijing Tongren Hospital, Capital Medical University, Beijing, China

S. Gong
Department of Otolaryngology Head and Neck Surgery, Beijing Friendship Hospital, Capital Medical University, Beijing, China

B. Yang
Department of Radiology, Beijing Tongren Hospital, Capital Medical University, Beijing, China

Z. Yu (ed.), *Ear Diseases and CT*, https://doi.org/10.1007/978-981-99-7220-3_6

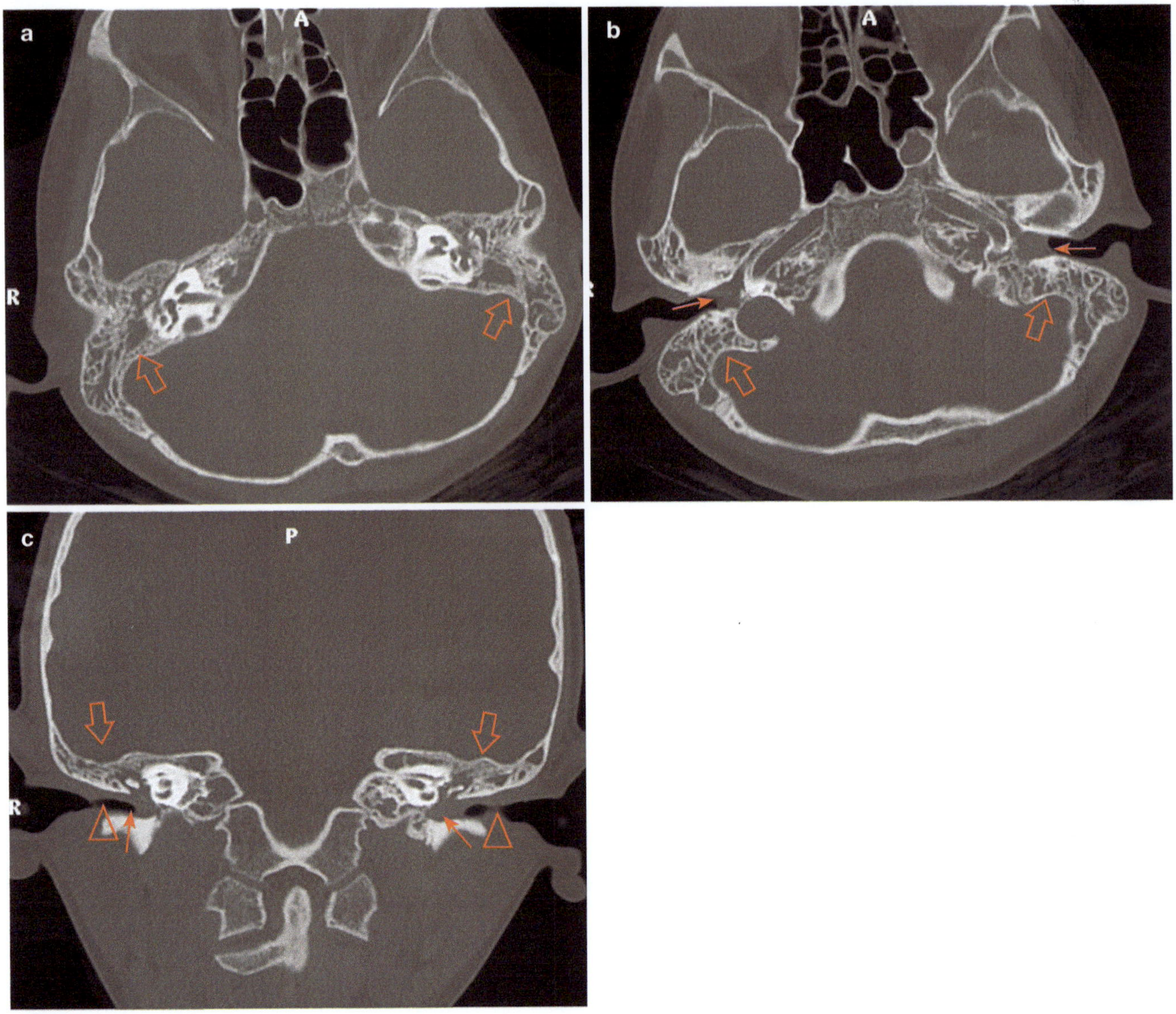

Fig. 6.1 Wegner's granuloma. (**a**, **b**). Axial CT; (**c**) Coronal CT. Female, 13 years old. Bilateral middle ear and mastoid were full of soft tissue shadow (⇧); tympanic membrane (↑) and superior wall soft tissue (△) of external auditory canal were swelling without obvious bone destruction.

Note: Wegener's granuloma, also known as granulomatous vasculitis, is a necrotizing granulomatous vasculitis, an autoimmune disease that mainly affects the upper and lower respiratory tracts and kidneys, and can also affect the ear. The mortality is high and relapses are a major cause of mortality and morbidity (Schilder 2010)

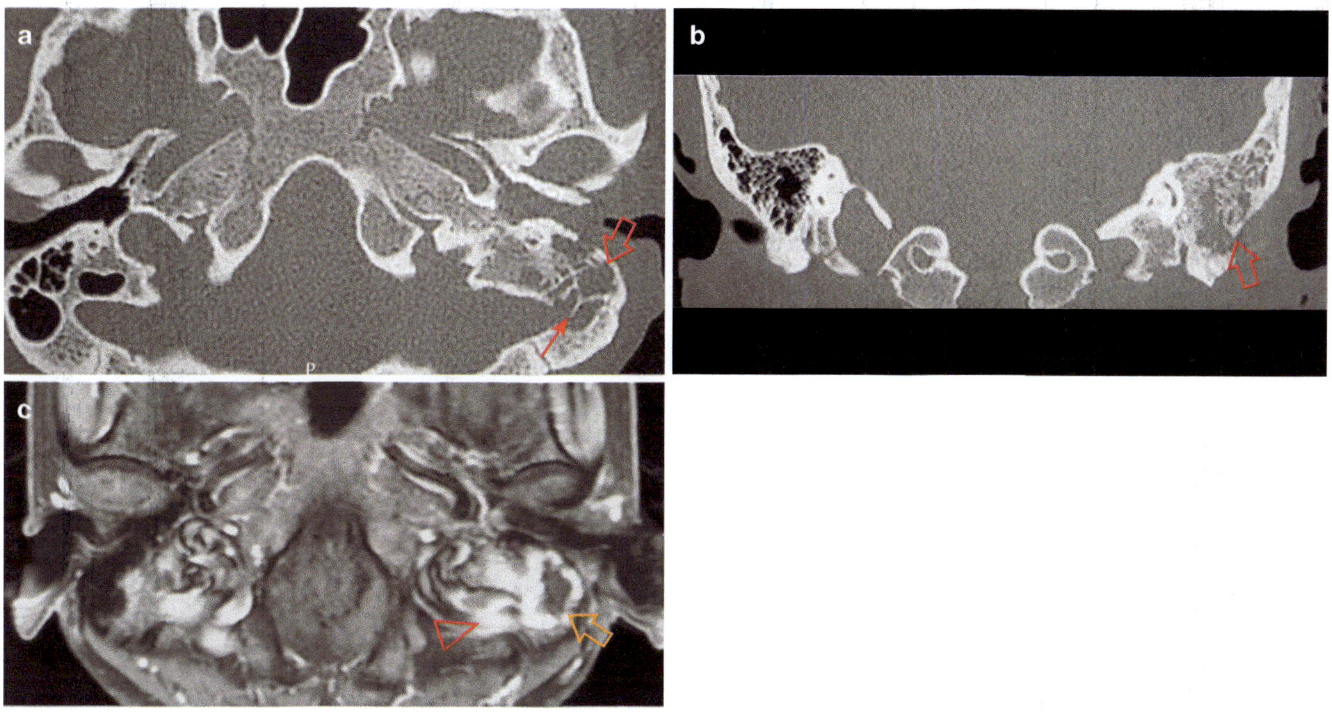

Fig. 6.2 Wegener granuloma of left ear. (**a**) Axial CT; (**b**) Coronal CT; (**c**) Axial MRI T_1MI postgadolinium. Female, 26 years old. (**a**, **b**) Mastoid bone cortex destruction (⇧), soft tissue shadow (↑) in mastoid process; (**c**) MRI T_1 WI enhancement sigmoid sinus wall hyperintense signal (△); central hypointense signal shadow with surrounding hyperintense signal in mastoid cavity (⇧)

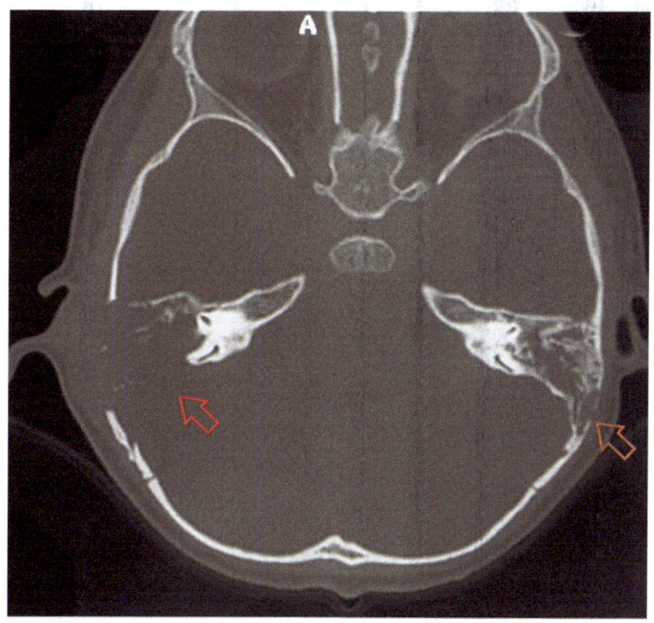

Fig. 6.3 Langerhans cell histiocytosis of temporal bone. Axial CT. Three years old boy. Horizontal CT shows the destruction and absorption of bone in bilateral temporal bone (right, ⇧; and left, ⇧), swelling of temporal soft tissue.

Note: The etiology of Langerhans cell histiocytosis, the most common histiocytic disorder, is still unclear, characterized by aberrant function and differentiation or proliferation of cells of the mononuclear phagocyte system, it has certain familial and tumor nature. The diagnosis is based on clinical, imaging, and pathological examination. The clinical manifestations are diverse and can involve multiple systems and organs, and have a particular affinity for bone, skin, the lungs, and the pituitary (Allen et al. 2018). The main manifestation of bone lesions is irregular osteolytic lesions at the edge, with skull lesions being the most common. The ear can show the swelling of the external auditory canal and postauricular soft tissue. The main symptom is ear discharge, soft tissue swelling, and conductive hearing loss. CT scan can show bone and soft tissue lesions.

The annual incidence of Langerhans cell histiocytosis has been reported to be 4.6 cases per one million children under 15 years of age, with a male-to-female ratio of 1.2:1 (Guyot-Goubin et al. 2008)

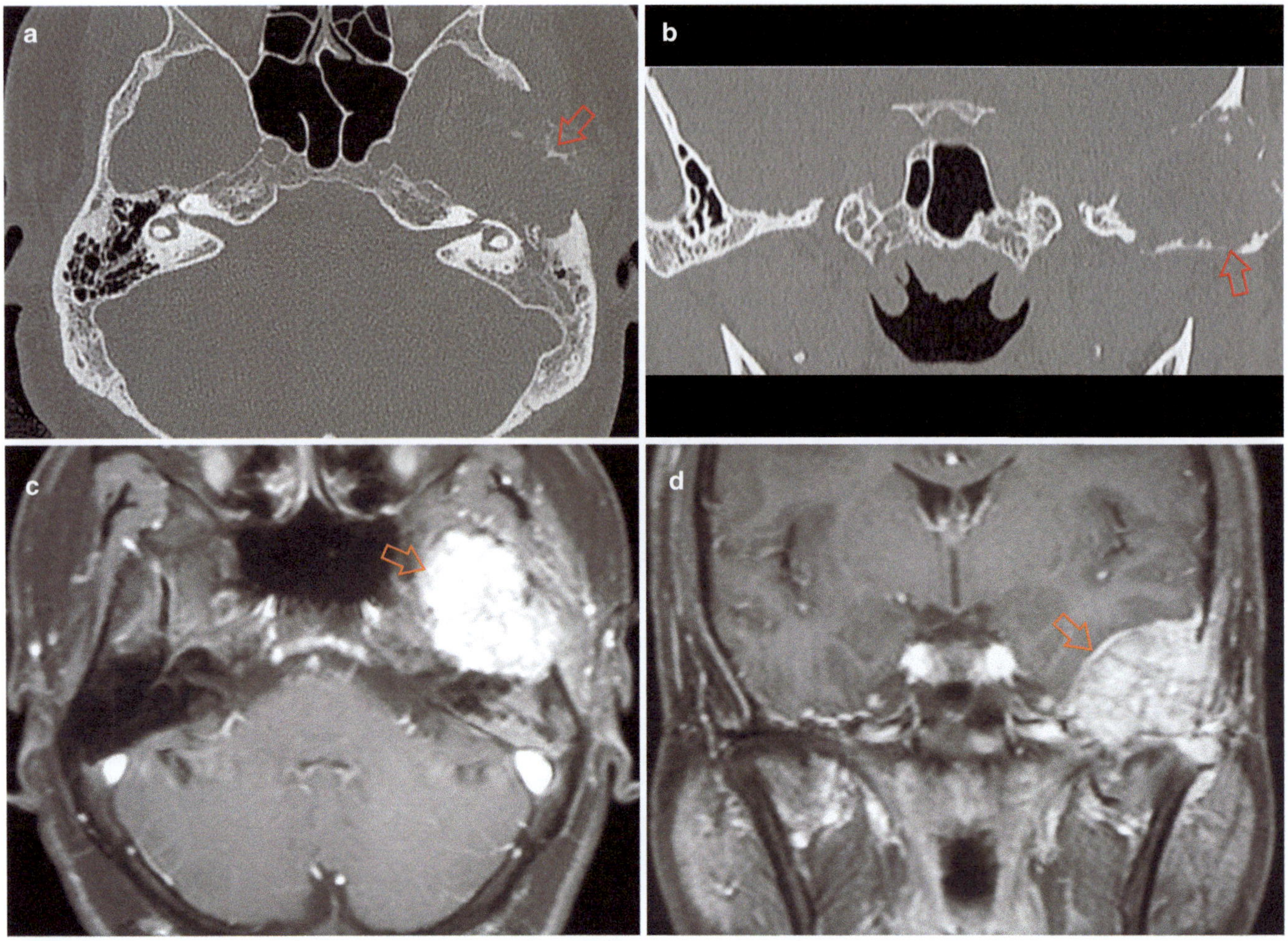

Fig. 6.4 Giant cell repair granuloma of left temporal bone. (**a**) Axial CT; (**b**) Coronal CT; (**c**) Axial MRI T_1MI postgadolinium; (**d**) Coronal MRI T_1MI postgadolinium. Male, 29 years old. (**a**, **b**) Squamous of portion of left temporal bone presented expansive bone destruction and absorb (⇧), residual bone sclerosis; (**c**, **d**) Slight hyperintense patch signal shadow at the center of the mass (⇧), uneven surrounding enhancement signal with relative clear edge in coronal view (⇧).

Note: Giant cell repair granuloma is a rare non-neoplastic benign disease, which is a proliferative repair reaction caused by traumatic intraosseous hemorrhage, but has local invasion. Trauma and inflammation are risk factors for giant cell repair granuloma (Maerki et al. 2012). It mainly occurs in the skull, and its clinical manifestations are local swelling, pain or tenderness. The imaging manifestation is single room shadow with clear boundary, and the CT scan often shows honeycomb or soap bubble

6.2 Fibrous Dysplasia of Temporal Bone

See Figs. 6.5 and 6.6.

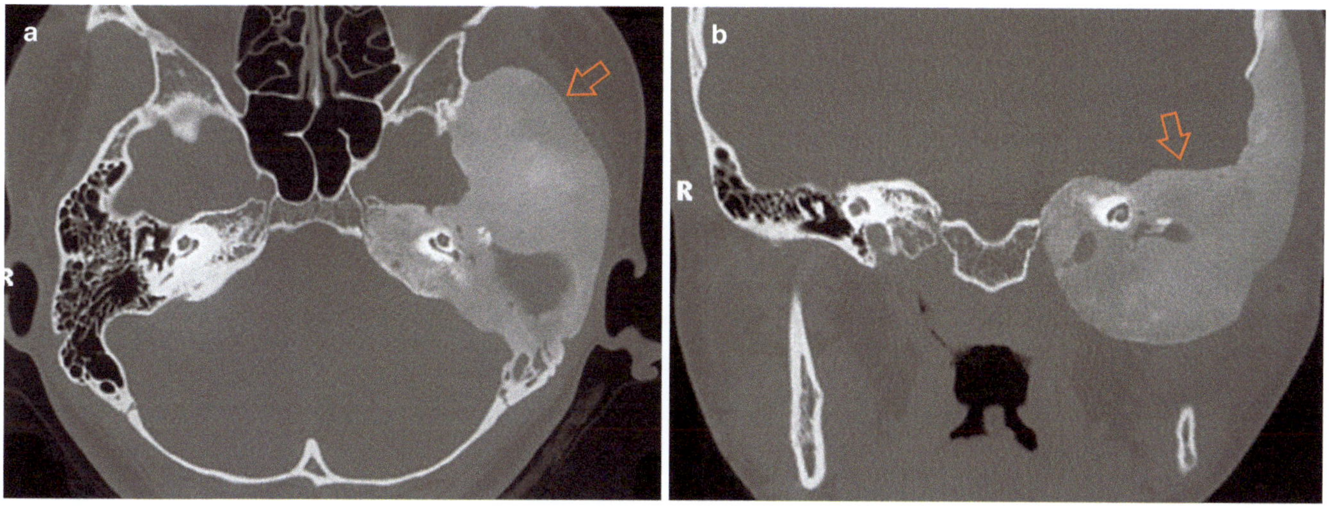

Fig. 6.5 Fibrous dysplasia of left temporal bone. (**a**) Axial CT; (**b**) Coronal CT. A 20-year-old female patient. CT shows fibrous hyperplasia (⇧) of bone with clear boundary of left temporal bone (frosted glass)

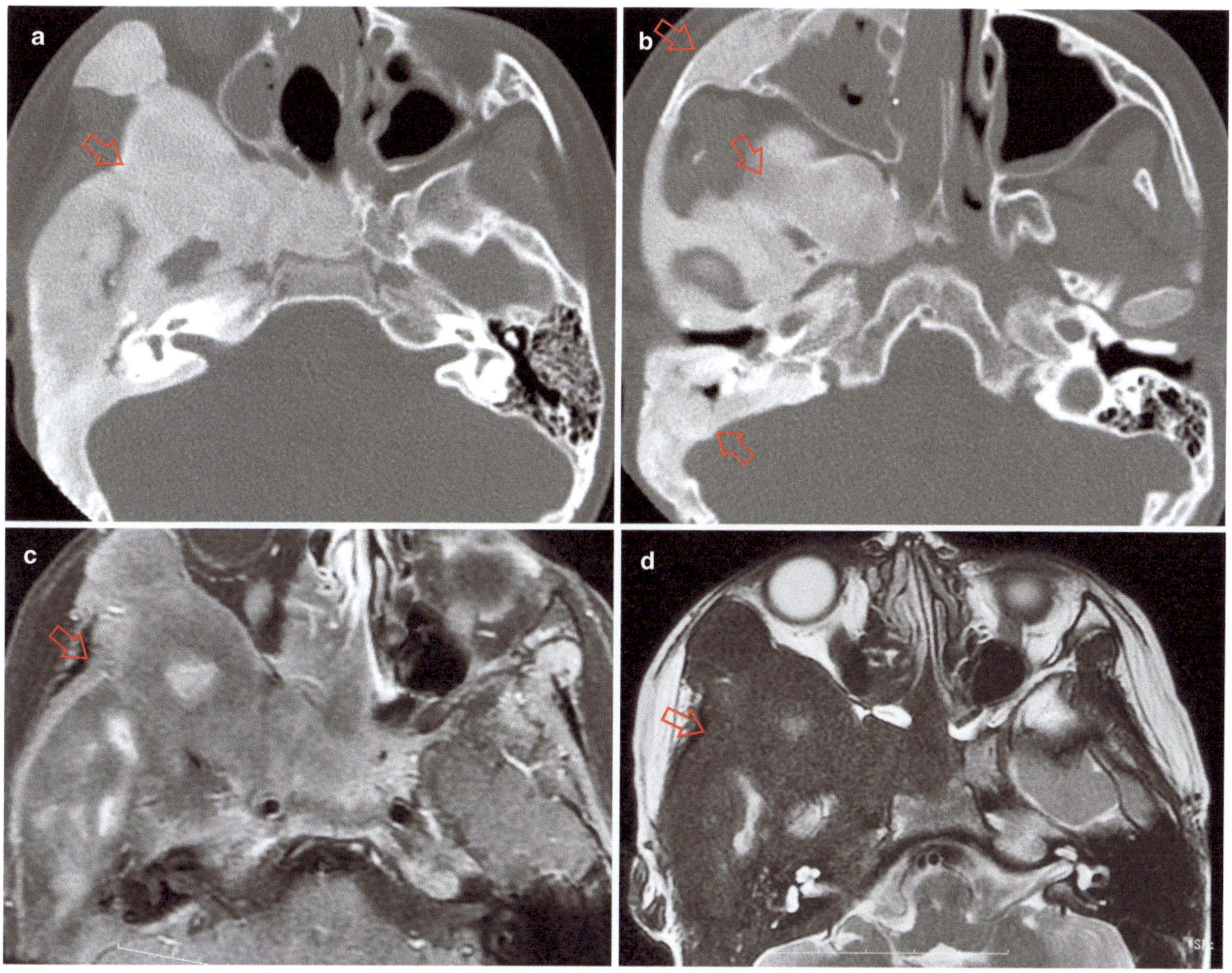

Fig. 6.6 Left cranial fibrous dysplasia. (**a**) Axial CT; (**b**) Coronal CT; (**c**) Axial MRI T_1 MI postgadolinium; (**d**). Axial MRI T_2 MI. Male, 6 years old. (**a**, **b**) Right skulls (temporal bone, sphenoid bone) proliferate, showing frosted glass (⇧); (**c**) MRI T_1 WI enhancement signal shadow showed uneven medium signal (⇧); (**d**) MRI T_2 WI showed hypointense signal shadow (⇧).

Note: Fibrous dysplasia of bone is a skeletal system disease characterized by fibrous deformation of bone. It is a developmental abnormality rather than a true tumor. It occurs in children and adolescents, and is more common in women. The disease develops slowly and can be divided into single bone type and multiple bone type

6.3 Benign Tumor of Temporal Bone

6.3.1 Osteofibroma of Temporal Bone

See Figs. 6.7 and 6.8.

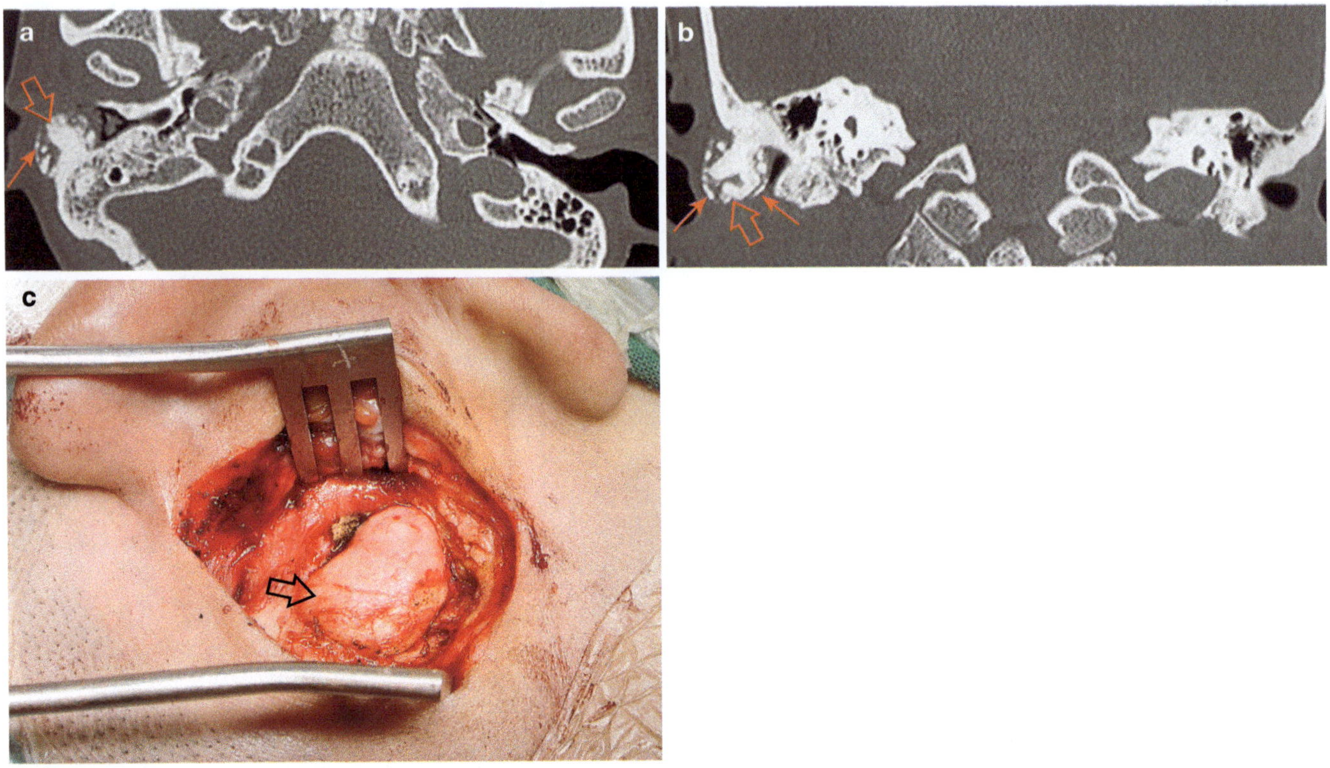

Fig. 6.7 Ossifying fibroma of right external auditory canal. (**a**) Axial CT; (**b**) Coronal CT; (**c**) Intraoperative finding**.** Female, 36 years old. (**a**, **b**) Mixed high-density irregular mass (⇧) at posteroinferior wall of right external auditory canal, covered incomplete bony capsule at the edge (↑); (**c**) Surface smooth irregular neo-mass on posteroinferior wall of external auditory canal (⇧), with clear boundary and broad base

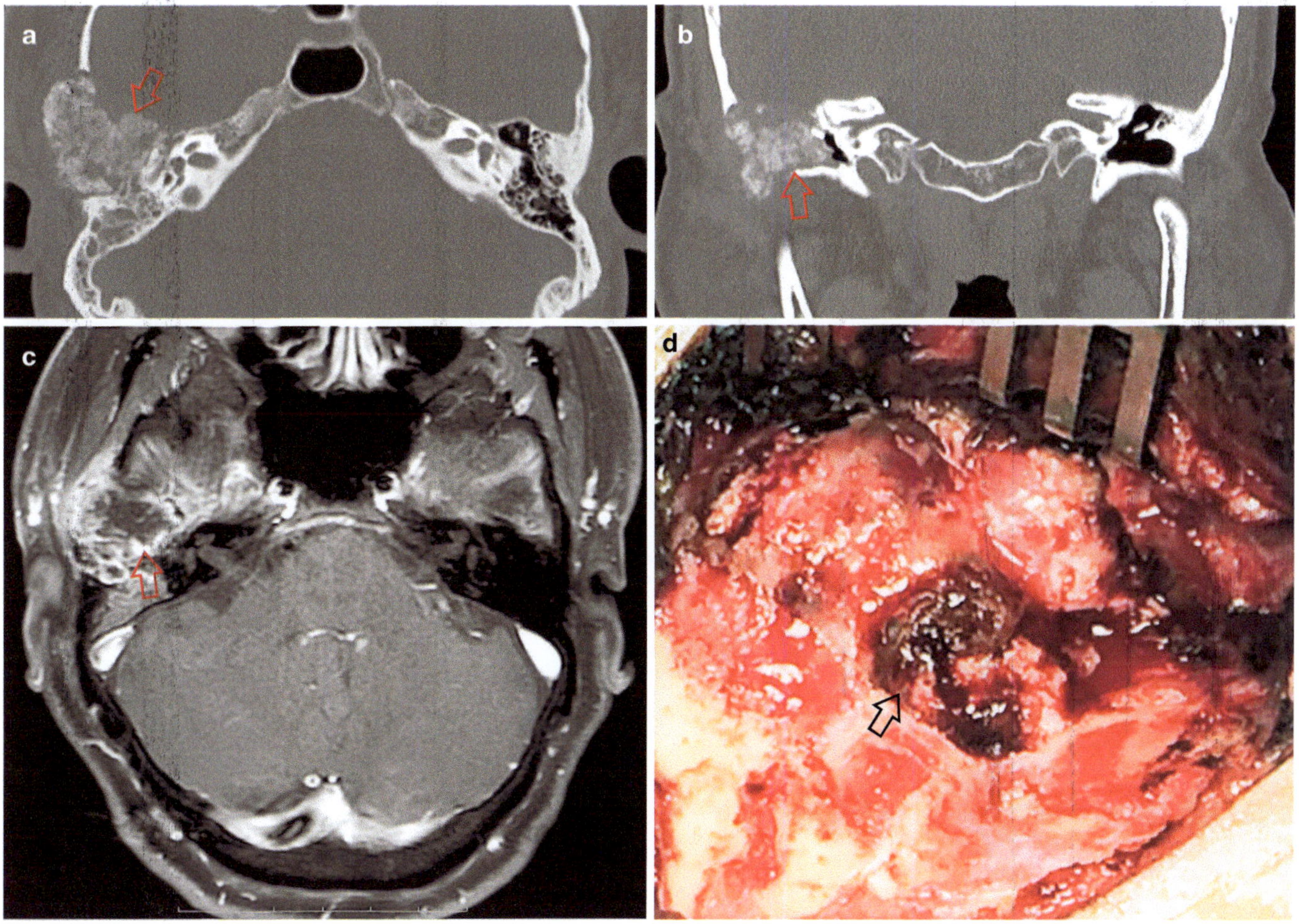

Fig. 6.8 Chondromyxoid Fibroma of Right Temporal Bone. (**a**) Axial CT; (**b**) Coronal CT; (**c**) Axial MRI T_1 MI postgadolinium; (**d**) Intraoperative finding. Male, 52 years old. (**a**, **b**) Squamous portion of temporal bone were replaced by fine granular, slightly high density and unevenly distributed cloud soft tissue shadow (⇧), with clear and scalpel like boundary, swelling of surrounding soft tissue, incomplete bone in middle cranial fossa, soft tissue shadow in the external auditory canal, complete bone canal of facial nerve in the tympanic segment; (**c**) After enhancement, tumor located at squamous portion of right temporal bone presented irregular soft tissue with uniformly enhanced and clear edge (⇧); (**d**) Tumor was bulbous, and the internal was yellow and white gravel, without obvious blood supply (⇧), the boundary was still clear.

Note: Chondromyxoid fibroma is a rare form of benign bone tumor and easily misdiagnosed as fibrosarcoma, comprising approximately 0.5% of primary bone tumors. It is common at osteoepiphysis end of long bone, and rarely occurs in the head and neck, especially in the temporal bone (LeMay et al. 1997; Tarhan et al. 2000)

6.3.2 Giant Cell Tumor of Temporal Bone

See Figs. 6.9.

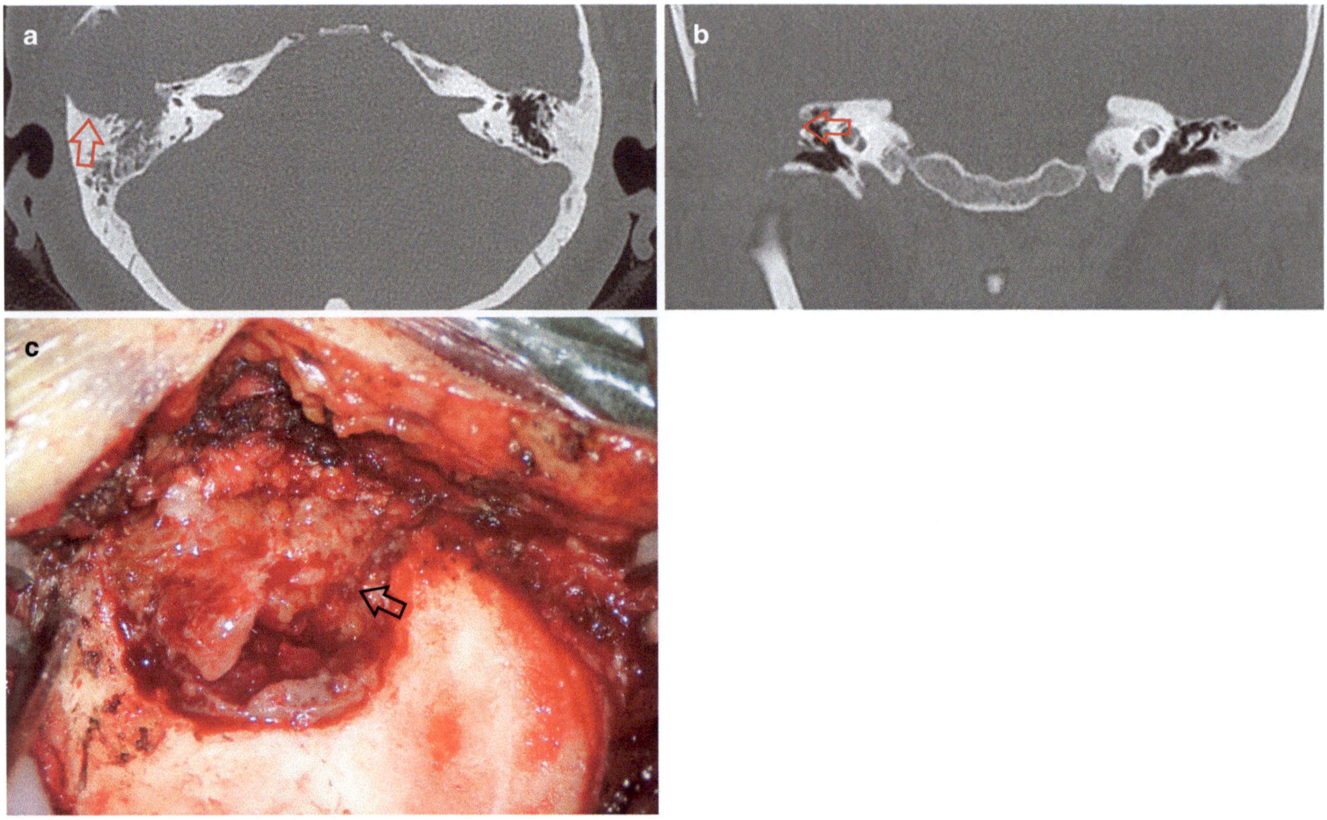

Fig. 6.9 Giant cell tumor of bone in right temporal bone. (**a**) Axial CT; (**b**) Coronal CT; (**c**) Intraoperative finding. Female, 39 years old. (**a**, **b**) Squamous portion of right temporal bone had uniform osteolytic bone destruction (⇧), with neat edges, bone destroy involved in middle cranial fossa and posterior walls of the external auditory canal, and the mastoid process was blocked; (**c**) Bone cortex of temporal bone was broken, gray-red, brittle tumor tissue (⇧) formatted under the temporal muscle, no new osteogenesis, no capsule, blood supply medium.

Note: Osteo-giant cell tumors, one of the common primary bone tumors, are characterized morphologically by the presence of numerous osteoclastic giant cells (Orosz et al. 2017). It is highly invasive and has a great effect on the dissolution and destruction of bone. It can penetrate through the bone to form soft tissue masses, can have local malignant changes. Therefore, it is a low-grade or potential malignant tumor, with a predisposing age of 20–40 years. CT scan showed osteolytic and expansive bone destruction with clear boundary

6.3.3 Osteoma of Temporal Bone

See Figs. 6.10, 6.11, 6.12, and 6.13.

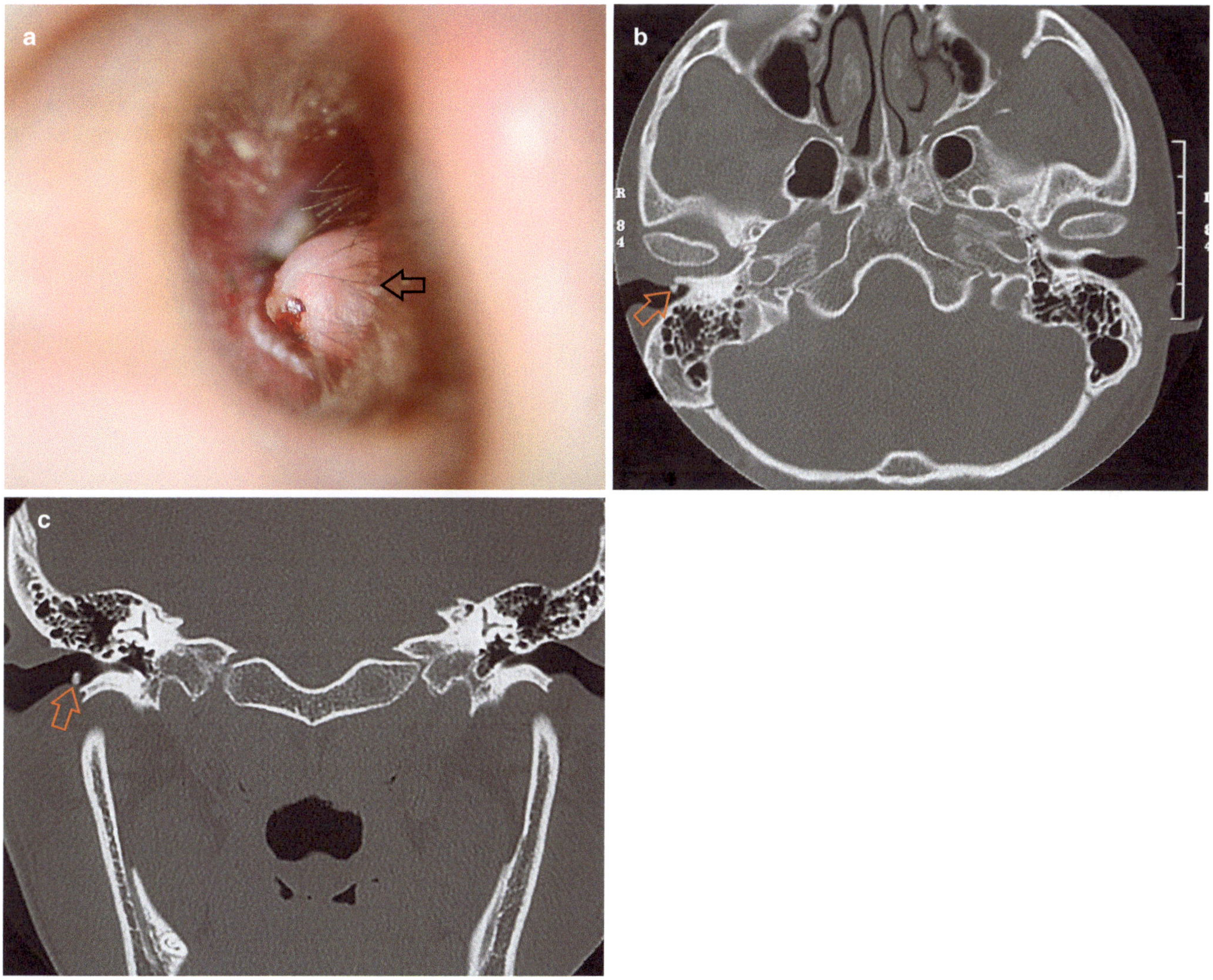

Fig. 6.10 Exogenic osteoma of right external auditory canal. (**a**) Microscopic view of tumor; CT; (**b**) Coronal CT; (**c**) Sagittal CT; Male, 26 years old. (**a**) Isolated neoformation (⇧) located at anteroinferior wall of right external auditory canal; (**b**, **c**) Fine pedicled exogenic bone tissue on anteroinferior wall of external auditory canal (⇧).

Note: Osteoma of the external auditory canal is one of the most common benign tumors in the external auditory canal. It is common in young and middle-aged people, and can be single or multiple. Multiple cases may be related to cold water stimulation

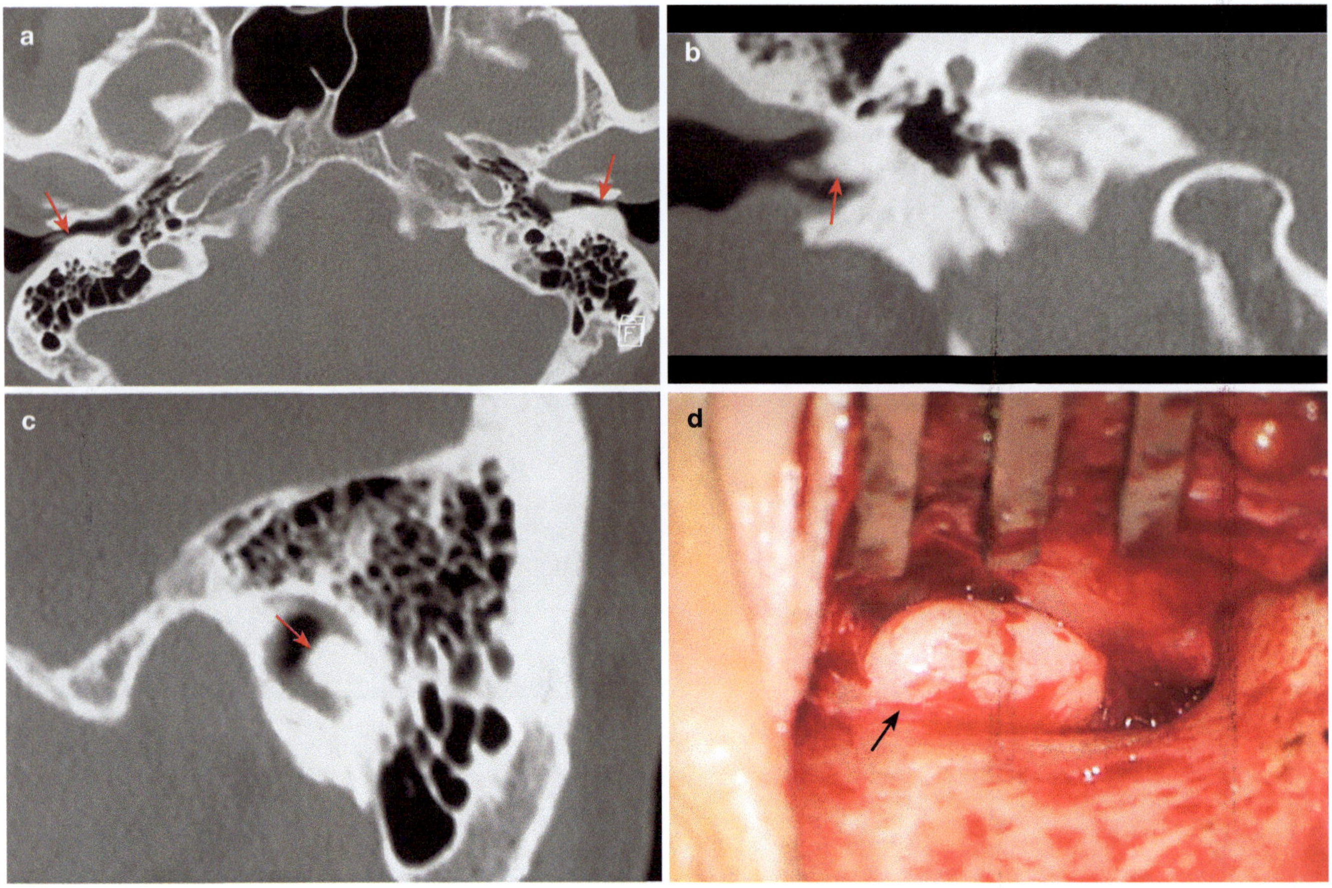

Fig. 6.11 Osteoma of external auditory canal in bilateral ears. (**a**) Axial CT; (**b**) Coronal CT. (**c**) Sagittal CT; (**d**) Intraoperative finding. Male, 61 years old. (**a, b**) Bony protuberances of posterior wall of bilateral external auditory canals (↑); (**c**) Bony and pedicled protuberances of posteroinferior wall of left external auditory canal (↑); (**d**) Pedunculated hard masses (↑) with smooth surface and clear boundary of left external auditory meatus

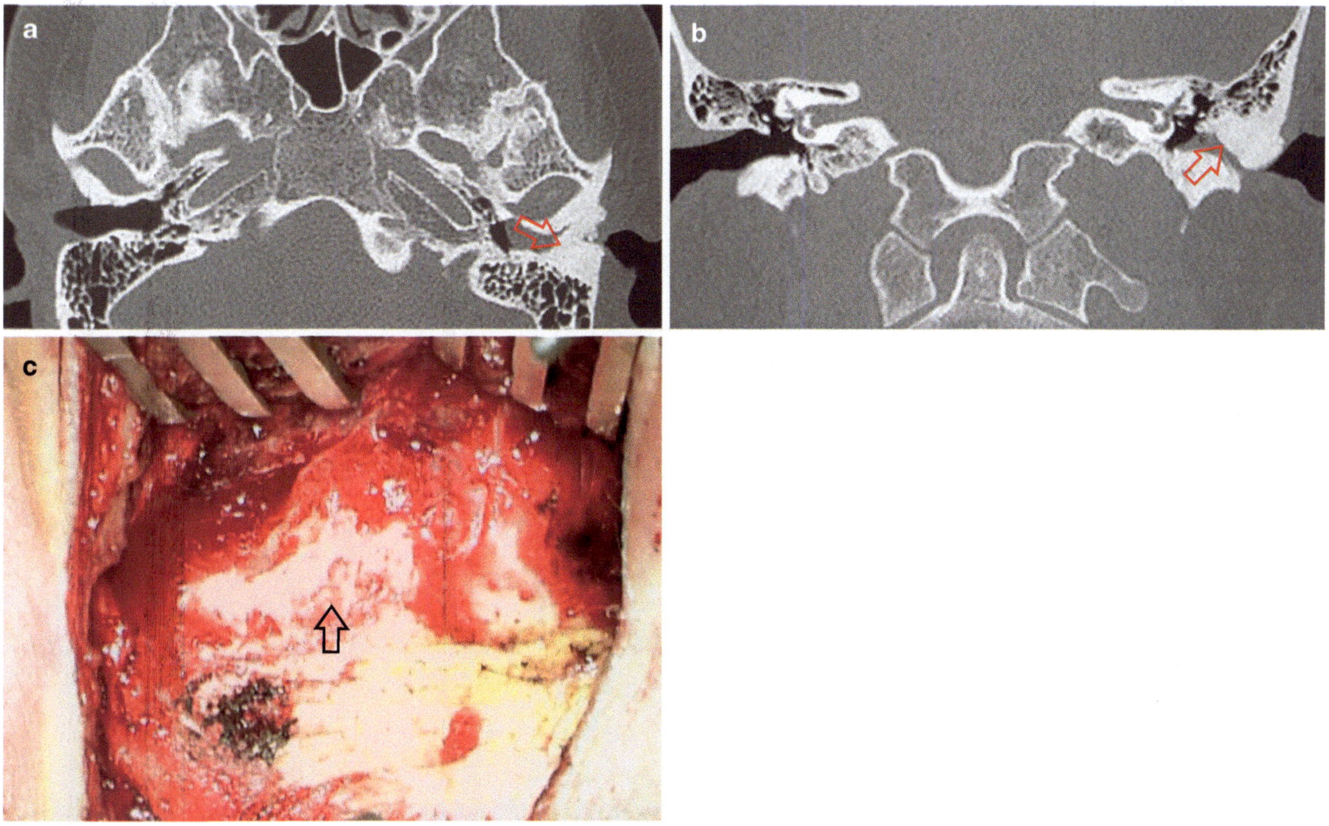

Fig. 6.12 Osteoma of left external auditory canal. (**a**) Axial CT; (**b**) Coronal CT. (**c**) Intraoperative finding. Male, 27 years old. (**a**, **b**) Uniformly dense, broad-based high dense eminence (⇧) with stenosis of external auditory canal(left); (**c**) External auditory canal orifice was blocked by a broad-based bony mass (⇧)

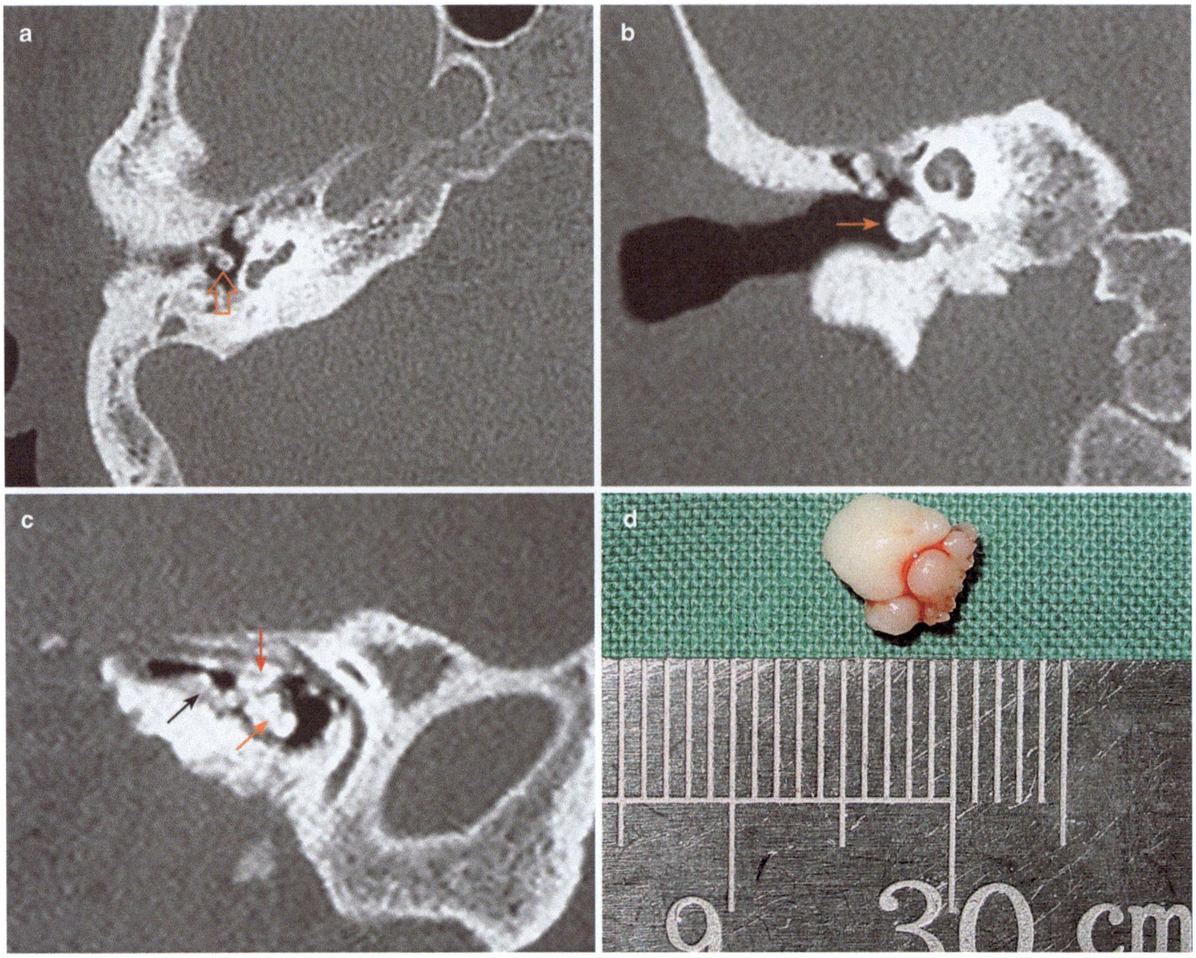

Fig. 6.13 Multiple osteomas of right middle ear. (**a**) Axial CT; (**b**) Coronal CT. (**c**) Sagittal CT; (**d**) Intraoperative finding. Male, 52 years old, with long-term chronic suppurative otitis media. (**a**) High density shadow at long crus of incus (⇧); (**b**) High density shadow at the lower part of promontory (↑); (**c**) High density shadows at semi-canal of tensor tympani muscle (↑), eustachian tube (↑), and promontory (↑); (**d**) Multiple small osteomas attached at the bottom of one bigger osteoma.

Note: Multiple osteomas in the middle ear are extremely rare and should be distinguished from the lamellar or punctate calcification of tympanosclerosis (Li et al. 2014)

6.3.4 Papilloma of External Auditory Canal

See Figs. 6.14.

6.3.5 Cerumen Adenoma of External Auditory Canal

See Fig. 6.15.

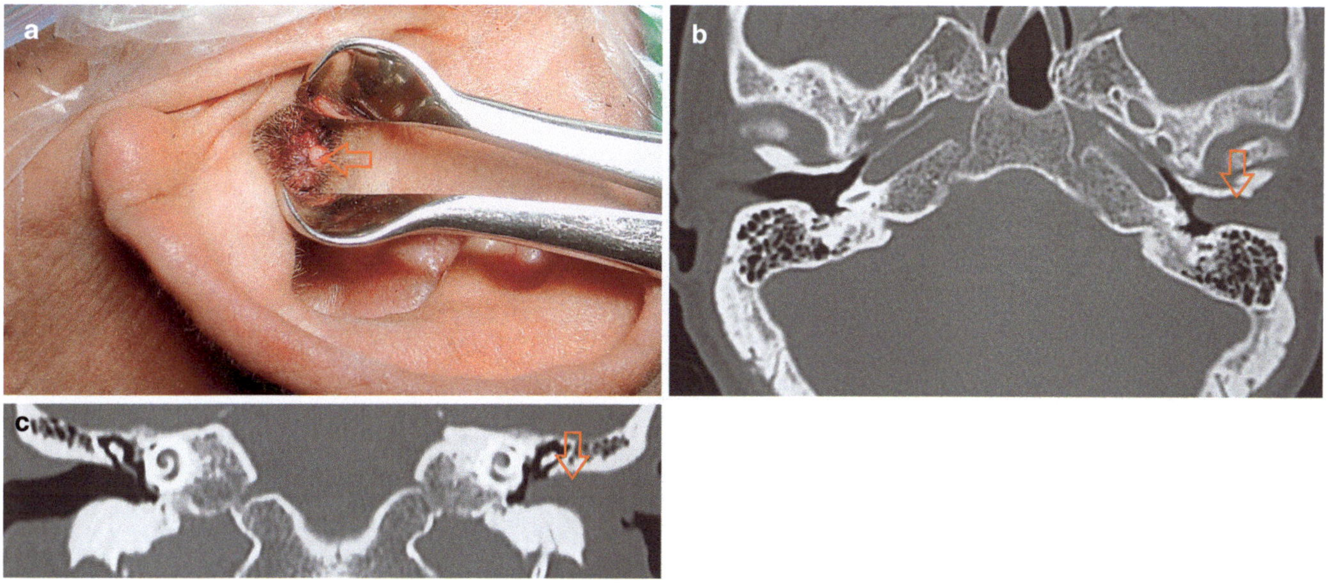

Fig. 6.14 Papilloma of left external auditory canal. (**a**) Intraoperative finding; (**b**) Axial CT; (**c**) Coronal CT. Male, 63 years old. Papillary neoformation of left external auditory canal (⇧); (**b**, **c**) Left external auditory canal (⇧) had blocked by soft tissue shadow with no obvious bone destruction.

Note: External auditory canal papilloma is a benign tumor occurring in the skin of the external auditory canal, which is the most common benign tumor of the ear

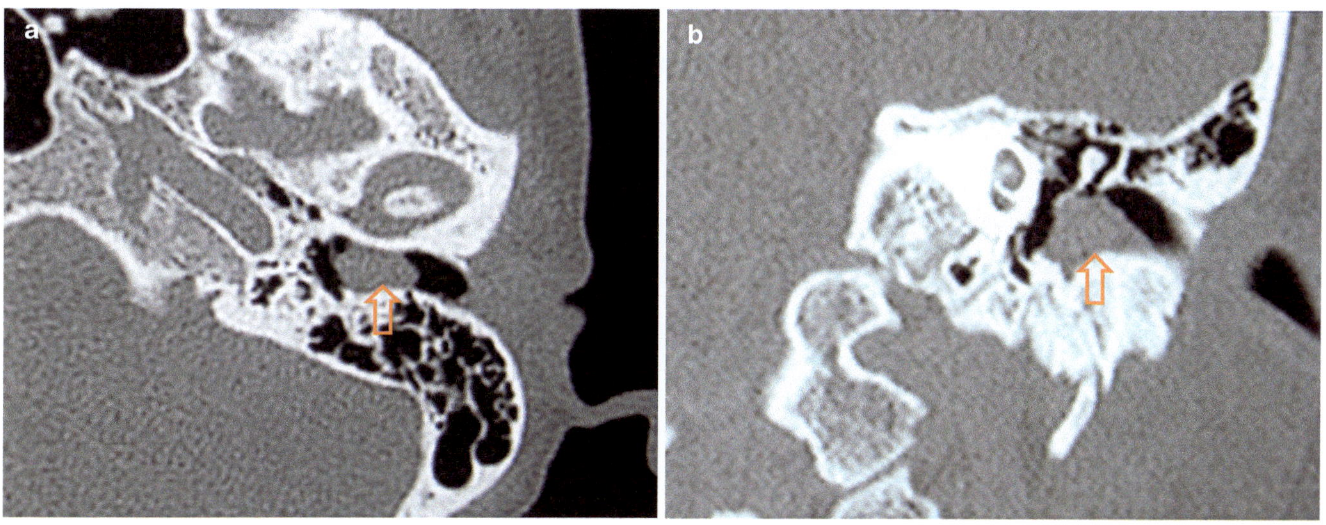

Fig. 6.15 Cerumen adenoma in left external auditory canal. (**a**) Axial CT; (**b**) Coronal CT. Female, 47 years old. A and B. Soft tissue shadow medial was located in segment of the left external auditory canal (⇧) with clear boundary.

Note: Cerumen adenoma is a benign tumor caused by hyperplasia of cerumen glands in the external auditory canal, which is prone to recur after surgery and has a tendency of malignant transformation. Malignant cases are called cerumen adenocarcinoma and/or adenoid cystic carcinoma

6.3.6 Paraganglioma of Temporal Bone

See Figs. 6.16, 6.17, 6.18, 6.19, 6.20, and 6.21.

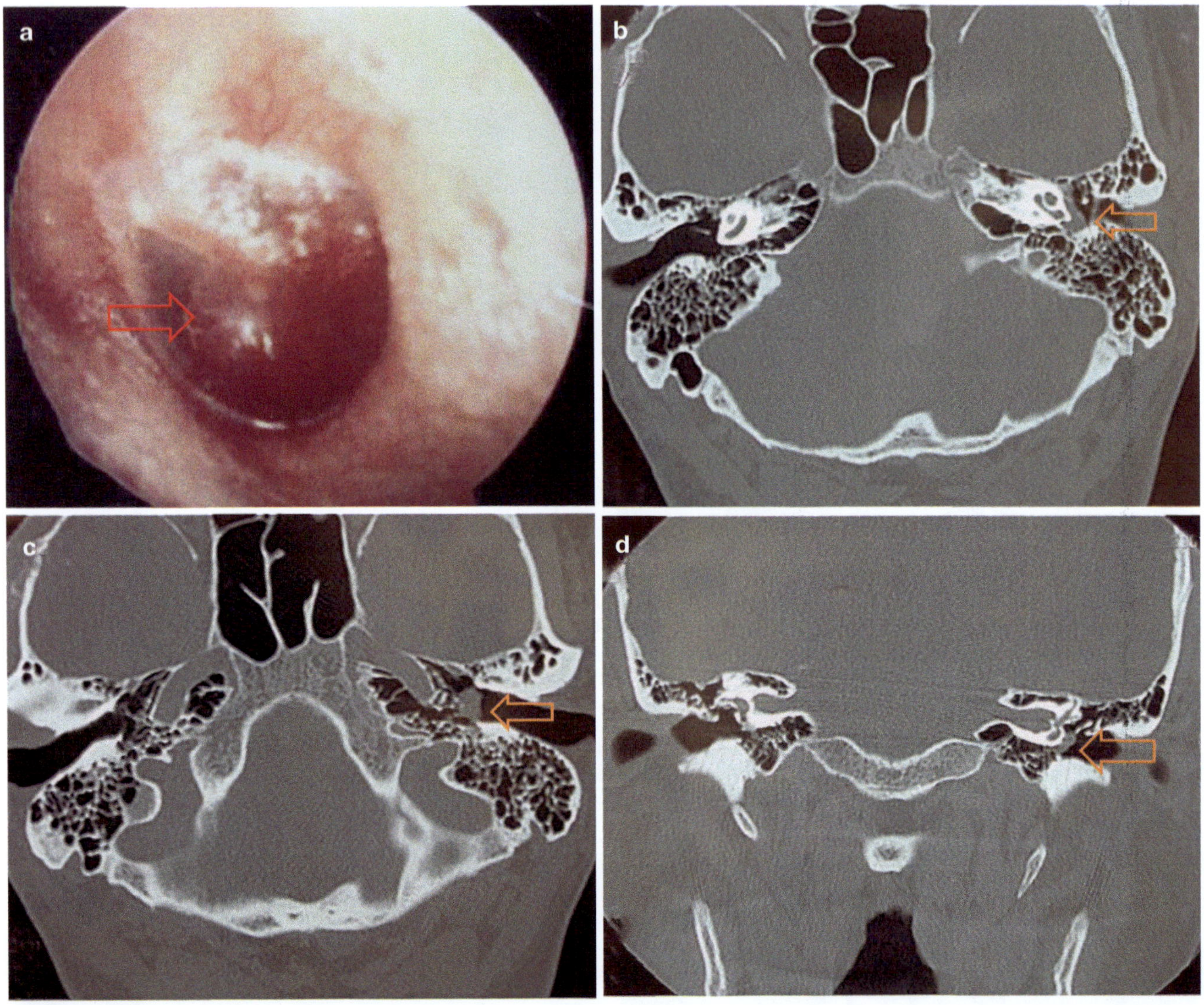

Fig. 6.16 Glomus tympani tumor of left ear. (**a**) Endoscopic view of ear; (**b**, **c**) Axial CT; (**d**) Coronal CT. Male, 35 years old. (**a**) Red neoformation could be seen in tympanic cavity through tympanic membrane (⇧); (**b**–**d**) Neoformation soft tissue shadow with clear boundary was originated from in hypotympanum and located on promontory (⇧).

Note: Glomus tympani tumor, a subset of paragangliomas located along the cochlear promontory, arises from the tympanic plexus of Jacobson's nerve (Sweeney et al. 2015). On CT imaging, these tumors appear as variably sized soft tissue masses (nodule) attaching the promontory, with or without destruction of the adjacent structures. Careful evaluation of such tumors on CT imaging is needed, as their appearance can be similar with that of an aberrant internal carotid artery (Nicolay et al. 2014)

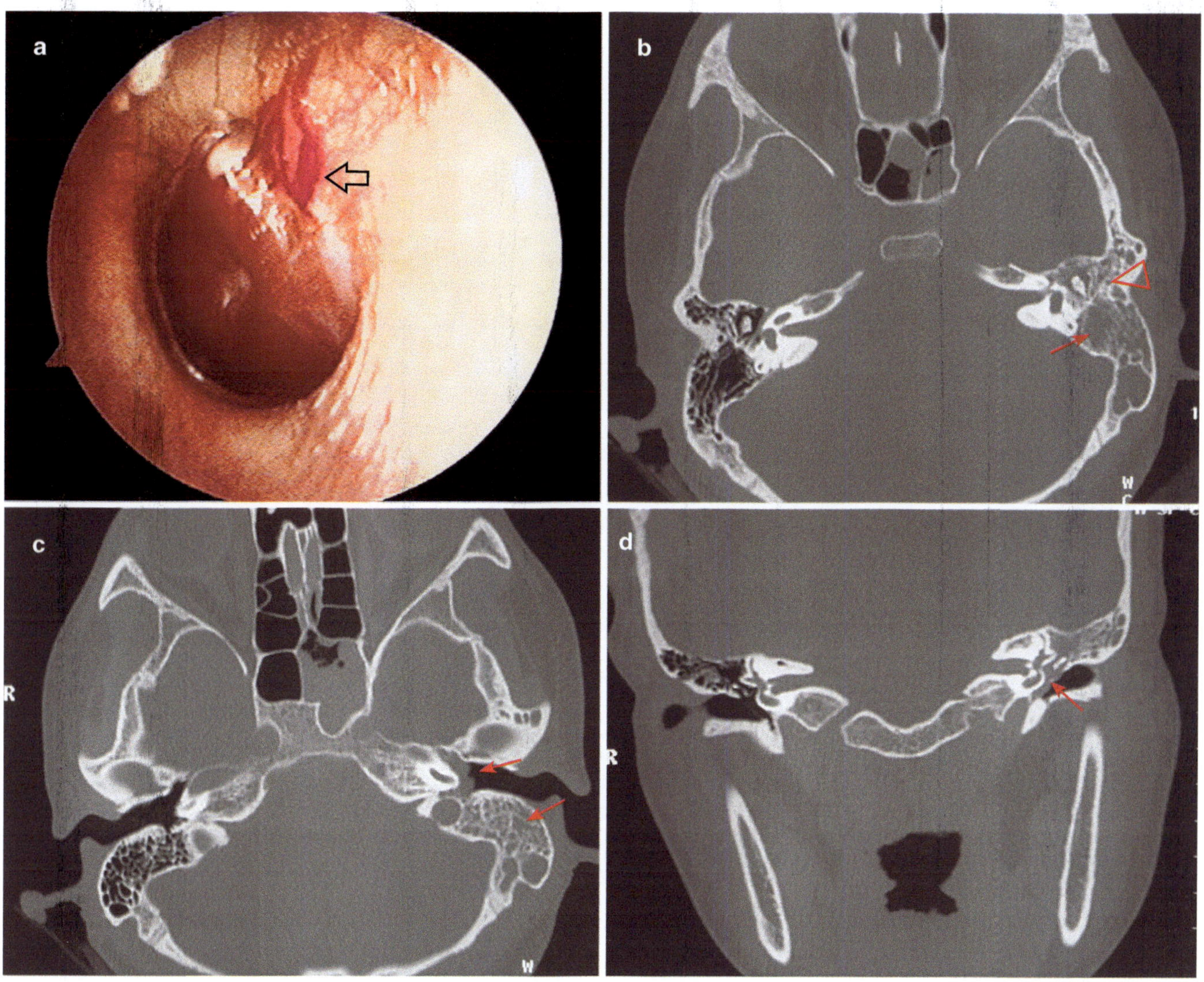

Fig. 6.17 Glomus tympani tumor of left ear. (**a**) Endoscopic view of ear; (**b**, **c**) Axial CT; (**d**) Coronal CT. Female, 31 years old. (**a**) Tympanic membrane in left ear presented red, dilated striae vascularis (⇧) could be seen in pars flaccida of tympanic membrane; (**b**–**d**). Soft tissue shadows (↑) could be seen in tympanic cavity and mastoid cavity, and auditory ossicles (△) were wrapped, but without obvious erosion, mastoid air cells were obstructive change

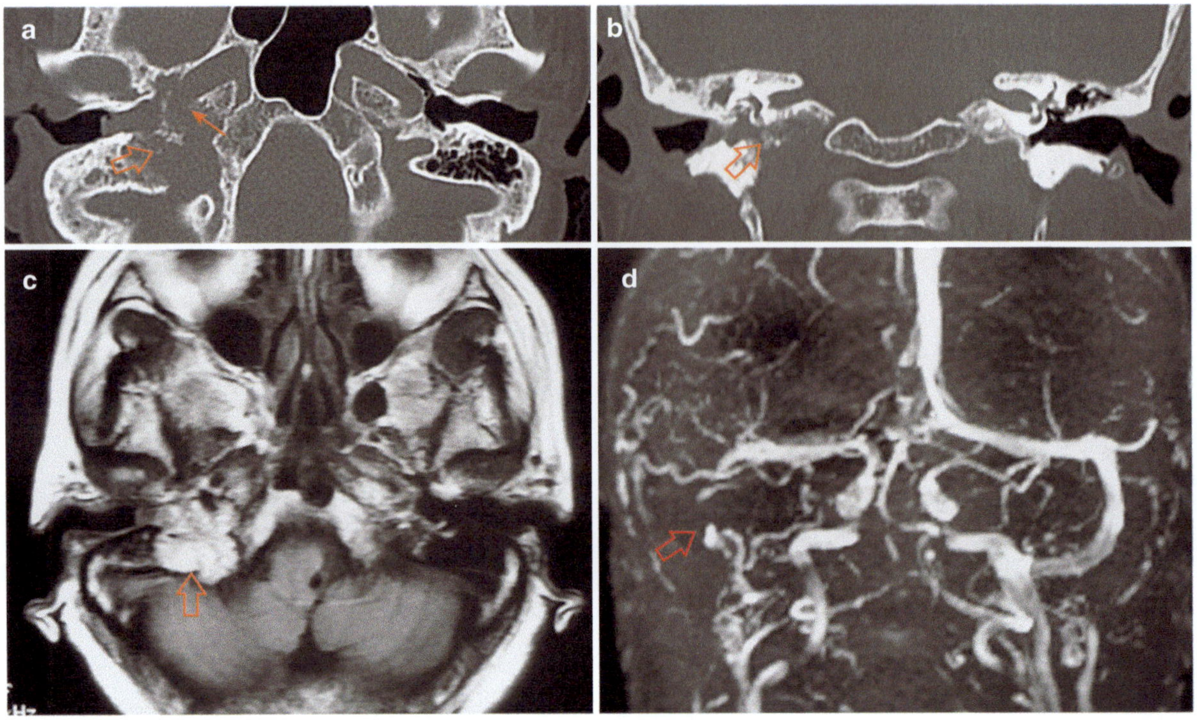

Fig. 6.18 Jugular glomus tumor of right ear. (**a**) Axial CT; (**b**) Coronal CT; (**c**) Axial MRI T_1 MI postgadolinium; (**d**) Coronal MRV. Female, 62 years old. (**a**, **b**) Bone destruction of right jugular foramen area (⇧) and posterior wall of carotid artery canal (↑), soft tissue invaded into external auditory canal; (**c**) Hyperintense signal mass of right jugular foramen area (⇧); (**d**) No signal existed in ipsilateral sigmoid sinus (⇧)

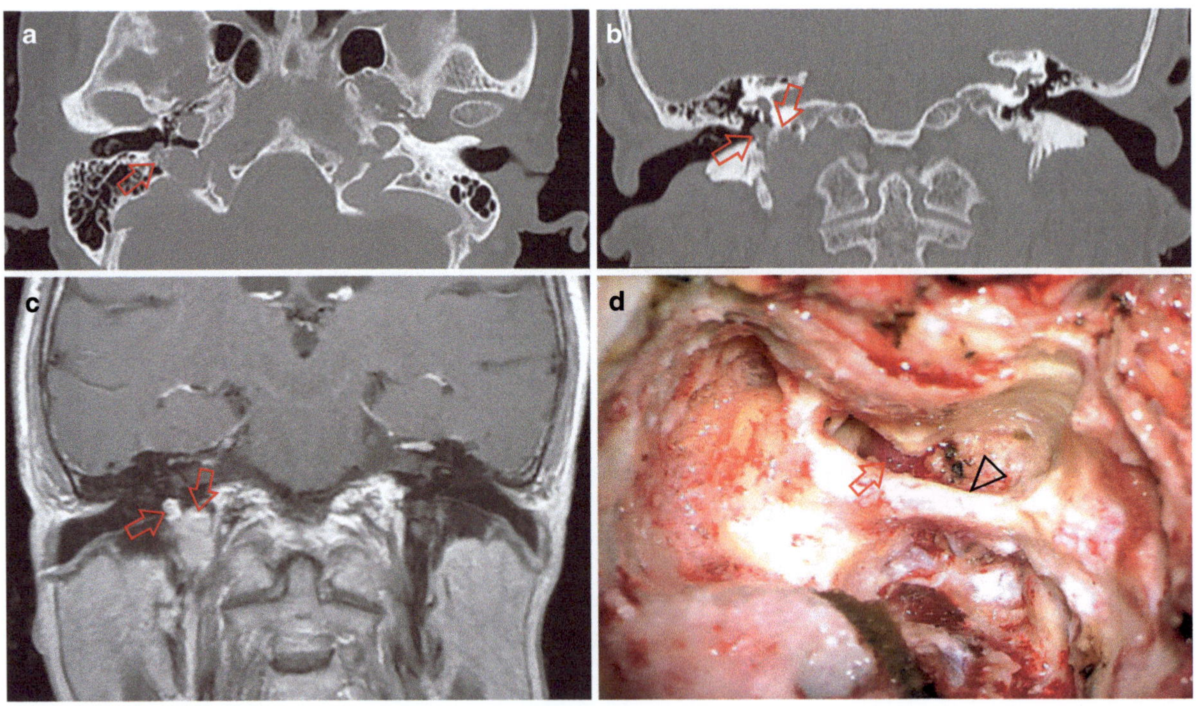

Fig. 6.19 Jugular glomus tumor of right ear. (**a**) Axial CT; (**b**) Coronal CT; (**c**) Axial MRI T_1 MI postgadolinium; (**d**) Intraoperative finding. Female, 28 years old, right ear pulsatile tinnitus for 7 years. (**a**, **b**) Anterolateral wall bone erosion of jugular foramen area, soft tissue shadow had invaded into posteroinferior tympanum (⇧); (**c**) Hyperintense signal shadow with clear boundary could be seen above the glomus jugular (⇧); (**d**) Fresh red and pulsative neoformation presented in the posteroinferior tympanum (⇧), posterior wall of external auditory canal (**Δ**)

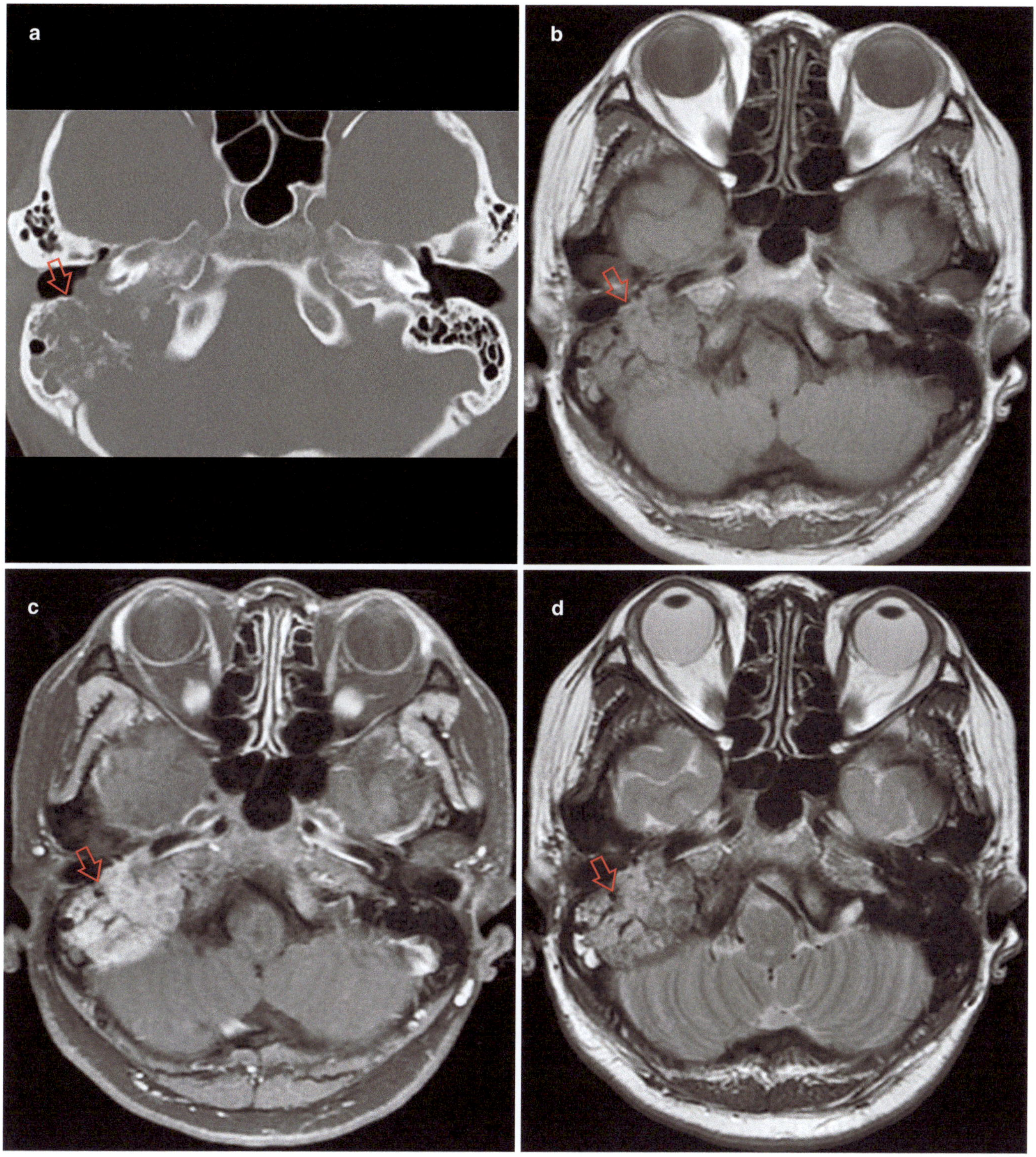

Fig. 6.20 Glomus jugular tumor of right ear. (**a**) Axial CT; (**b**) Axial MRI T_1MI; (**c**) Axial MRI T_1 MI postgadolinium. (**d**) Axial MRI T_2 MI. Female, 32 years old. (**a**) Osteolytic change (⇧) in right jugular foramen area, neoformation had extensively invaded surrounding structure (cochlea, facial nerve canal and posterior wall of external auditory canal); (**b**) Mass (⇧) showed uneven and equal signals, and flow void signal shadow could be seen inside; (**c**) Center of mass (⇧) was uneven and significantly enhanced signal, and flow void signal shadow could be seen inside (pepper and salt signs); (**d**) Center of mass was uneven and moderately enhanced (⇧), and the flow void signal shadow could be seen inside

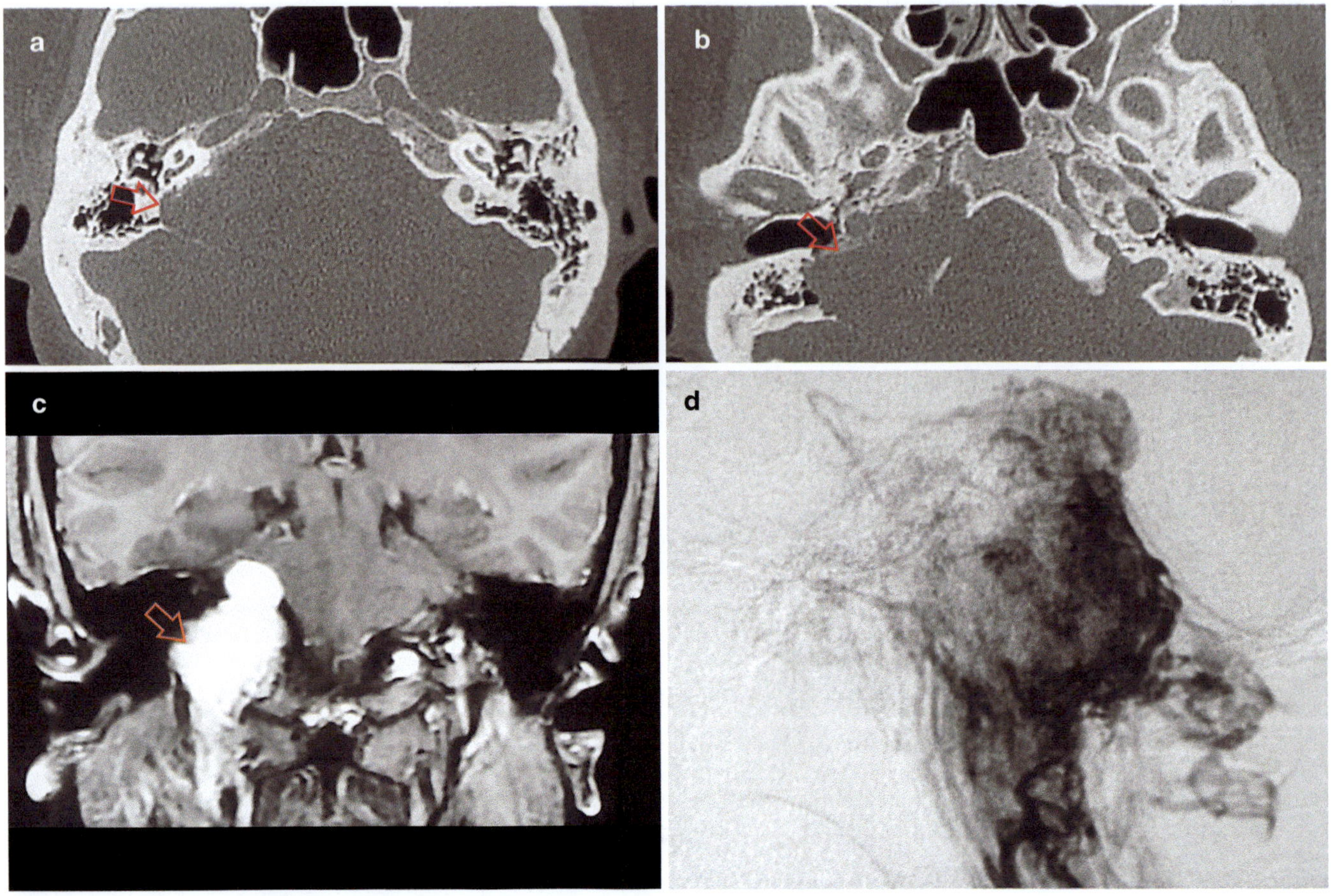

Fig. 6.21 Glomus jugular tumor of right ear. (**a**) Axial CT; (**b**) Coronal CT; (**c**) Axial MRI T_1 MI postgadolinium; (**d**) DSA. Female, 34 years old. (**a, b**). Bone destruction (⇧) of jugular foramen area in right ear; there was little residual bone in mass; (**c**) hyperintense signal shadow (⇧) could be seen up to the brain stem and down to the parapharyngeal space (**d**) Digital subtraction showed abundant blood supply of the tumor.

Note: Glomus jugular tumor, also known as non-chromaffin paraganglioma or chemoreceptor tumor, is tumor rich in blood vessels. The glomus jugular from the outer membrane of the top of the glomus jugular is a chemoreceptor similar to the carotid body tissue

6.3.7 Hemangioma of Temporal Bone

See Figs. 6.22 and 6.23.

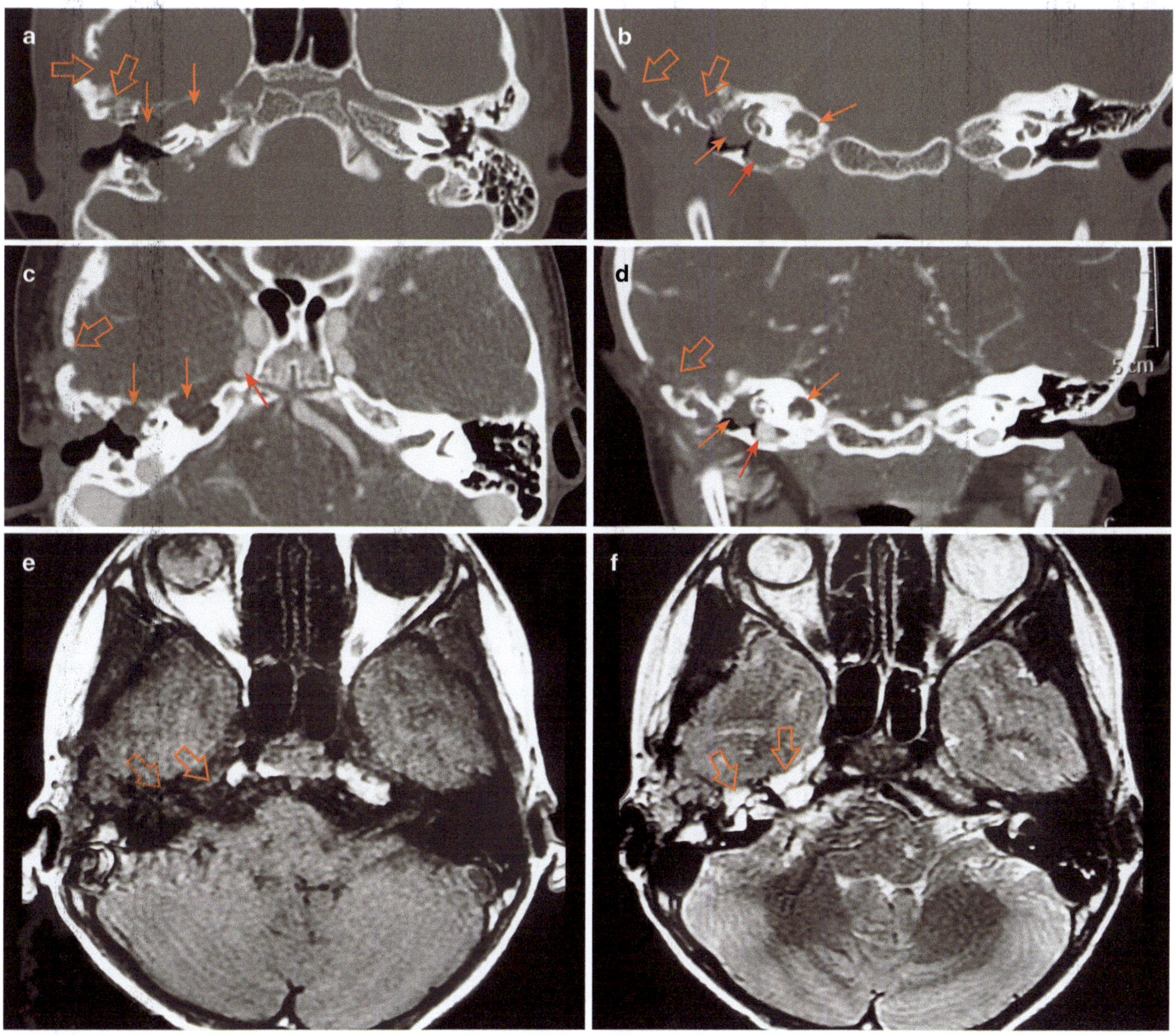

Fig. 6.22 Meningoencephalocele of right ear with infantile capillary hemangioma. (**a**) Axial CT; (**b**) Coronal CT; (**c**, **d**) Brain CT postgadolinium; (**e**) Axial MRI T_1 MI; (**f**) Axial MRI T_2 MI. Male, 7 years old. (**a–d**) Bone defect and destruction of right temporal bones (⇧), soft tissue (↑) invading cochlea and petrous apex, high position and bare of jugular glomus (↑), internal carotid artery (↑); (**e**) Tumor mass showed hypointense signal (⇧); (**f**) Tumor tissue showed hyperintense signal shadow (⇧)

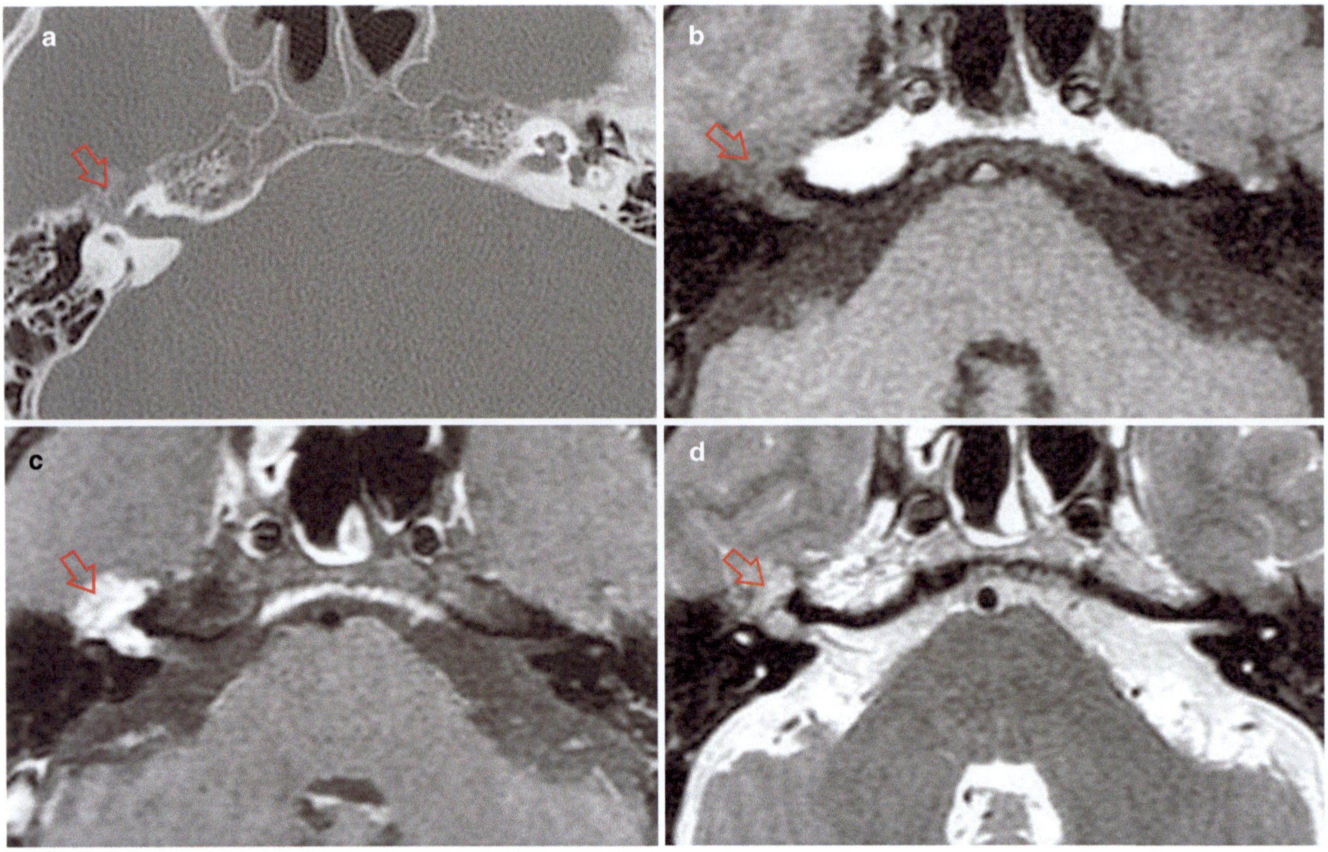

Fig. 6.23 Facial neurohemangioma of right temporal bone. (**a**) Axial CT; (**b**) Axial MRI T_1 MI; (**c**) Axial MRI T_1 MI postgadolinium; (**b**) Axial MRI T_2 M. Male, 59 years old. (**a**) Bone canal expansion in geniculate ganglion and widened labyrinth segment of right facial nerve (⇧); (**b**) Tumor was uneven and hypointense signal (⇧); (**c**) Tumor (⇧) was uneven and significantly enhanced; (**d**) Tumor was visible in geniculate ganglion and labyrinth segment with uneven and medium signal shadow (⇧)

6.3.8 Intratemporal Facial Neuroma

Facial schwannoma is most common in facial neurinoma, and neurofibroma is rare. Facial nerve schwannomas are benign peripheral nerve sheath tumors that arise from Schwann cells, and most commonly present with facial paresis and/or hearing loss (Quesnel et al. 2018). HRCT scan and MRI are critical to diagnosis.

Facial schwannoma can occur in all segments of facial nerve, but it usually occurs in the geniculate ganglion, or in the vertical segment of facial nerve. The typical manifestation is slow progressive facial nerve paralysis, which can also be manifested as sudden onset of facial nerve paralysis, recurrent intermittent facial nerve paralysis and hemifacial spasm. Differentiation between facial neurilemmoma and acoustic neurinoma occurring in the internal acoustic meatus: facial neurilemmoma has bone destruction in the anterosuperior wall of internal acoustic meatus, which is manifested as a mass in the middle cranial fossa communicating the labyrinthine segment of facial nerve with internal acoustic meatus, while acoustic neurinoma is manifested as a mass in internal acoustic meatus and cerebellopontine angle, which does not involve the labyrinthine segment of facial nerve (Figs. 6.24, 6.25, 6.26, and 6.27).

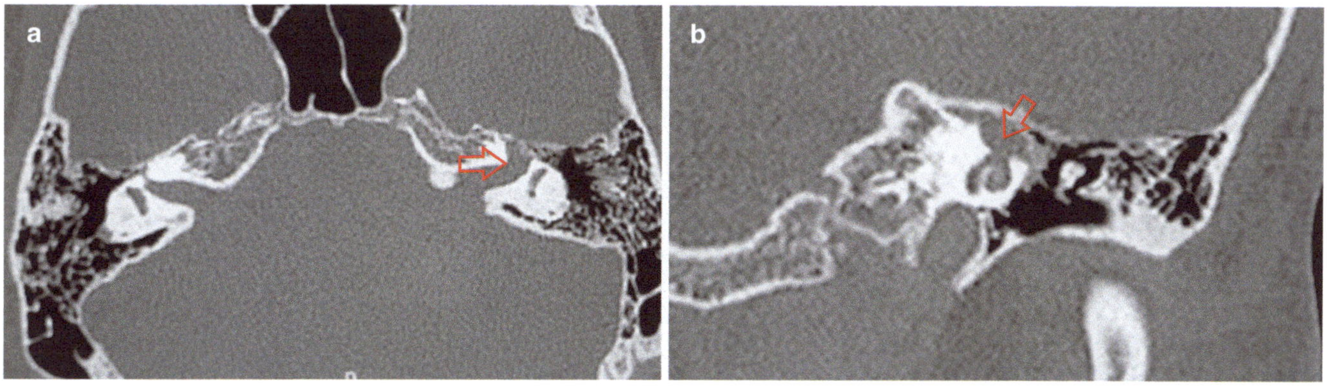

Fig. 6.24 Facial nerve schwannoma in labyrinthine segment and geniculate ganglion of left facial nerve. (**a**) Axial CT; (**b**) Coronal CT. Male, 26 years old. Facial nerve labyrinthine segment and geniculate ganglion (⇧) in the temporal bone of the left ear were enlarged and invaded into the cochlea, resulting in total deafness

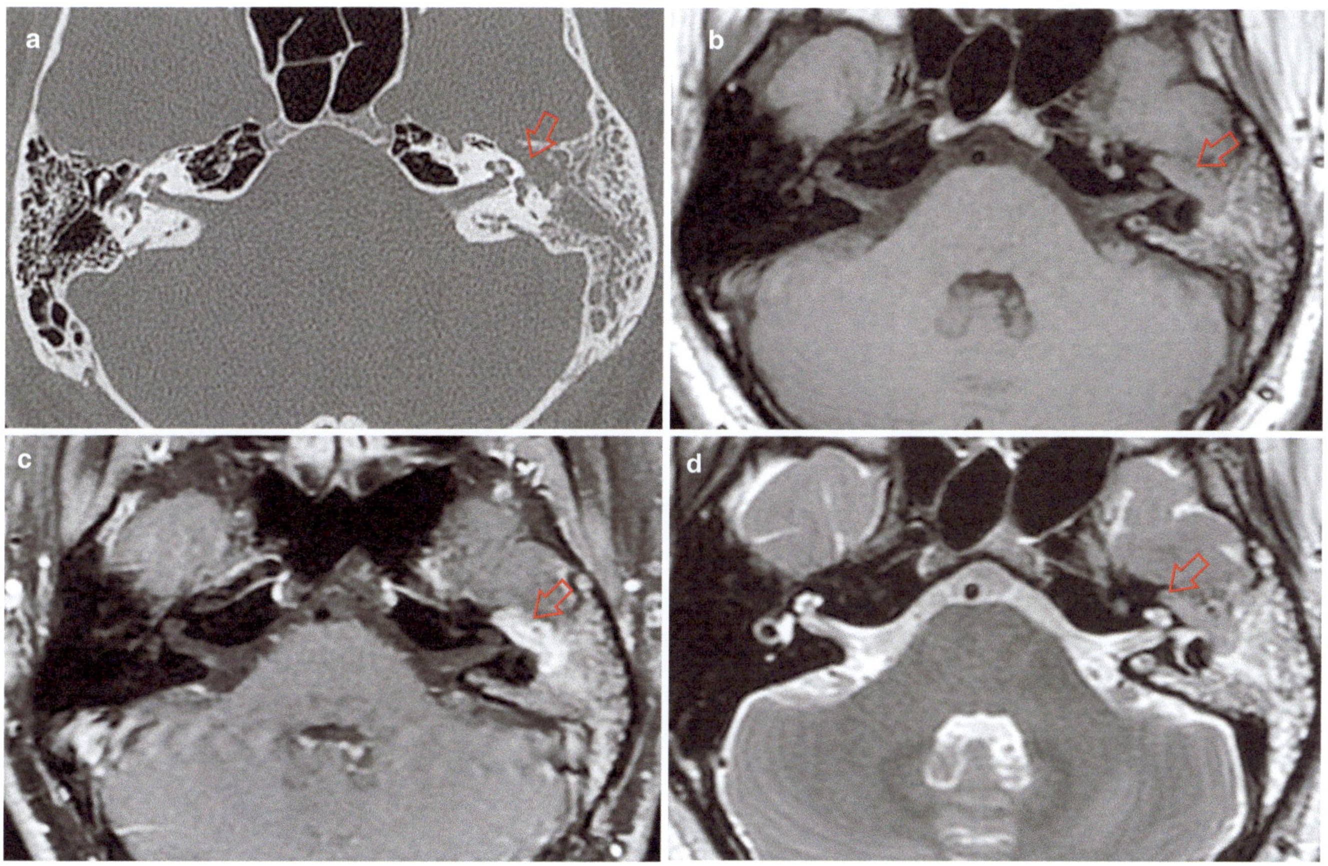

Fig. 6.25 Facial nerve schwannoma of right ear. (**a**) Axial CT; (**b**) Axial MRI T_1 MI; (**c**) Axial MRI T_1 MI postgadolinium; (**d**) Axial MRI T_2 MI. Male, 25 years old. (**a**) Tympanic segment (⇧) of facial nerve was widened, middle ear and mastoid was filled with soft tissue shadow; (**b**) Tympanic segment of left facial nerve presented shuttle-shaped mass (⇧), uniform and equal signal, middle ear mastoid soft tissue shadow was scattered slight hyperintense signal; (**c**) Mass (⇧) was uniform and significantly enhanced comparison with mastoid cavity shadow, which was inflammatory change; (**d**) Tympanic segment of left facial nerve was uniform and equal signal shadow (⇧), middle ear mastoid soft tissue shadow was scattered hyperintense signal shadow

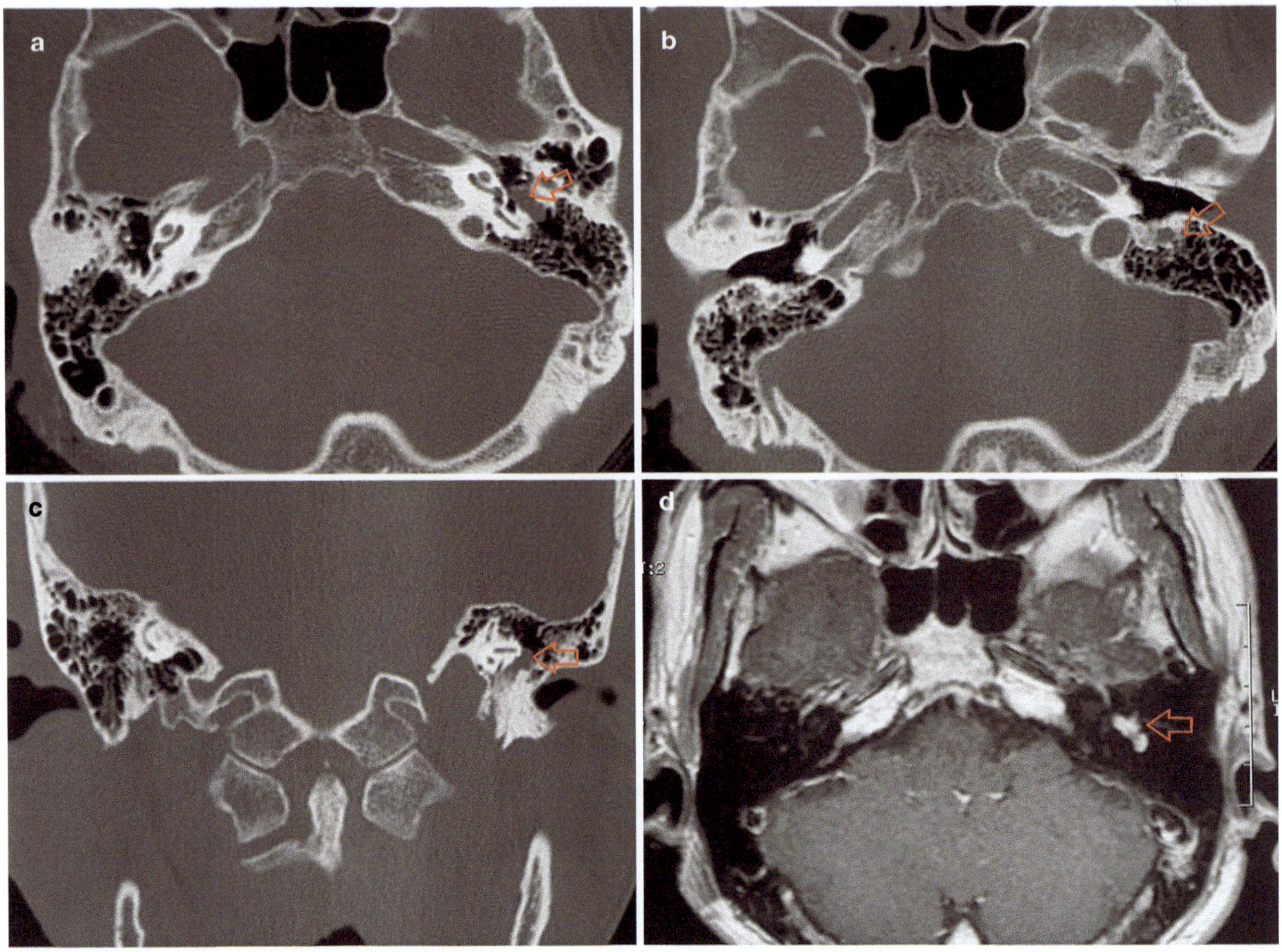

Fig. 6.26 Facial nerve schwannoma of left ear. (**a**, **b**) Axial CT; (**c**) Coronal CT; (**d**) Axial MRI T_1 MI postgadolinium. Male, 46 years old. (**a**, **c**) Facial nerve schwannoma at (thicken) second genu of facial nerve (⇧); (**b**) Schwannoma at (thicken) vertical segment of facial nerve (⇧); (**d**) Hypointense signal shadow at second genu of facial nerve (⇧)

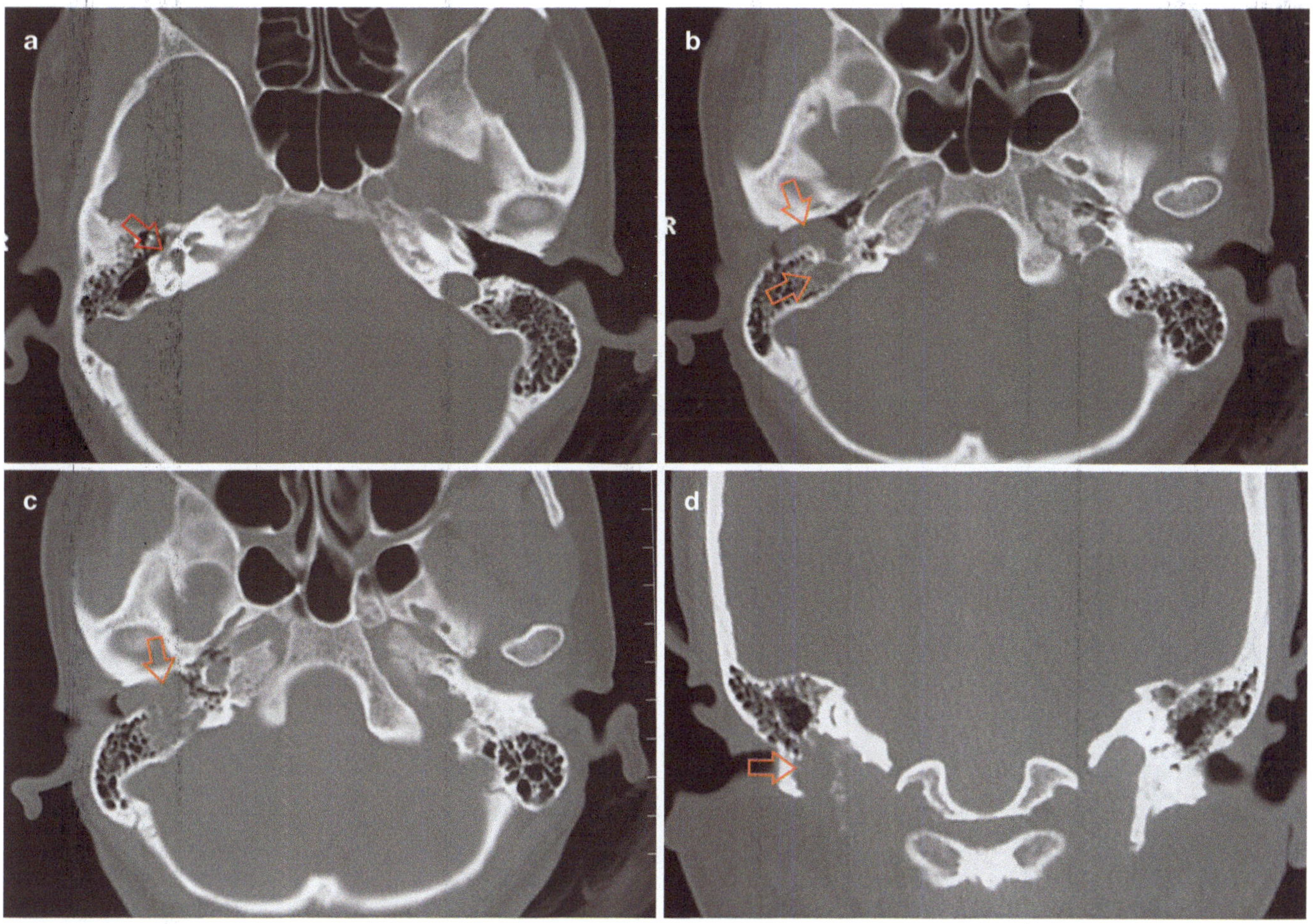

Fig. 6.27 Facial nerve schwannoma of right ear. (**a**, **b**) Axial CT; (**c**) Coronal CT. Female, 43 years old. (**a**) Without obvious abnormality in horizontal segment (⇧) of facial nerve; (**b–d**) Tumor tissue was located at vertical segment (⇧) of facial nerve, and had protruded into external auditory canal and retrotympanum (⇧)

6.4 Malignant Tumor of Temporal Bone

Ear malignant tumors can occur in the auricle, external auditory canal, middle ear and inner ear (including the internal acoustic meatus). In terms of primary region of cancer, most of the tumors occur in the auricle, followed by the external auditory canal, and then in the middle ear. The tumors in the inner ear are rare. Most patients with middle ear cancer have a history of chronic otitis media. According to the nature of cancer, the most common cancer of the ear is squamous cell carcinoma, followed by basal cell carcinoma, adenocarcinoma, sarcoma and melanoma. Metastatic cancers are rare, occasionally from the breast, thyroid, and prostate. The cancer of adjacent organs, such as nasopharyngeal carcinoma, may sometimes invade the middle ear through the eustachian tube, parotid gland carcinoma may invade the external auditory canal, and tumors of clivus and pituitary may also affect the petrous part of temporal bone. All ulcers, "granulation tissue" prone to bleeding, and "inflammatory" pain of ear that cannot be controlled by anti-inflammatory treatment should be suspected as malignant tumors. Malignant tumors of temporal bone, prone to facial nerve, posterior cranial nerves and others, are not easy to be diagnosed early, CT and MRI examination are really necessary.

6.4.1 Myofibroblastoma of Temporal Bone

See Fig. 6.28.

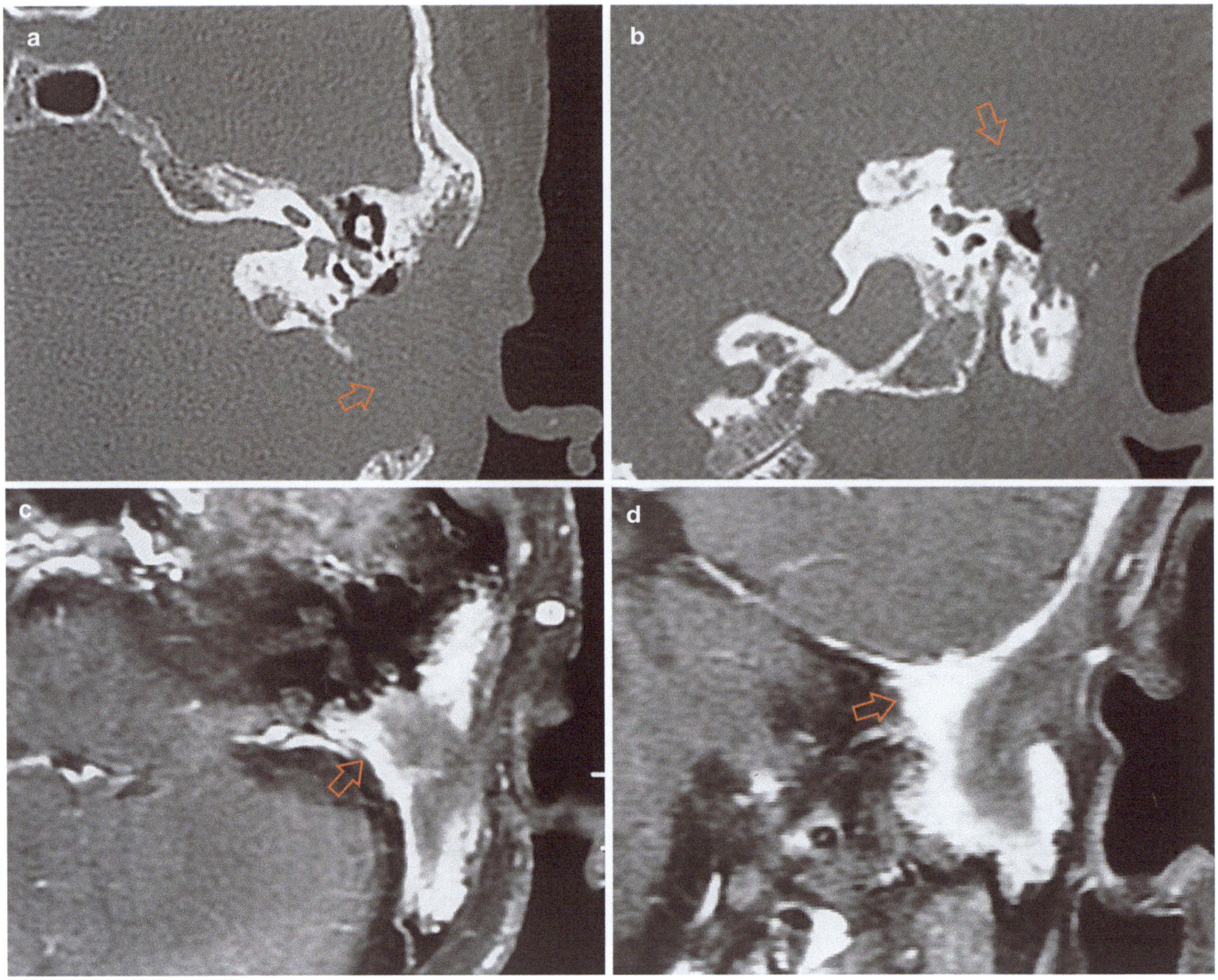

Fig. 6.28 Myofibroblastoma of left temporal bone. (**a**) Axial CT; (**b**) Coronal CT; (**c**) Axial MRI T_1 MI postgadolinium; (**d**) Coronal MRI T_1 MI postgadolinium. Female, 54 years old. (**a, b**) Occupied soft tissue of squamous portion, petrous portion and mastoid portion of temporal bone and large bone destruction disappearance (⇧); (**c, d**). Enhanced irregular soft tissue signals shadow (⇧) occupied squamous portion, petrous portion and mastoid portion of temporal bone, with clear boundary, obvious uniform enhancement of the lesion edge (⇧), and no enhancement of the central part of the lesion.

Note: Pathology: Myofibroblastic tumor (low grade malignant)

6.4.2 Adenoid Cystic Carcinoma

Adenoid cystic carcinoma (ACC) of the external auditory canal is a rare primary malignancy, and surgery is the primary management strategy (Wang et al. 2023). Otalgia is the most common manifestation of adenoid cystic carcinoma of the external auditory canal, and misdiagnosis is frequently encountered. ACC is a commonly encountered salivary gland malignancy, whose clinical course is burdened by local recurrence and distant dissemination. The adenoid cystic carcinoma is neurophilic and can grow along the facial nerve (Figs. 6.29 and 6.30)

6.4.3 Squamous Cell Carcinoma of Temporal Bone

Squamous cell carcinoma of the temporal bone is a rare malignancy accounting for only 0.2% of head and neck cancers (Lechner et al. 2021) (Figs. 6.31 and 6.32).

6.4.4 Temporal Osteosarcoma

Rhabdomyosarcoma, the most common soft tissue sarcoma of childhood, involves the temporal bone in approximately 7% of reported cases, the prognosis remains poor for disease involving temporal bone and other parameningeal sites (Wiatrak et al. 1989; Viswanatha 2007) (Fig. 6.33).

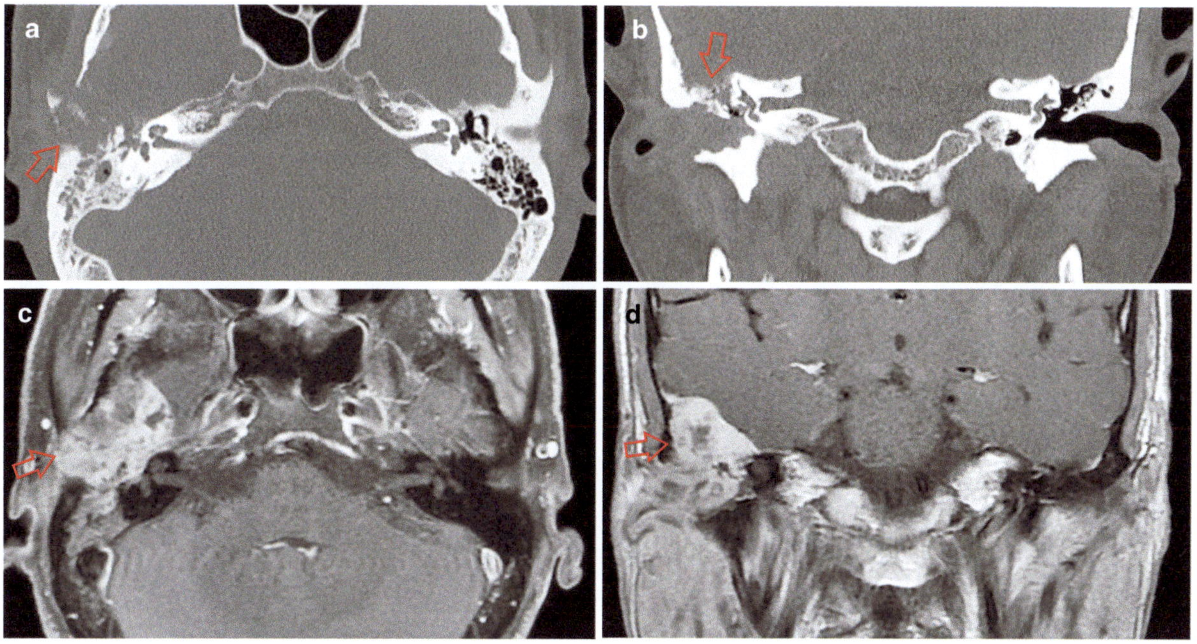

Fig. 6.29 Adenoid cystic carcinoma of left ear. (**a**) Axial CT; (**b**) Coronal CT; (**c**) Axial MRI T_1 WI postgadolinium; (**d**) Axial MRI T_1 WI postgadolinium**.** Male, 45 years old. (**a, b**) Squamous portion and tympanic portion of right temporal bone (⇧) were destroyed and absorbed, residual bone could be seen inside tumor; (**c, d**) Enhanced masses (⇧) presented mixed hyperintense signal, with clear boundary, and invaded ipsilateral temporal lobe and external auditory canal and tympanic cavity. The mastoid process showed obstructive changes

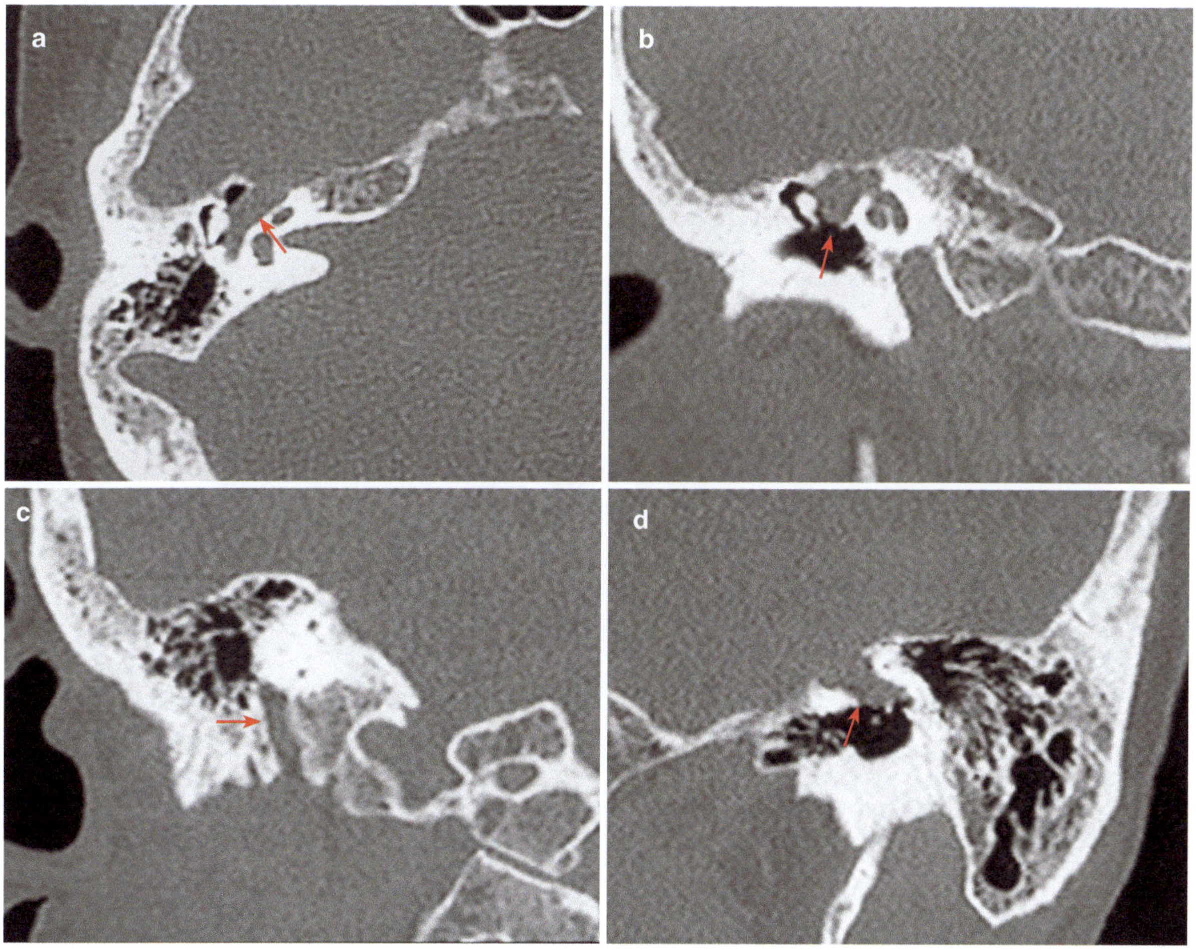

Fig. 6.30 Adenoid cystic carcinoma of facial nerve in right ear. (**a**) Axial CT; (**b, c**) Coronal CT; (**d**) Sagittal CT. Female, 66 years old. Bone canal of facial nerve in temporal bone thickens (⇧)

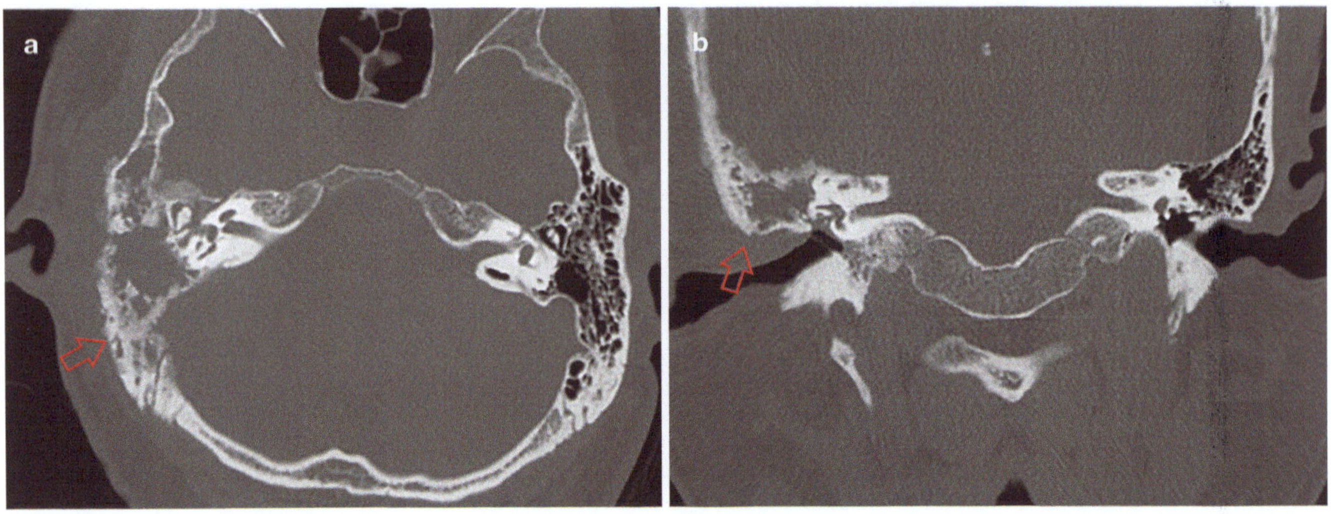

Fig. 6.31 Squamous cell carcinoma of right temporal bone. (**a**) Axial CT; (**b**) Coronal CT. Male, 40 years old. Erosive lesion and absorb of right temporal bone (⇧) with rough margin and hyperosteogeny; no clear boundary could be found between the lesion and the surrounding soft tissue, and lateral soft tissue of temporal bone and superior wall soft tissue of external auditory canal were swollen

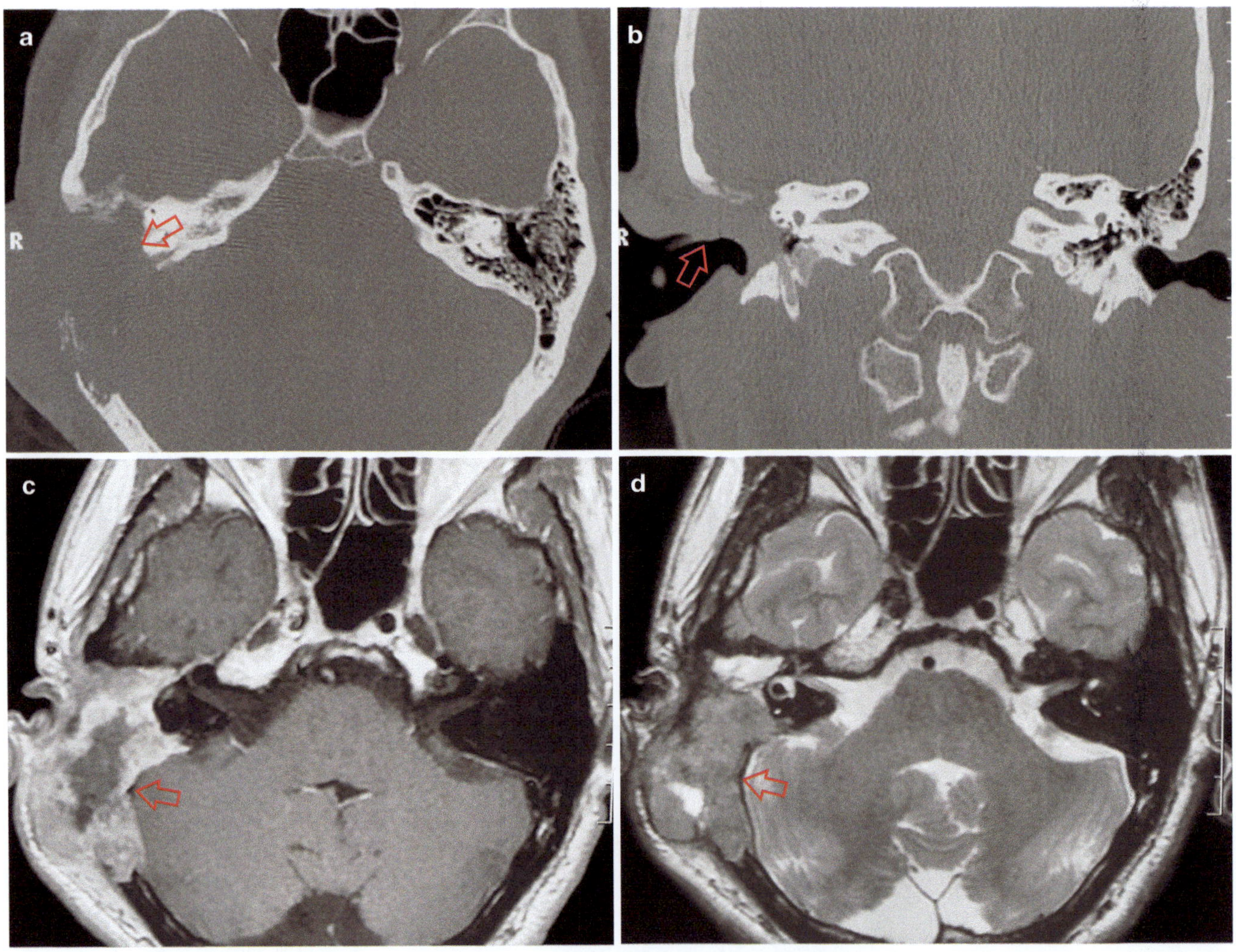

Fig. 6.32 Squamous cell carcinoma of right temporal bone. (**a**) Axial CT; (**b**) Coronal CT; (**c**) Axial MRI T_1MI postgadolinium; (**d**) Axial MRI T_2 MI. Male, 43 years old. (**a, b**) Right tympanomastoid bone destruction (⇧), involving tympanic segment of facial nerve canal and middle skull base; (**c**) Enhancement irregular mass of right tympanomastoid cavity (⇧), peripheral moderate enhancement, internal equal signal (liquefaction); facial nerve and adjacent brain tissue were involved; (**d**) Right tympanomastoid cavity irregular signal (⇧), peripheral uneven signal, part of internal areas strengthened

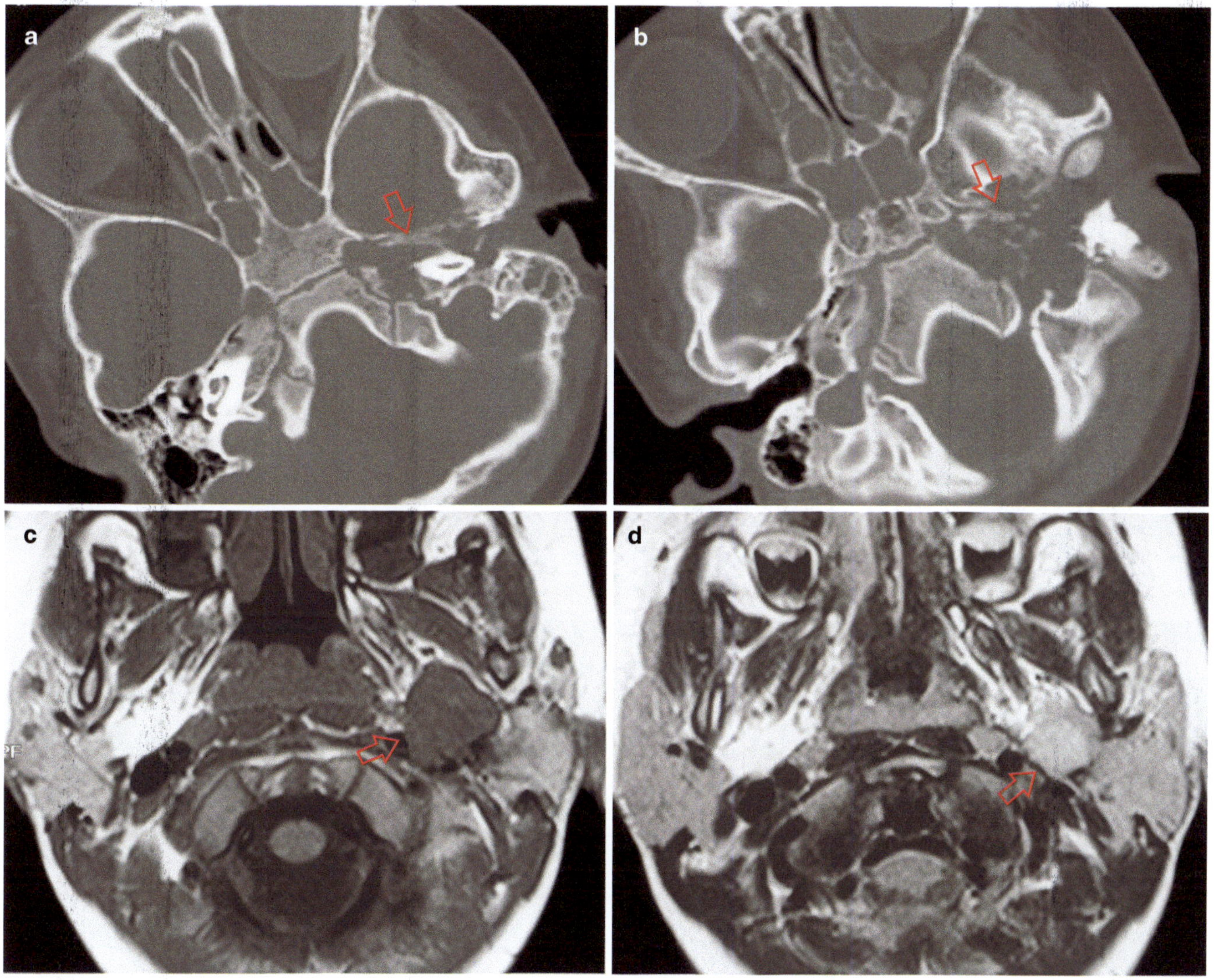

Fig. 6.33 Rhabdomyosarcoma of left temporal bone. (**a**, **b**) Axial CT; (**c**) Axial MRI T_1MI; (**d**) Axial MRI T_2 MI. Female, 3 years old. (**a**, **b**) Right petrous apex, petrous portion (⇧) of temporal bone were destroyed, ascending and horizontal part of carotid artery canal was also involved; (**c**) Equal signal soft tissue shadow (⇧); (**d**) Slight hyperintense signal soft tissue shadow (⇧) in petrous apex with relative clear boundary

6.4.5 Melanoma of Temporal Bone

Temporal bone mucosal melanomas (MMs) are rare, and patients may experience delays in diagnosis and treatment. Chronic serous otitis media patients with bloody otorrhea or an associated cranial nerve palsy should be suspected temporal bone MM, the acquisition of a biopsy or imaging studies should not be delayed (Young et al. 2023) (Fig. 6.34).

6.4.6 Cartilaginous Tumor of Temporal Bone

Cartilage-producing tumor most commonly occurred in the epiphyses of growing patients. Temporal bone chondroblastoma is a rare, accounts for less than 1% of primary bone tumors, locally aggressive tumor originating from immature cartilage, which recurs to a high degree. The diagnosis is based on detailed imaging and histopathological examination (Fig. 6.35).

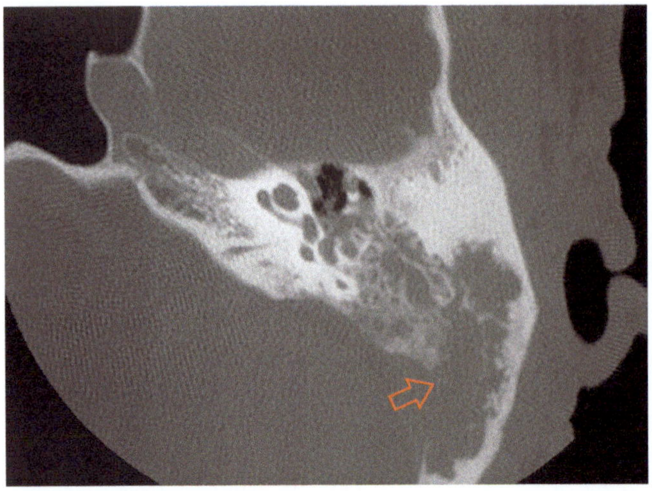

Fig. 6.34 Melanoma of left temporal bone on axial CT view. Male, 67 years old. Erosive lesion of middle ear and mastoid process, partial absorption of bone trabecula, destruction of anterolateral wall of sigmoid sinus (⇧)

6.4.7 Endolymphatic Sac Tumor

Endolymphatic sac tumor (classified according to the 2017 WHO) is a low-grade malignant epithelial tumor originated from the endolymphatic sac, also known as low-grade malignant adenocarcinoma of the endolymphatic sac, adenoid cystic carcinoma of the endolymphatic sac, papillary adenocarcinoma of the endolymphatic sac, and papillary endolymphatic sac tumor. It is rare, slow in progression, and can be diagnosed bilaterally. Patients may have dizziness, tinnitus, hearing loss in a short time, or even total deafness.

The tumor can cause a characteristic appearance on CT consisting of expansile, motheaten, lytic destruction of the retrolabyrinthine temporal bone including the margins of the vestibular aqueduct, with a thin peripheral rim of calcification that represents the expanded cortex of the petrous bone. Intratumoral spicules are often seen (Juliano 2018) (Fig. 6.36).

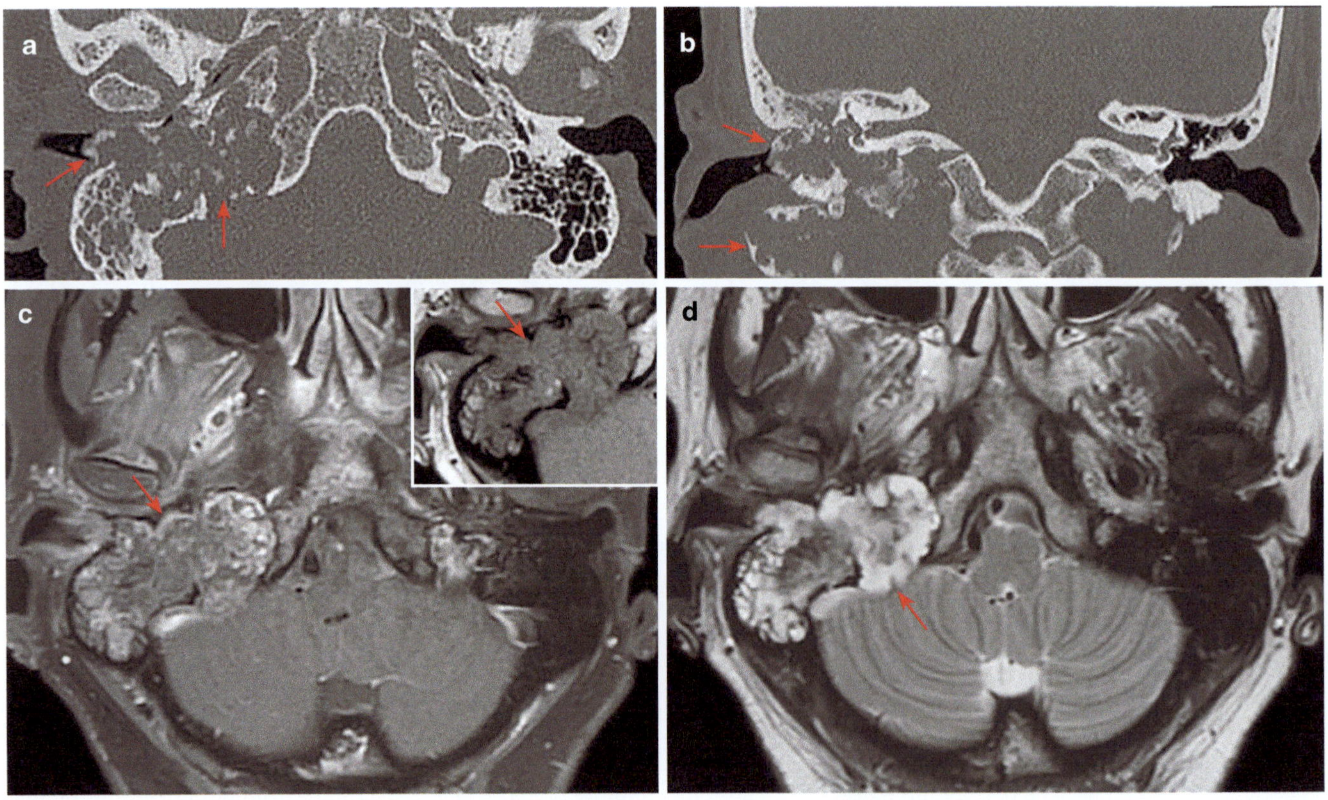

Fig. 6.35 Cartilaginous tumor of right temporal bone. (**a**) Axial CT; (**b**) Coronal CT; (**c**) Axial MRI T_1MI postgadolinium; (**d**) Axial MRI T_2 MI. Female, 47 years old, right facial paralysis for 10 years. (**a, b**) Occupying lesions was centered on the jugular foramen (↑), mixed density, with calcification and bone destruction coexisted, mass had protruded into external auditory canal and tympanum and neck; Facial nerve mastoid segment, internal carotid artery and jugular foramen were also involved; (**c**) Enhancement mixed hyperintense signal mass (↑) had surrounding internal jugular vein and partial posterior cranial nerve; inset (T_1): Mass (↑) showed mixed equal signal; (**d**) Mass (↑) showed mixed strong hyperintense signal, internal flow void

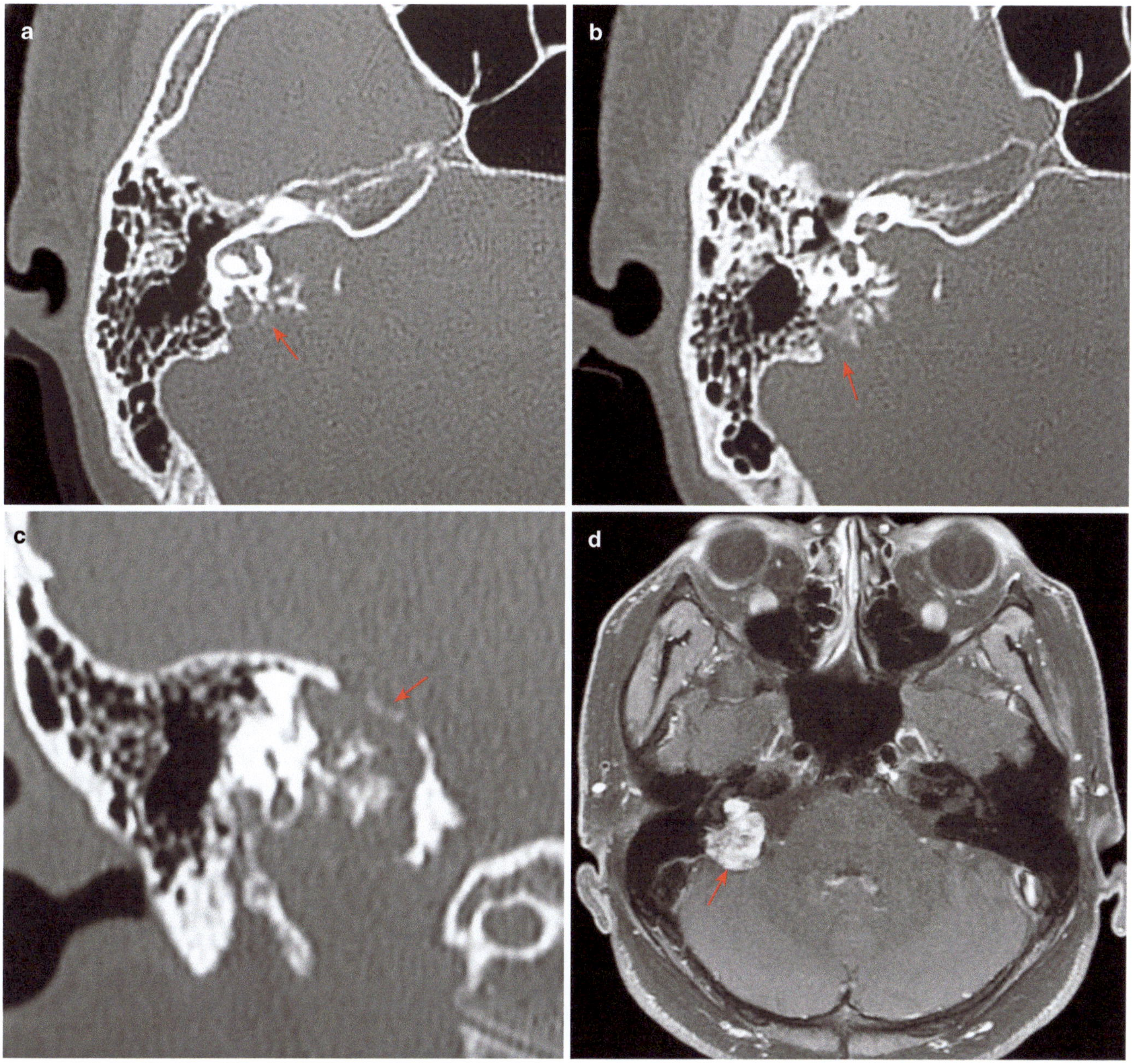

Fig. 6.36 Endolymphatic sac tumor of right ear. (**a, b**) Axial CT; (**c**) Coronal CT; (**d**) Axial MRI T_1 MI postgadolinium. Male, 26 years old. (**a–c**) Bone destruction (↑) in right endolymphatic sac area, patchy or needle-like erosive bone destruction in center with incomplete bone shell in the periphery; (**d**) Uneven and significant enhancement signal in center of mass (↑) (suggesting calcification, cystic change, and subacute hemorrhagic necrosis area in tumor rich in blood vessels), and flow void signal shadow could be seen inside.

Note: This disease needs to be differentiated from the following diseases:

1. Inflammatory pseudotumor of the endolymphatic sac: The incidence rate of inflammatory pseudotumor of the endolymphatic sac is only 1% of its tumor. The clinical manifestations (hearing loss, dizziness) and imaging are similar to the tumor, which depends on pathological differentiation;
2. Schwannoma: Schwannoma (CT imaging) in this area shows that the adjacent compressed bone is incomplete, with sharp edges, and no bone marrow cavity is involved;
3. Glomus jugular tumor: Glomus jugular tumor originates from the glomus jugular, mainly manifested by nerve paralysis, pulsating tinnitus, hearing loss and worm-bitten osteolytic destruction of CT imaging, can involve the tympanum, external auditory canal, internal acoustic meatus, carotid canal, etc., and can pass through the inside and outside of the skull along the jugular vein. MRI can have salt and pepper signs

7 Cerebellopontine Angle Diseases

Yong Li, Zilong Yu, Shubin Chen, Jie Wang, and Bentao Yang

The cerebellopontine angle area is surrounded by the medial brainstem, the posterior cerebellomedullary angle and cerebellum, the anterior petrous part of the temporal bone, the lower IX, X, XI cranial nerves, and the upper cerebellar tentorium. In addition to the V, VII, and VII cranial nerves, there are also anteroinferior cerebellar artery and internal auditory artery in this area. The nerves, blood vessels, bone, cartilage, and embryonic residual tissues in this area may have pathological changes, and there may also be distant metastatic tumors.

Acoustic neuroma and meningioma are the most common tumors in the cerebellopontine angle. In addition, there are neurogliomas, ependymomas, basilar artery varicose aneurysms, and metastatic carcinomas, which have different clinical manifestations due to different origins of tumors in this region. Taking acoustic neuroma as an example, according to its degree of development, it can appear as follows: unilateral sensorineural hearing loss, gradually increasing high-pitched tinnitus, dizziness or vertigo, facial numbness (involving the fifth cranial nerve), facial weakness, and facial paralysis (involving the seventh cranial nerve), gait instability and path deviation (involving cerebellar function), dysphagia and dysphonia (involving the ninth and tenth cranial nerve), and later headache symptoms such as optic papilla edema (intracranial hypertension) (Wang, 1994).

Y. Li
Department of Neurosurgery, Beijing Tongren Hospital, Capital Medical University, Beijing, China

Z. Yu (✉) · S. Chen · J. Wang
Department of Otolaryngology Head and Neck Surgery, Beijing Tongren Hospital, Capital Medical University, Beijing, China

B. Yang
Department of Radiology, Beijing Tongren Hospital, Capital Medical University, Beijing, China

7.1 Acoustic Neuroma

Acoustic neuroma, also known as acoustic neuromeningioma, mostly comes from vestibular nerve, and about 70%–80% of the tumors originate in the internal acoustic meatus, accounting for 8%–10% of intracranial tumors, accounting for 80%–90% of cerebellopontine angle, mostly seen in adults, slightly more in women, more in unilateral cases (95%), without family history and heredity, and most of the tumors are unilateral solitary; bilateral cases are rare (called NF2, neurofibromatosis) (5%). They are autosomal dominant hereditary diseases, which are manifested as bilateral acoustic neuromas, and age of onset is relatively young.

The posterior wall of the internal acoustic meatus is relatively thin. The benign tumors in the internal acoustic meatus, like acoustic neuromas, are more likely to cause the posterior wall of the internal acoustic meatus to become blunt and its acute angle to disappear, resulting in the conical expansion of the internal acoustic meatus. Therefore, the temporal bone CT horizontal (axial) scanning is more advantageous when observing the changes of the internal acoustic meatus.

It is difficult to recognize soft tissue masses within the IAC on CT. However, if the IAC is dilated and smoothly scalloped with a focally expansile appearance, an underlying mass should be suspected, most commonly a vestibular schwannoma. A meningioma tends to be centered at the cerebellopontine angle cistern (CPA) rather than the IAC, and does not cause expansion of the porus acusticus or IAC, although the surrounding bone might be involved with a mixed permeative/sclerotic/hyperostotic appearance (Juliano, 2018) (Figs. 7.1, 7.2, 7.3, 7.4, 7.5,7.6, and 7.7).

Z. Yu (ed.), *Ear Diseases and CT*, https://doi.org/10.1007/978-981-99-7220-3_7

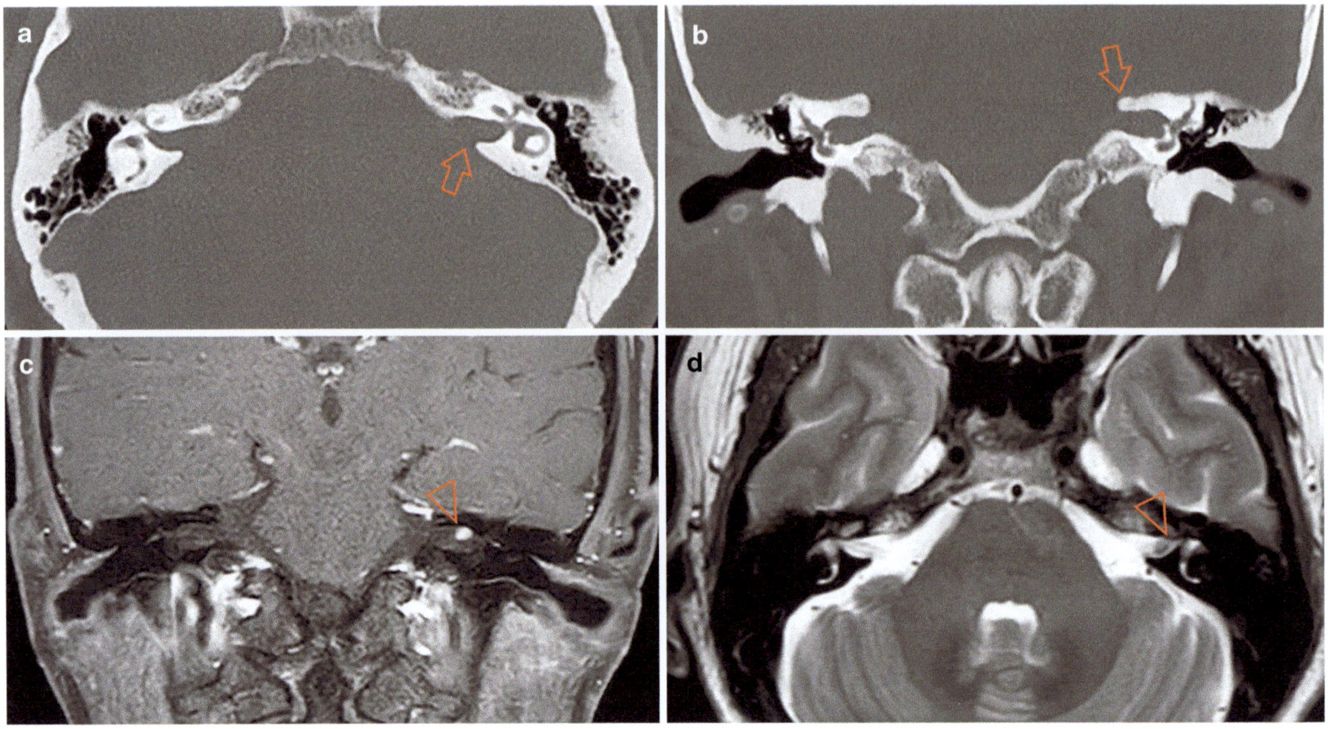

Fig. 7.1 Microacoustic neuroma (intraductal type) in left ear. (**a**) Axial CT; (**b**) Coronal CT; (**c**) Coronal MRI T_1 MI postgadolinium; (**d**) Axial MRI T_2 MI. Female, 53 years old. (**a, b**) There is no obvious abnormality in bone wall and lumen of internal acoustic meatus of bilateral ears (⇧); (**c**) MRI enhancement showed abnormal hyperintense signal shadow near fundus of internal acoustic meatus (△); (**d**) MRI T_2 showed equal signal or slightly hypointense signal shadow at fundus of internal acoustic meatus of left ear (△), the boundary is clear.

Note: When the diameter of acoustic neuroma is smaller than the diameter of internal acoustic meatus, it is difficult to find the small acoustic neuroma in its canal by bone window CT scan, the advantage of MRI is that it can detect small tumors in the bone canal when the bone wall has not changed (Jäger, 2001)

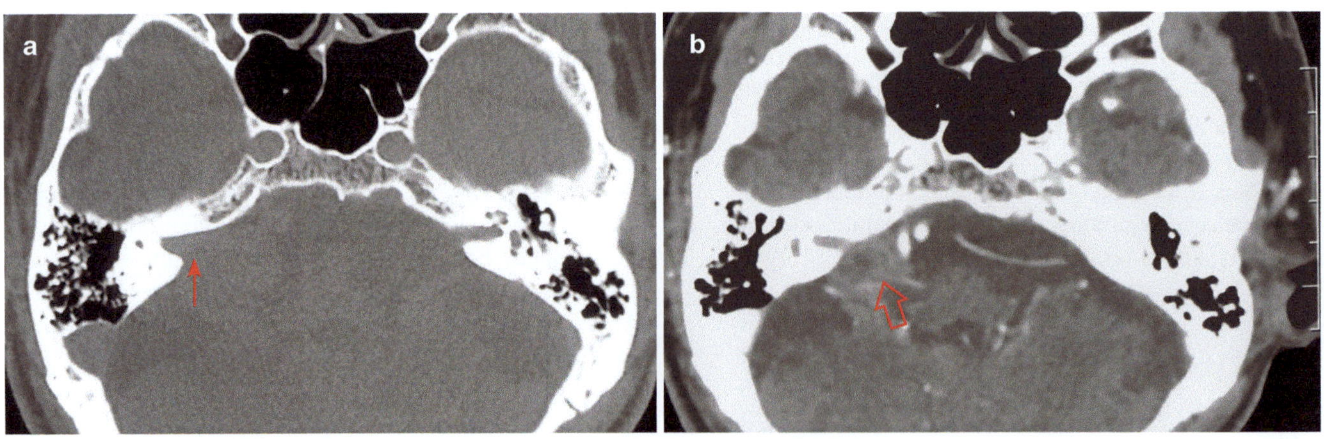

Fig. 7.2 Acoustic neuroma of right ear (**a**) Axial CT; (**b**) Brain CT postgadolinium**.** Male, 75 years old. (**a**) Conical enlargement of right internal acoustic meatus (↑); (**b**) Brain CT enhancement showed soft tissue mass (⇧) in cerebellopontine angle

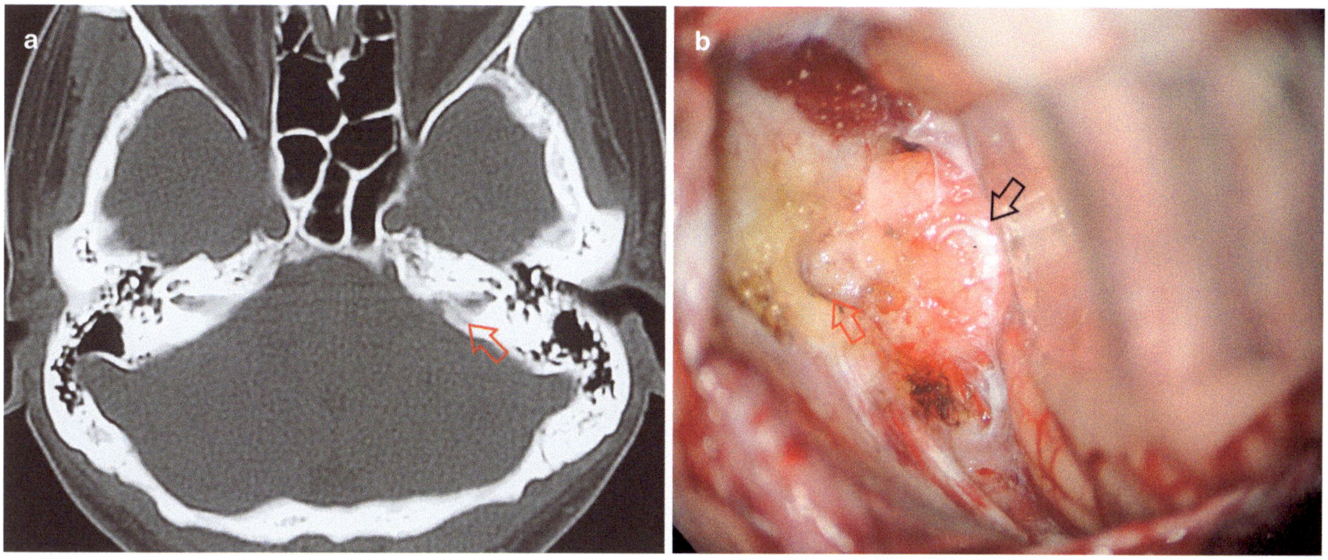

Fig. 7.3 Acoustic neuroma of left ear. (**a**) Axial CT; (**b**) Intraoperative finding. Female, 48 years old. (**a**) Left internal acoustic meatus showed conical expansion (⇧); (**b**) When partial superior wall of internal acoustic meatus removal, internal acoustic meatus was found to be enlarged (⇧), and a neoformation was seen in cerebellopontine angle area (⇧) (middle cranial fossa approach)

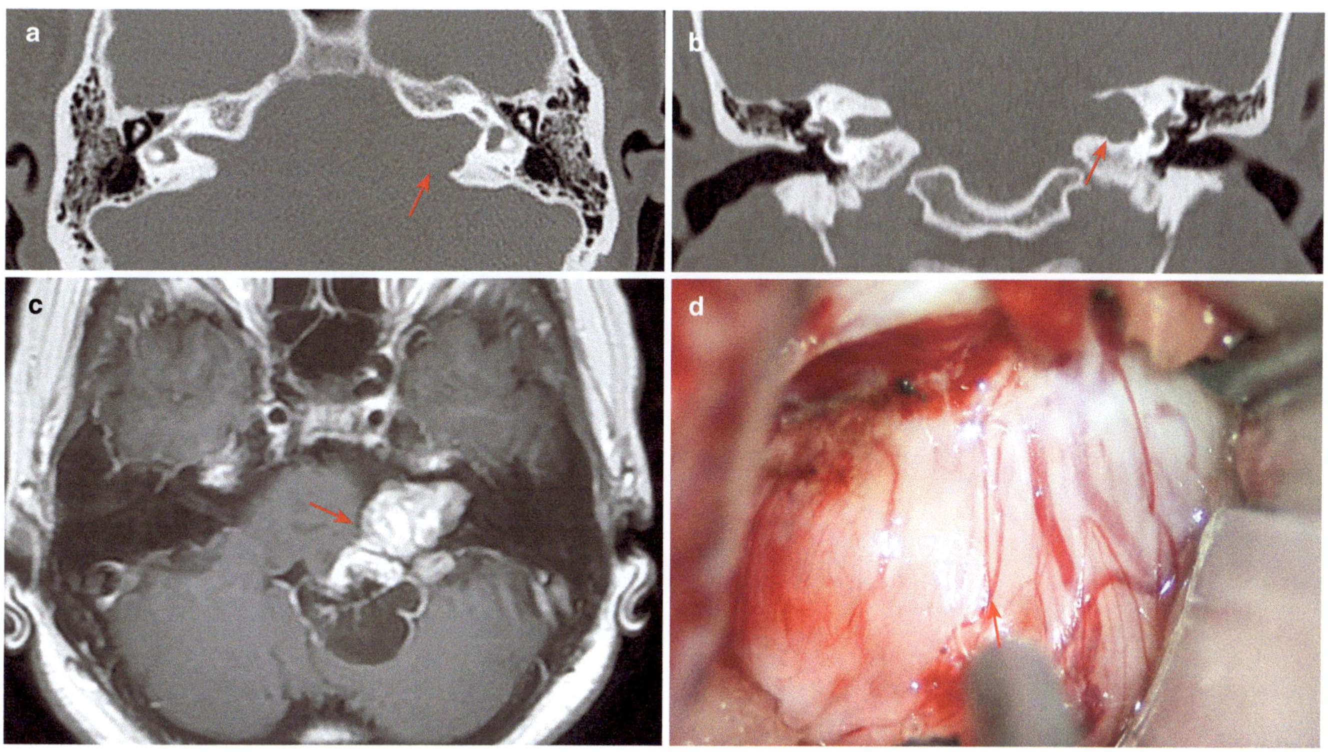

Fig. 7.4 Large acoustic neuroma in left ear. (**a**) Axial CT; (**b**) Coronal CT; (**c**) Axial MRI T_1 WI postgadolinium; (**d**) Intraoperative finding. Female, 25 years old. (**a, b**) Internal acoustic meatus of left ear presented conical expansion (↑); (**c**) Enhancement soft tissue mass in left cerebellar pontine angle showed mixed hyperintense and flow void signal shadow (↑), tumor had significantly compressed brainstem and cerebellum; (**d**) Tumor mass with abundant blood supply (↑) was clearly defined during surgery

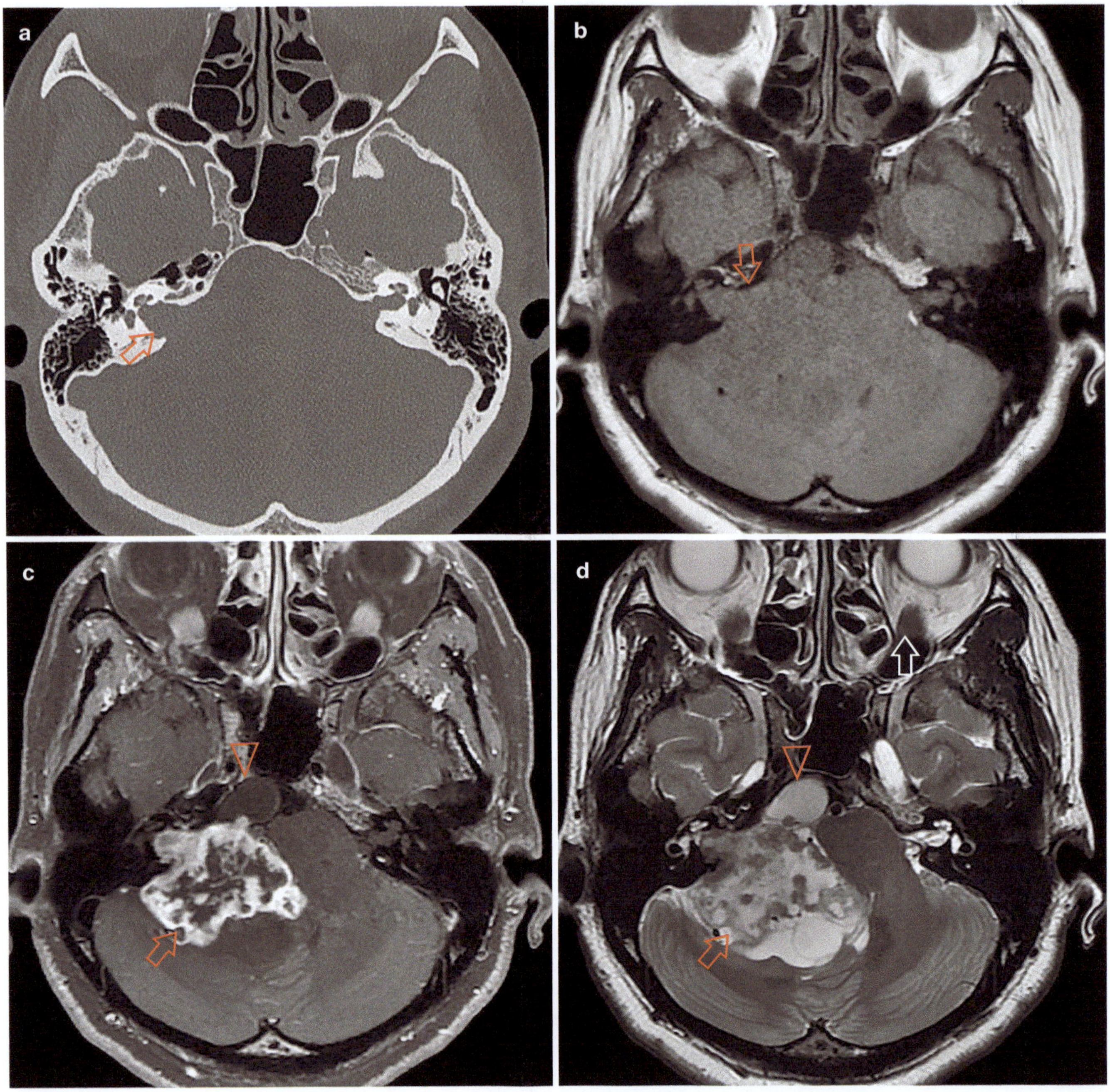

Fig. 7.5 Right giant acoustic neuroma. (**a**) Axial CT; (**b**) Axial MRI T_1 WI; (**c**) Axial MRI T_1 WI postgadolinium; (**d**) Axial MRI T_2 WI. Female, 29 years old. (**a**) Internal acoustic meatus of right ear was conical expansion (⇧); (**b**) Right cerebellopontine angle area showed slightly hypointense signal shadow (⇧); (**c**) Right cerebellopontine angle area and internal acoustic meatus presented irregular strong hyperintense signal shadow (⇧), central hypointense signal shadow (liquefied) (cystic acoustic neuroma), tumor tissue had crossed midline causing brainstem compression and displacement, fatty tissue of petrous apex (▲); (**d**) Right cerebellopontine corner area and internal acoustic meatus showed hyperintense and medium mixed signal shadow (⇧), fatty tissue of petrous apex (▲)

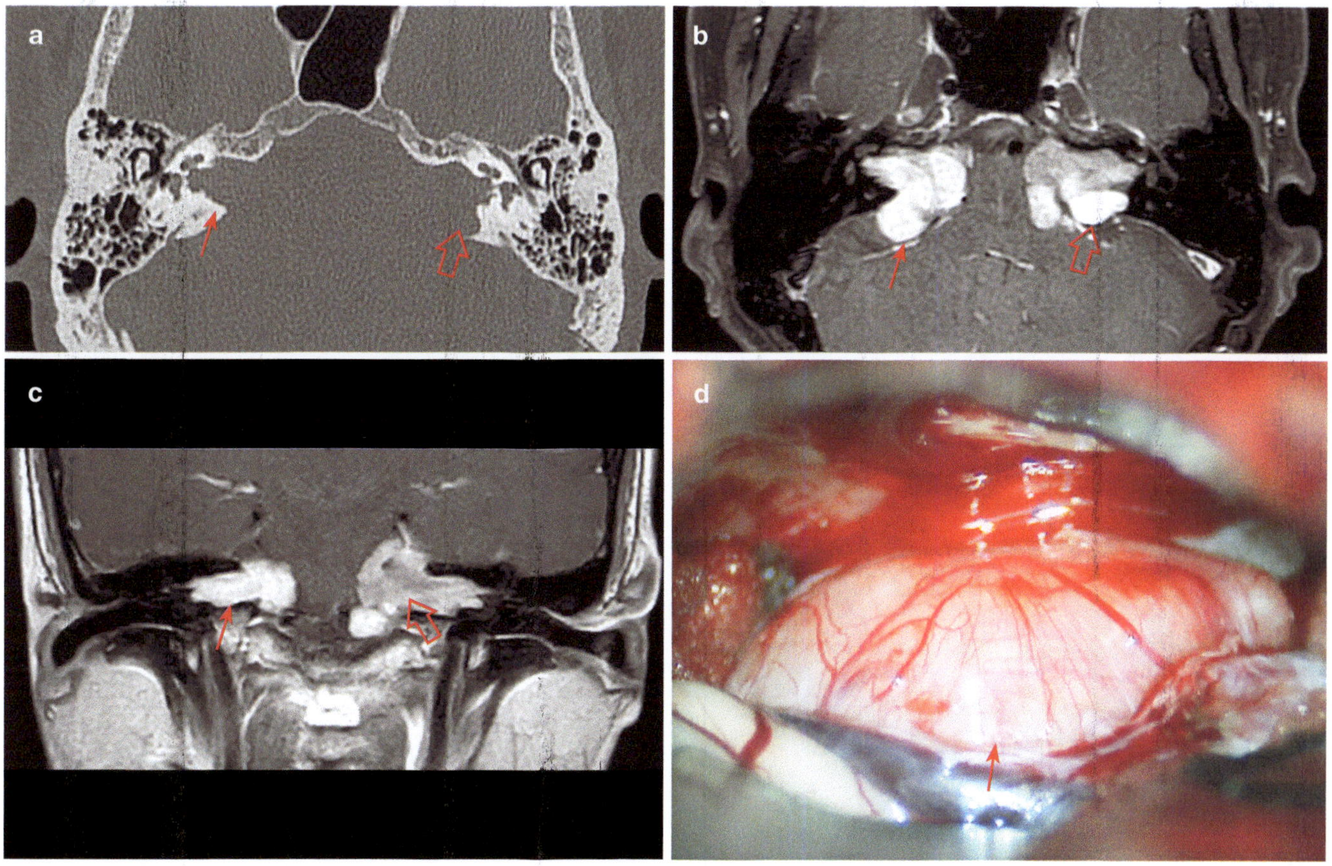

Fig. 7.6 Auditory neurofibromatosis (bilateral ears). (**a**) Axial CT; (**b**) Axial MRI T_1 WI postgadolinium; (**c**) Axial MRI T_1 WI postgadolinium; (**d**) Intraoperative finding. Male, 33 years old. (**a**) Internal acoustic meatus of bilateral ears was conical expansion (right ↑, left ⇧); (**b**, **c**) Right ear mass showed gourd-like hyperintense signal shadow (↑), left ear postoperative change (⇧); (**d**) Tumor mass (↑) with clear boundaries, rich blood supply

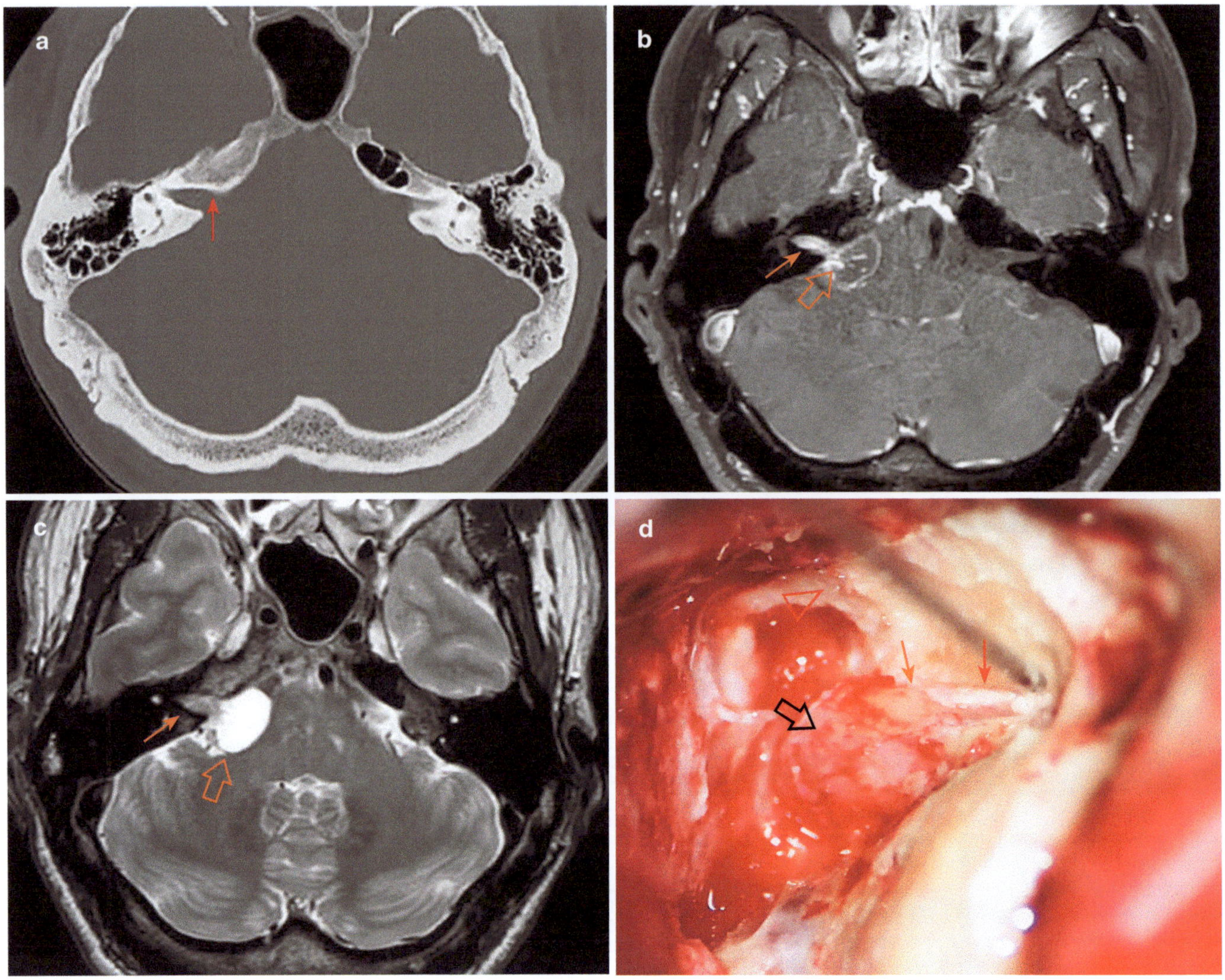

Fig. 7.7 Right ear acoustic neuroma. (**a**) Axial CT; (**b**) Axial MRI T_1 WI postgadolinium; (**c**) Axial MRI T_2 WI; (**d**) Intraoperative finding. Male, 47 years old, right tinnitus and hearing loss for 10 years. (**a**) Right internal acoustic meatus was conical enlarged (↑); (**b**) Enhanced MRI showed hyperintense signal shadow in right internal acoustic meatus(↑) and extended to cerebellopontine angle area (⇧), which was flask-shaped, center of tumor body was hypointense signal (liquefaction), and the surrounding was hyperintense signal; (**c**) Tumor mass showed slightly hyperintense signal in internal acoustic meatus (↑) and hyperintense signal in tumor body (⇧); (**d**) Enlarged labyrinthine approach showed tumors (⇧) in cerebellopontine angle area and internal acoustic meatus (↑) and petrous apex (△), which had adhesion with surrounding brain tissue

7.2 Meningioma

See Fig. 7.8.

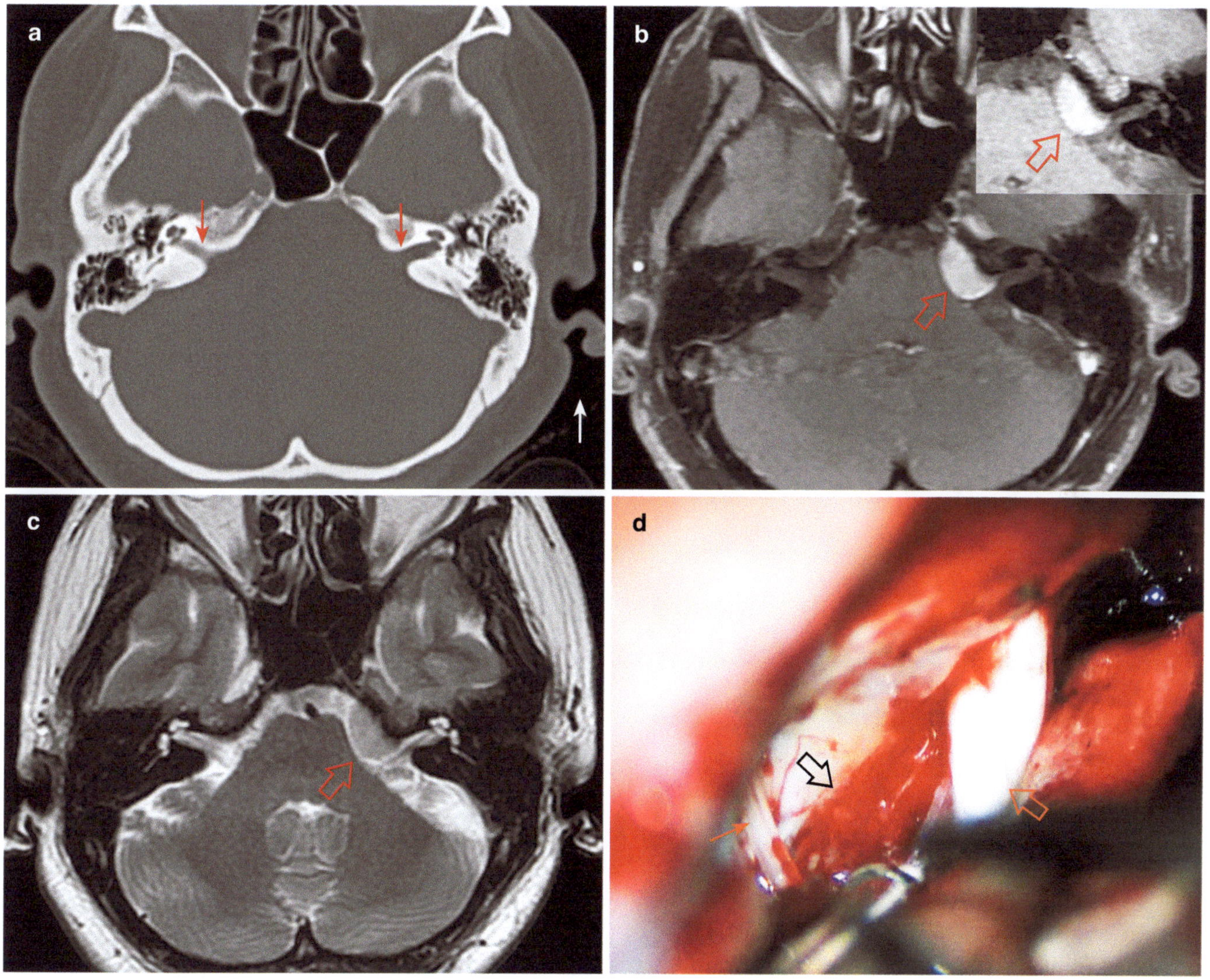

Fig. 7.8 Left cerebellopontine angle meningioma. (**a**) Axial CT; (**b**) Axial MRI T_1 WI postgadolinium; (**c**) Axial MRI T_2 WI; (**d**) Intraoperative finding. Female, 43 years old. (**a**) Bilateral internal acoustic meatus bone (↑) was normal; (**b**) Enhancement cerebellopontine angle tumor (⇧) showed semi-moon hyperintense signal shadow, internal acoustic meatus hypointense signal. Inset (T_1WI): Tumor (⇧) showed equal signal shadow, internal acoustic meatus showed hypointense signal shadow; (**c**) Tumor slightly hypointense signal shadow (⇧), internal acoustic meatus showed equal signal shadow; (**d**) Tumor (⇧) was grayish red, rich blood supply, base of tumor was located in the deep part of facial nerve in internal acoustic meatus (⇧), glossopharyngeal nerve (↑).

Note: Typical findings of meningioma of cerebellopontine angle are differentiated them from acoustic neuromas as follows: (1) (MRI) Meningiomas are sessile, possessing a broad base against the petrous face, whereas acoustic neuromas are globular; They are often extrinsic and eccentric to the internal auditory canal (IAC); when involving the IAC, they usually do not erode the IAC; (2) (CT)Meningiomas of cerebellopontine angle demonstrate hyperostosis of the subjacent bone and possess intratumoral calcification (Fig. 9.1); (3) Meningiomas of cerebellopontine angle involve adjacent intracranial spaces and structures, and they are characterized by a distinctive dural "tail" extending away from the tumor surface (Lalwani et al. 1993).

MR is often more helpful for diagnosis of neuromas, epidermoid cysts, exophytic gliomas, and vascular lesions, while CT is usually more informative for diagnosis of meningiomas, metastases in cerebellopontine angle. MRI with high accuracy in lesion detection, characterization, and localization, is a suitable primary diagnostic modality for evaluating patients with suspected cerebellopontine angle lesions (Lalwani et al. 1993)

7.3 Cholesteatoma

See Fig. 7.9.

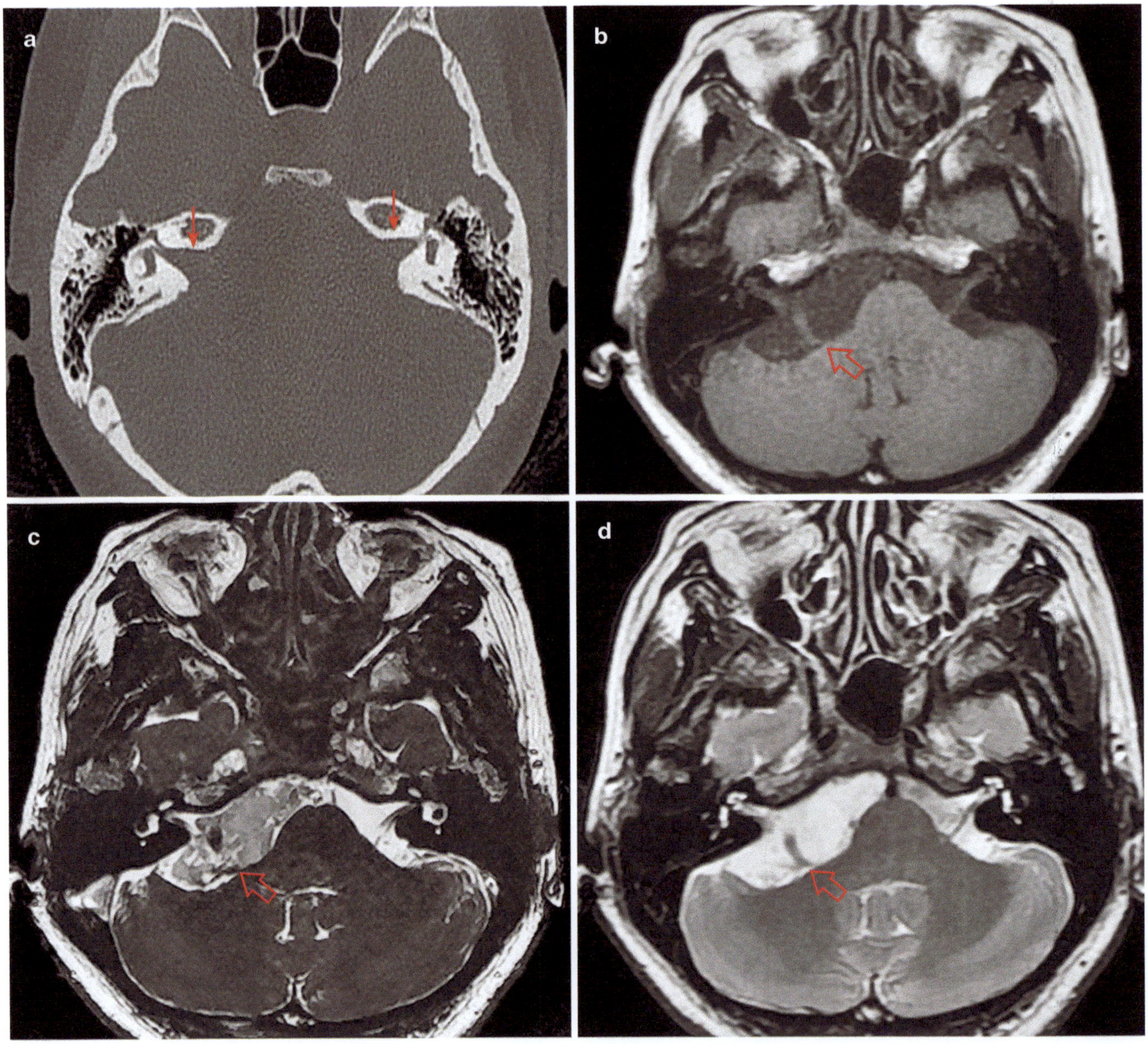

Fig. 7.9 Cholesteatoma of cerebellopontine angle. (**a**) Axial CT; (**b**) Axial MRI T_1 WI; (**c**) Axial MRI T_1 WI postgadolinium; (**d**) MRI T_2 WI. Female, 40 years old. (**a**) No abnormality was found in bilateral internal acoustic meatus (↑); (**b**) Cerebellopontine angle hypointense signal shadow (⇧); (**c**) Peripheral hyperintense signal shadow, central hypointense and mixed hyperintense signal area in enhanced cerebellopontine angle (⇧); (**d**) Cerebellopontine angle hyperintense signal shadow (⇧).

Note: Cholesteatoma MRI T1 WI shows relatively homogeneous hypointense signal, MRI T2 WI shows homogeneous hyperintense signal, this can be distinguished from cholesterol granuloma (Fig. 8.2) which MRI T1 WI and MRI T2 WI are both hyperintense signal areas.

Figures. 7.1, 7.7, and 7.8, suggest that when the symptoms of unilateral ear cannot be explained by the results of bone window CT scan, further examination should be performed, including MRI and enhanced brain CT

8 Petrous Apex Disease

Yong Li, Bentao Yang, and Zilong Yu

The petrous apex, which is the most medial portion of the temporal bone, is also a complex region of the central skull base. Lesions arising in or spreading to the petrous apex can cause varied and severe sequelae, which may result from mass effect or direct invasion of the cranial nerves, brainstem, or internal carotid artery. Because the petrous apex is not amenable to direct examination, HRCT and MR imaging plays an important role in diagnosis and characterization of lesions occurring there, and in aiding surgical planning.

Cholesterol granuloma is the most common primary disease of the petrous apex. Other diseases include cephaloceles, primary cholesteatoma, aneurysm, chordoma, benign and malignant chondroma and osteoma, metastatic cancer, and petrous apex syndrome caused by otitis media. Reduced diffusivity without associated enhancement is pathognomonic for a cholesteatoma (epidermoid). Intrinsic T_1 hyperintensity is diagnostic of a cholesterol granuloma (Connor et al. 2008; Pisaneschi et al. 2000; Razek et al. 2012; Schmalfuss, 2009; Tringali et al. 2010).

Y. Li
Department of Neurosurgery, Beijing Tongren Hospital, Capital Medical University, Beijing, China

B. Yang
Department of Radiology, Beijing Tongren Hospital, Capital Medical University, Beijing, China

Z. Yu (✉)
Department of Otolaryngology Head and Neck Surgery, Beijing Tongren Hospital, Capital Medical University, Beijing, China

Z. Yu (ed.), *Ear Diseases and CT*, https://doi.org/10.1007/978-981-99-7220-3_8

8.1 Cerebrospinal Fluid Otorrhea Caused by Petrous Apex Deformity

See Fig. 8.1.

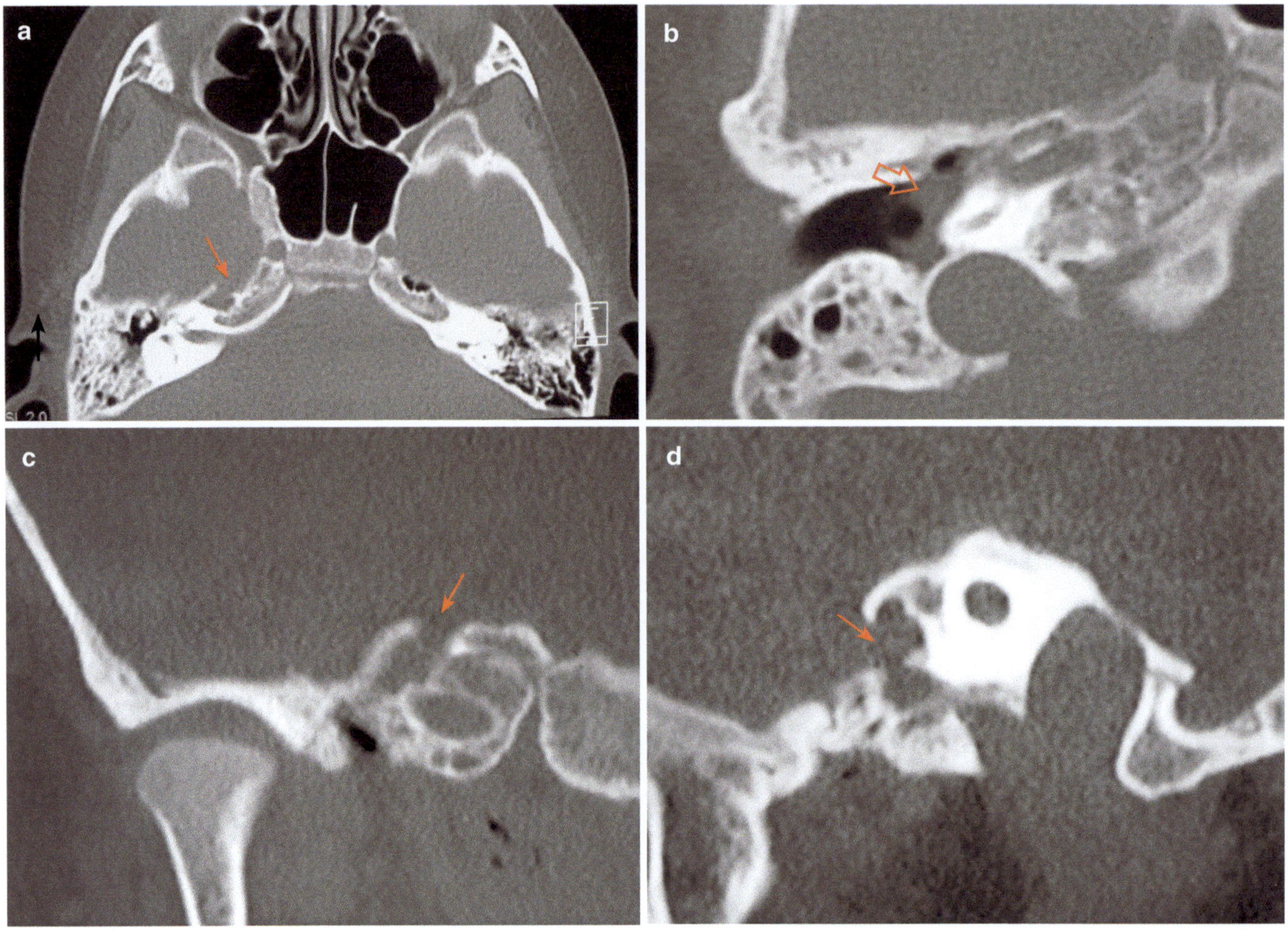

Fig. 8.1 Right petrous apex bone loss and meningoencephalocele and cerebrospinal fluid otorrhea. (**a**, **b**) Axial CT; (**c**) Coronal CT; (**d**) Sagittal CT. Male, 10 years old, multiple meningitis. (**a**) Bone absence of petrous apex (↑); (**b**) Soft tissue shadow (⇧) (cerebrospinal fluid otorrhea) in tympanic cavity and mastoid cavity; (**c**) Bone absence of petrous apex above eustachian tube and meningoencephalocele (↑); (**d**) Bone absence of petrous apex (↑).

Note: When cerebrospinal fluid otorrhea is suspected, MR hydrography examination is needed

8.2 Inflammatory Disease of Petrous Apex and Cholesteatoma

See Figs. 8.2 and 8.3.

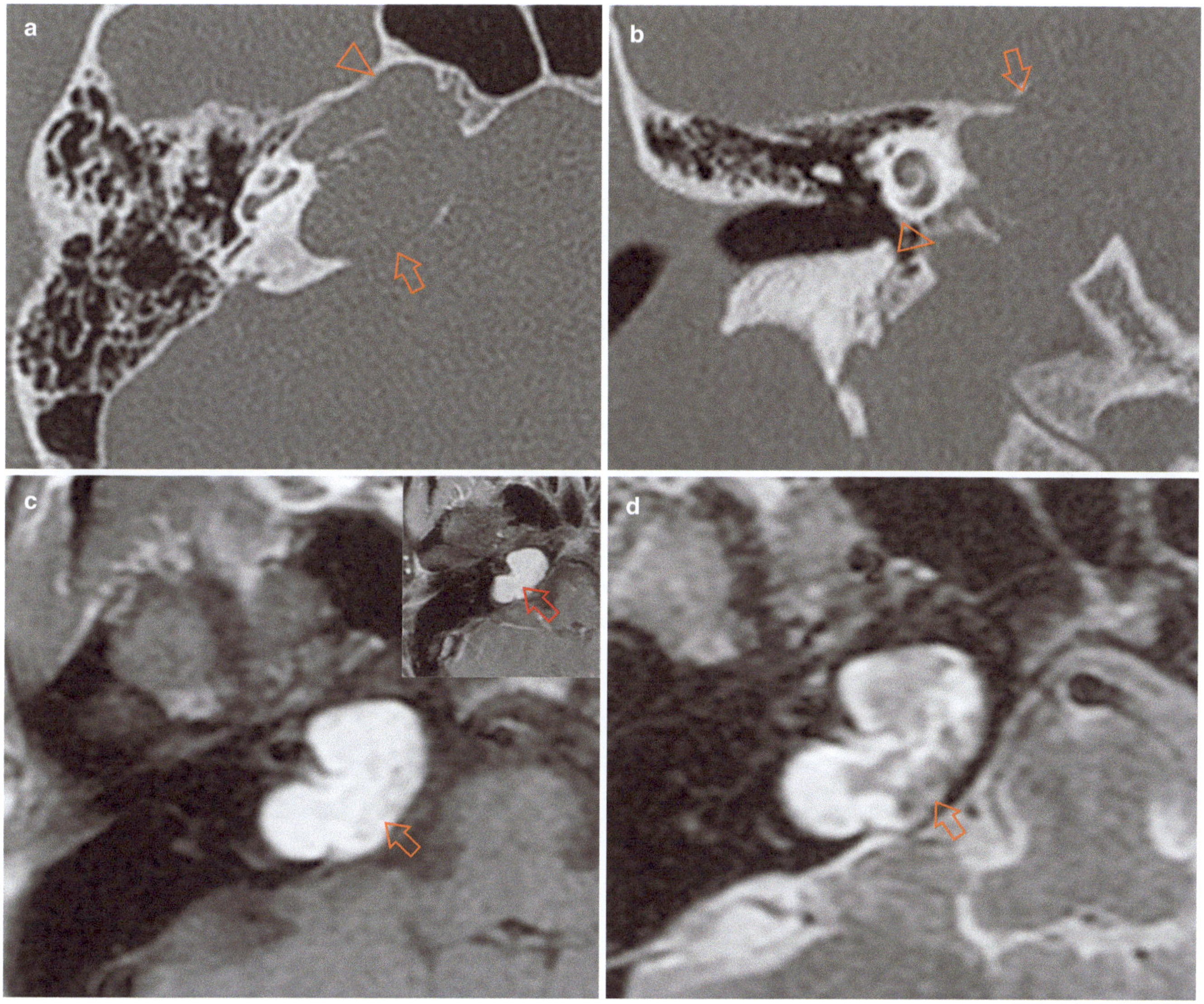

Fig. 8.2 Cholesterol granuloma at right petrous apex. (**a**) Axial CT; (**b**) Coronal CT; (**c**) Axial MRI T_1 WI; (**d**) Axial MRI T_2 WI. Female, 40 years old. (**a**, **b**) Right ear petrous apex showed expansive bone destruction (⇧), indistinct boundary with carotid artery duct (△); (**c**) MRI T_1 and MRI T_1 enhancement (insert) showed hyperintense signal shadow (⇧), clear boundary; (**d**) Mixed signal shadow (⇧), surrounding of mass was hyperintense signal shadow, center was hypointense signal shadow.

Note: Cholesterol granuloma may be the reaction of multinucleated giant cells to foreign bodies to the stimulation of cholesterol crystals, followed by inflammation, small vessel proliferation, rupture, and then repeated bleeding of granulation tissue, forming expansive damage at the petrous apex. The hyperintense signal of MRI T1 WI and MRI T2 WI is the manifestation of hemorrhage, blood decomposition products and cholesterol crystals, and the hypointensive signal can be interpreted as the deposition of hemosiderin. MRI T1 WI postgadolinium is not significantly enhanced further (note the difference with cholesteatoma Fig. 7.8), that means MRI T1 WI, MRI T1 WI postgadolinium and MRI T2 WI show hyperintense signals in the meantime. Because cholesterol granuloma has no squamous epithelium, it is different from the treatment of petrous apex cholesteatoma: cholesterol granuloma mainly needs unobstructed drainage, while cholesteatoma has to be completely cleared

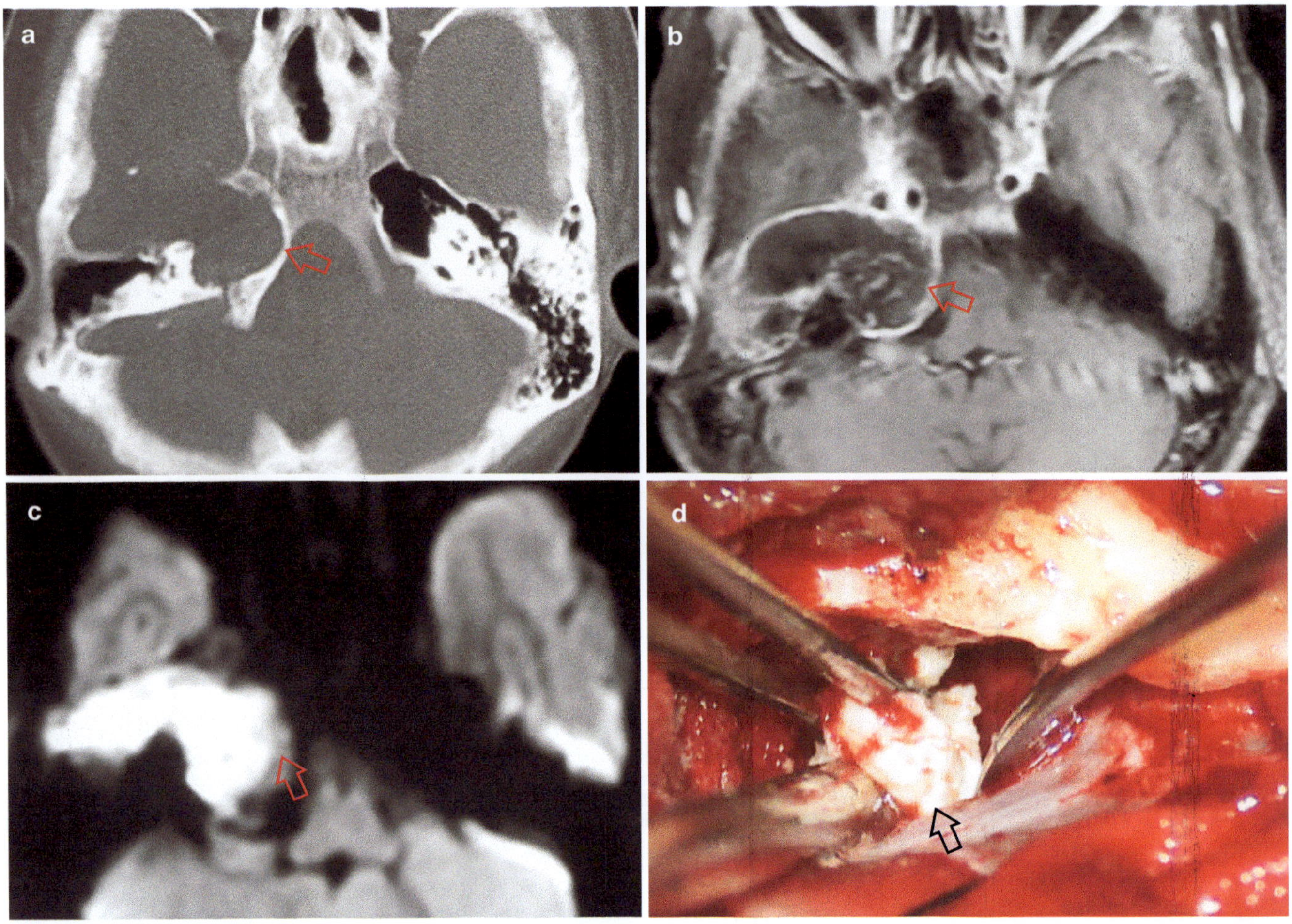

Fig. 8.3 Petrous apex cholesteatoma in right ear. (**a**) Axial CT; (**b**) Axial MRI T_1 WI postgadolinium; (**c**) Axial MRI DWI. Female, 52 years old. (**a**) Right ear petrous apex showed expansive bone destruction (⇧) and bone loss, and communicated with middle cranial fossa; (**b**) MRI T_1 enhanced peripheral hyperintense signal, central hypointense signal shadow (⇧); (**c**) MRI DWI (diffusion-weighted imaging) hyperintense signal shadow (⇧); (**d**) Petrous apex cholesteatoma epithelial mass (⇧).

Note: Petrous apex cholesteatoma accounts for about 2% of all temporal bone cholesteatomas, which may originate from aberrant embryonic epithelial nest. CT scan cannot differentiate petrous apex cholesterol granuloma from cholesteatoma

8.3 Petrous Apex Tumor

See Fig. 8.4.

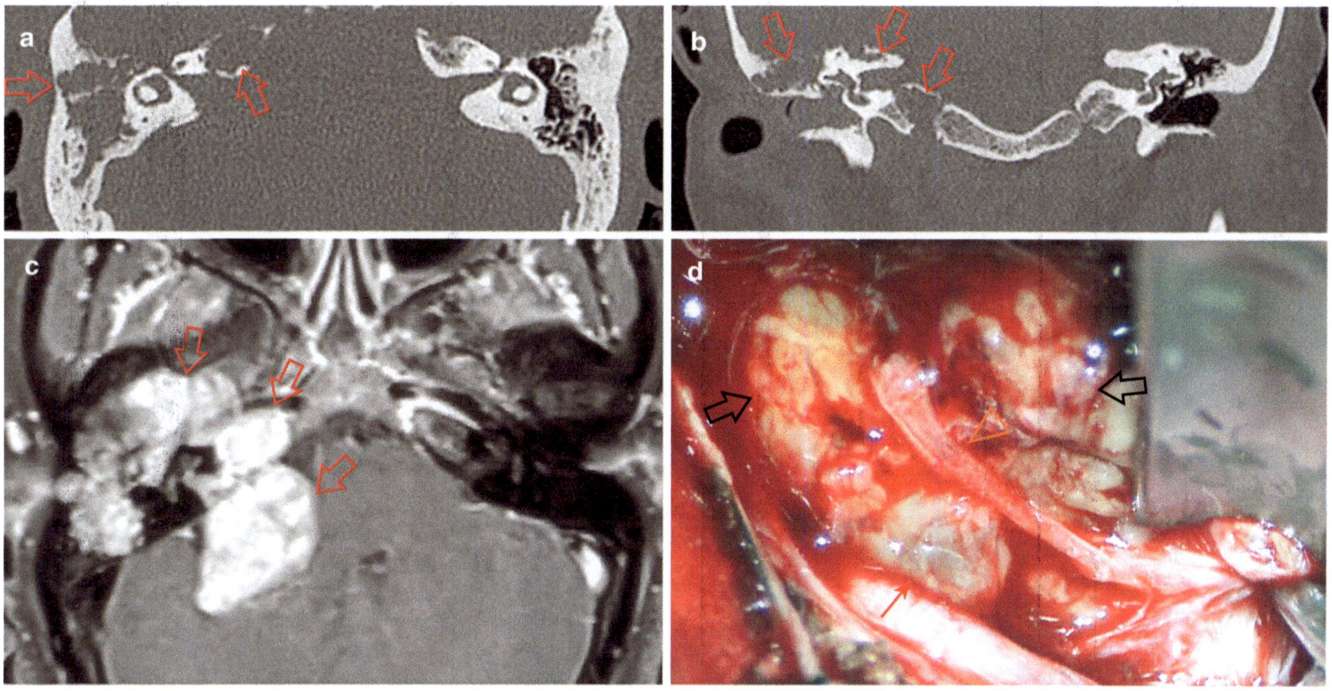

Fig. 8.4 Right petrous apex neurilemmoma. (**a**) Axial CT; (**b**) Coronal CT; (**c**) Axial MRI T_1 WI postgadolinium; (**d**) Intraoperative findings. Female, 46 years old. (**a**, **b**) Irregular bone destruction in squamous portion, tympanic portion, petrous portion and petrous apex of right temporal bone (⇧), ipsilateral expansive internal acoustic meatus; (**c**) Petrous apex, middle cranial fossa, cerebellopontine angle, middle ear and mastoid process with mixed hyperintense signal shadow (⇧), flow void signal shadow in the tumor; (**d**) Tumor was lobulated (⇧), enveloped, gray white, brittle, local cystic change (↑), trigeminal nerve root (△) was surrounded by tumor

Adjacent Diseases Invading Temporal Bone and Metastatic Carcinoma of Temporal Bone

9

Bentao Yang, Yong Li, and Zilong Yu

The temporal bone joined the anterior sphenoid bone and the posterior occipital bone together to forms the lateral skull base, upward adjacent to brain tissue, downward connected to neck, and it houses abundant cranial nerves and blood vessels. Therefore, temporal bone diseases can damage and spread to adjacent tissues and organs, and lesions in adjacent structures can also affect the temporal bone. Remote malignant tumors can reach the temporal bone through blood flow, on the contrary malignant tumors of temporal bone can also metastasize to distant organs.

9.1 Adjacent Diseases Invading Temporal Bone

9.1.1 Temporal Lobe Meningioma Invading Temporal Bone

See Fig. 9.1.

9.1.2 Pituitary Tumor Invading Temporal Bone

See Fig. 9.2.

9.1.3 Clival Chordoma Invading Temporal Bone

See Fig. 9.3, 9.4.

B. Yang
Department of Radiology, Beijing Tongren Hospital, Capital Medical University, Beijing, China

Y. Li
Department of Neurosurgery, Beijing Tongren Hospital, Capital Medical University, Beijing, China

Z. Yu (✉)
Department of Otolaryngology Head and Neck Surgery, Beijing Tongren Hospital, Capital Medical University, Beijing, China

Z. Yu (ed.), *Ear Diseases and CT*, https://doi.org/10.1007/978-981-99-7220-3_9

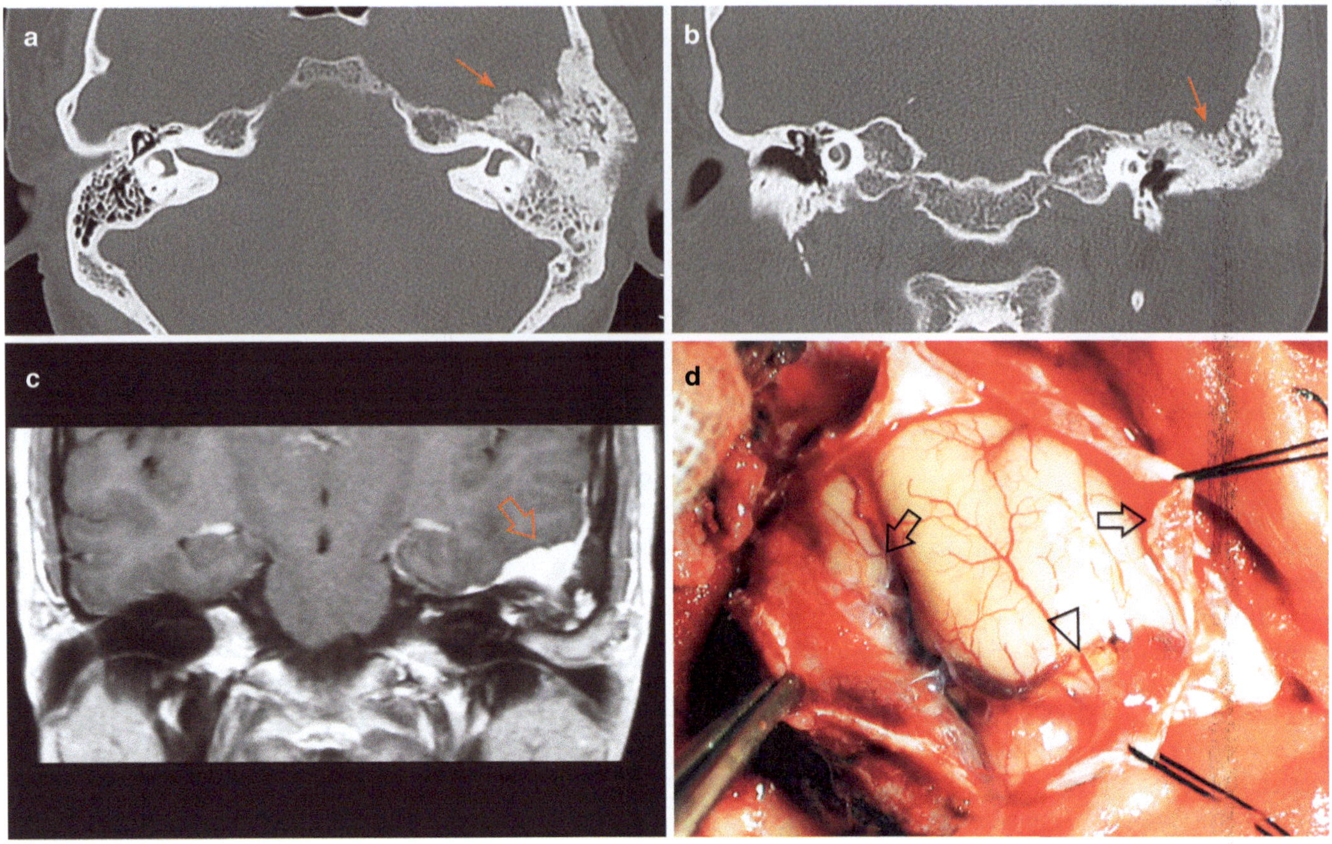

Fig. 9.1 Left flat meningioma with temporal bone hyperplasia and middle ear mastoiditis, (**a**) Axial CT; (**b**) Coronal CT; (**c**) Coronal MRI T_1 WI postgadolinium; (**d**) Intraoperative findings. Female, 48 years old. (**a, b**) Left temporal bone hyperosteogeny, uneven density, rough surface, irregular fine cracks extending into the bone (↑); (**c**) Ipsilateral temporal meningeal thickening with hyperintense signal shadow (⇧), accompanying compression of brain tissue and immersion of temporal bone; (**d**) Tumor (⇧) located in dura mater of skull base, creeping growth in subdural cavity, gray-red color, medium blood supply, slight adhesion with temporal lobe brain tissue (△)

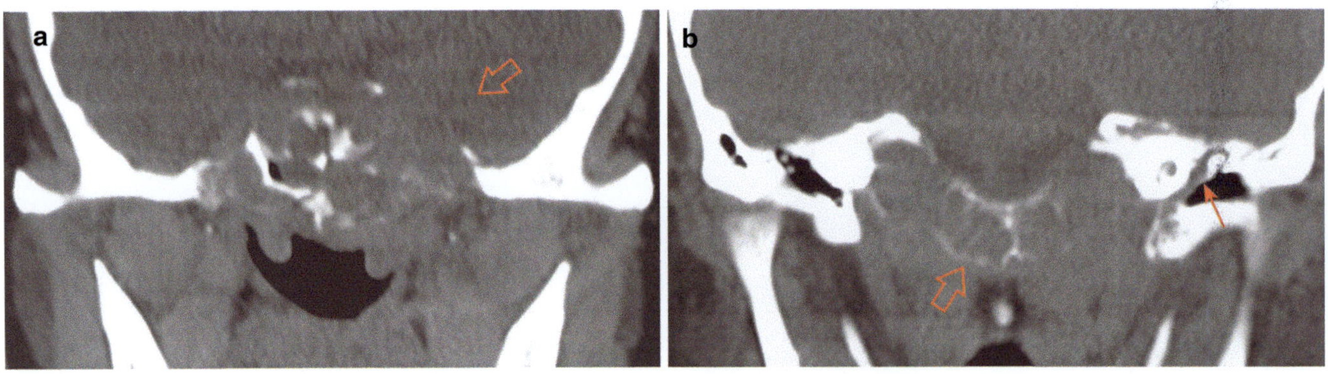

Fig. 9.2 Pituitary tumor with secretory otitis media in right ear. (**a, b**) Coronal CT. Female, 61 years old. (**a**) Irregular destruction and absorption of bone in pituitary fossa (⇧); (**b**) Dissolution of bone in clivus (⇧), involvement of left eustachian tube, left tympanic effusion (↑)

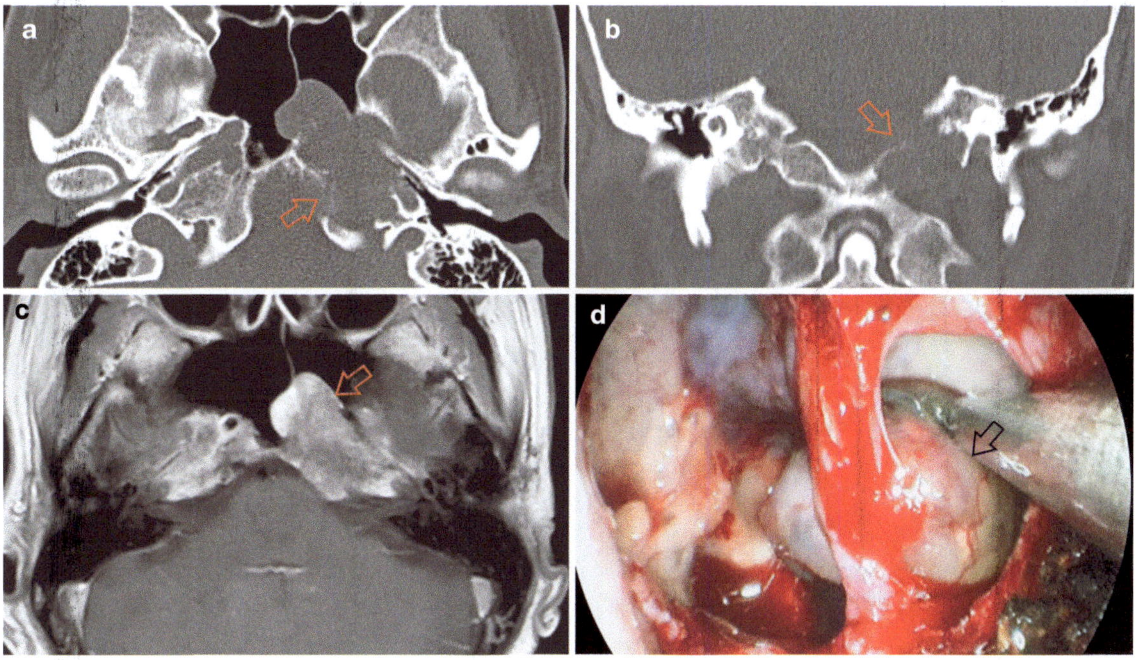

Fig. 9.3 Left clival chordoma invading petrous apex. (**a**) Axial CT; (**b**) Coronal CT; (**c**) Axial MRI T_1 WI postgadolinium; (**d**) Intraoperative finding. Female, 47 years old. (**a, b**) Left clivus, foramen lacerum bone destruction and absorption (⇧), mass protruded into ipsilateral sphenoid sinus; (**c**) Enhanced mass showed medium signal to hyperintense signal shadow (⇧) protruded into sphenoid sinus; (**d**) Endoscopic view of smooth, solid, light red mass (⇧) via anterior wall of sphenoid sinus.

Chordoma is a rare intracranial bone cancer that is aggressive, locally invasive, and has a poor prognosis, which originate from the residual notochord, and the nodular residual of the notochord can be seen throughout the interior of each vertebral body of the spine, The clivus and coccygeal region are the most common (Walcott et al. 2012) (Figs. 9.3 and 9.4)

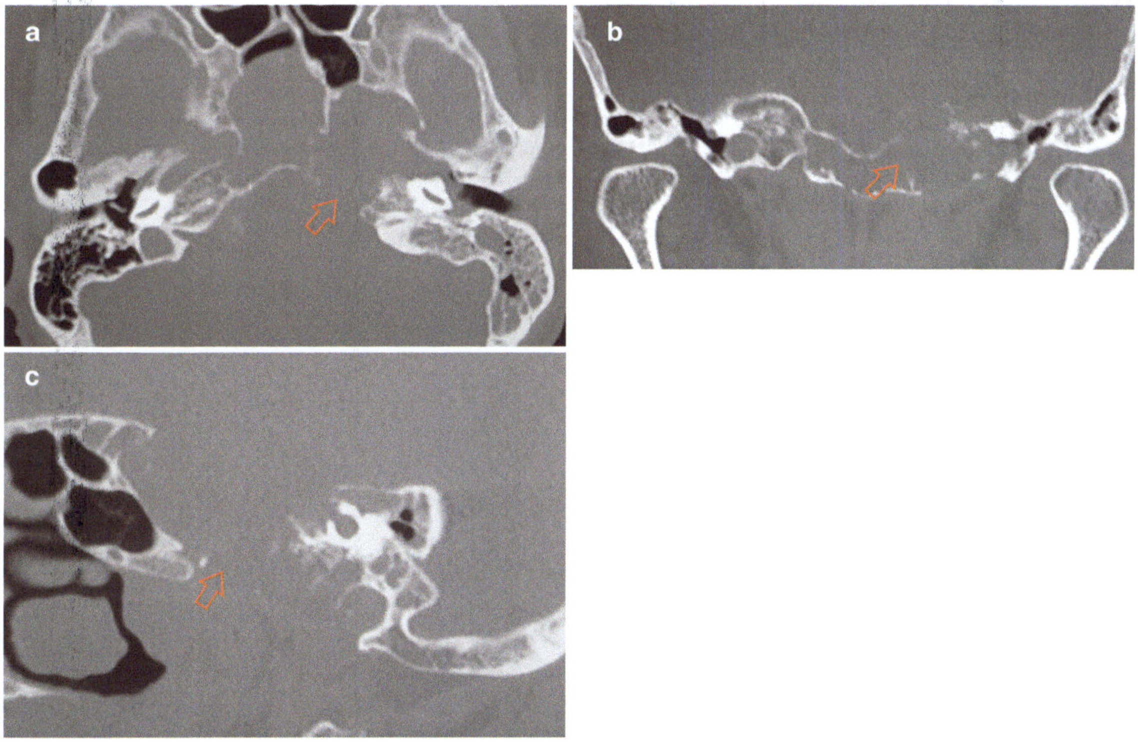

Fig. 9.4 Left clivus-middle cranial fossa occupied with ipsilateral abducent nerve palsy and middle ear mastoiditis, (**a**) Axial CT; (**b**) Coronal CT; (**c**) Sagittal CT. Female, 64 years old. (**a**) Bone destruction of left clivus and petrous apex of temporal bone (⇧); (**b**) Mass enveloping internal carotid artery, invading eustachian tube and bilateral sphenoid sinuses, causing ipsilateral secretory otitis media (⇧); (**c**) Bone destroyed of clivus and petrous apex (foramen lacerum enlarged) (⇧), penetrating skull base

9.1.4 Nasopharyngeal Teratoma Invading Temporal Bone

See Fig. 9.5.

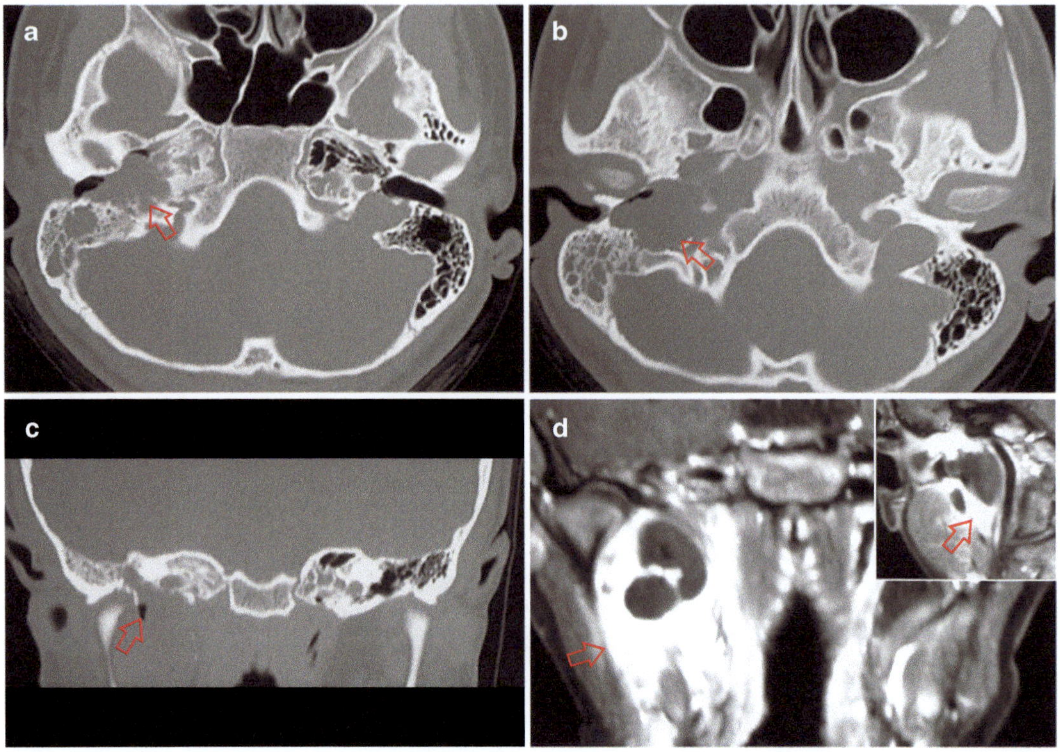

Fig. 9.5 Right parapharyngeal teratoma with hypotympanic cholesteatoma and parapharyngeal abscess. (**a**) Axial CT; (**b**) Axial CT; (**c**) Coronal CT; (**d**) Coronal MRI T_1 WI postgadolinium. Female, 16 years old. (**a, b**) Right lateral skull base, petrous apex was destroyed and absorbed, and replaced by soft tissue (⇧), internal carotid artery and jugular vein were surrounded; (**c**) Right nasopharyngeal soft tissue swelling (⇧), and containing air; (**d**) Right parapharyngeal space soft tissue swelling (⇧), mixed signal shadow, surrounding hyperintense signal, central regular hypointense signal shadow(pus formation) with irregular separation; Insert (coronal MRI T_2 WI): Swelled parapharyngeal space soft tissue with hyperintense signal shadow (⇧) and flow void signal of blood vessel.

Note: Surgical finding: Cholesteatoma was in external auditory meatus and middle ear, abscess cavity had formatted and contained hair in deep neck swelling tissue

9.1.5 Nasopharyngeal Carcinoma Invading Temporal Bone

See Fig. 9.6.

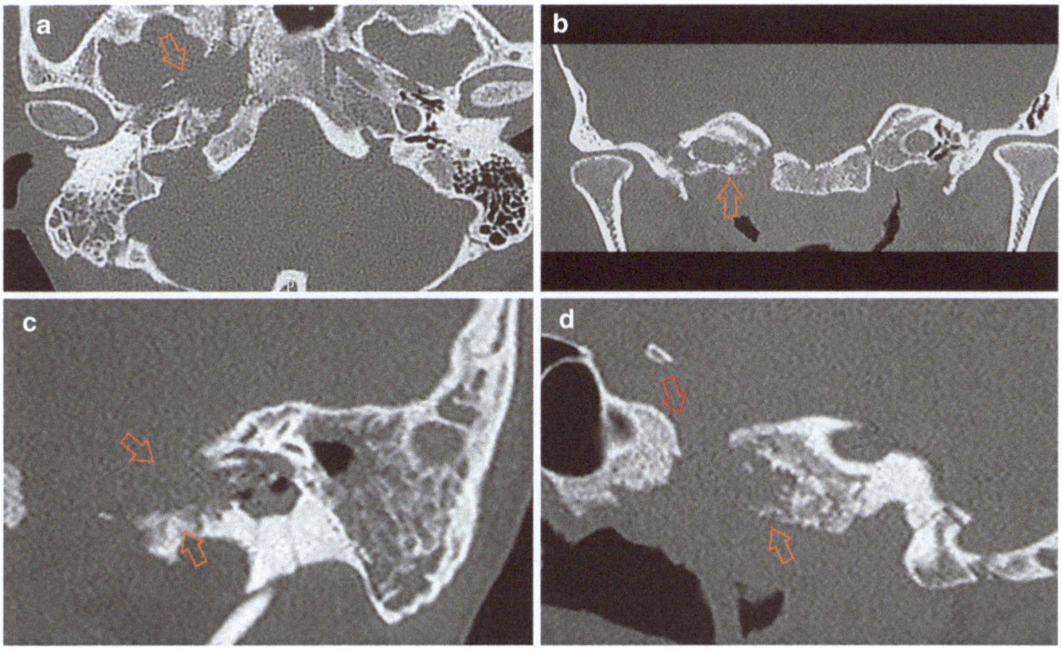

Fig. 9.6 Right nasopharyngeal carcinoma with middle ear mastoiditis and abducent nerve paralysis. (**a**) Axial CT; (**b**) Coronal CT; (**c**, **d**) Sagittal CT. Female, 28 years old. (**a**) Foramen lacerum enlarged, bone destruction (⇧); (**b**) Carotid artery canal erosion (⇧); (**c**) Bony eustachian tube destruction (⇧); (**d**) Extracranial bone of petrous apex destruction (⇧), foramen lacerum enlarged (⇧).

Please note. The differences between Fig. 9.4c with significant intracranial bone destruction and Fig. 9.6d with significant extracranial bone destruction

9.1.6 Rhabdomyosarcoma of Nasopharynx Invading Temporal Bone

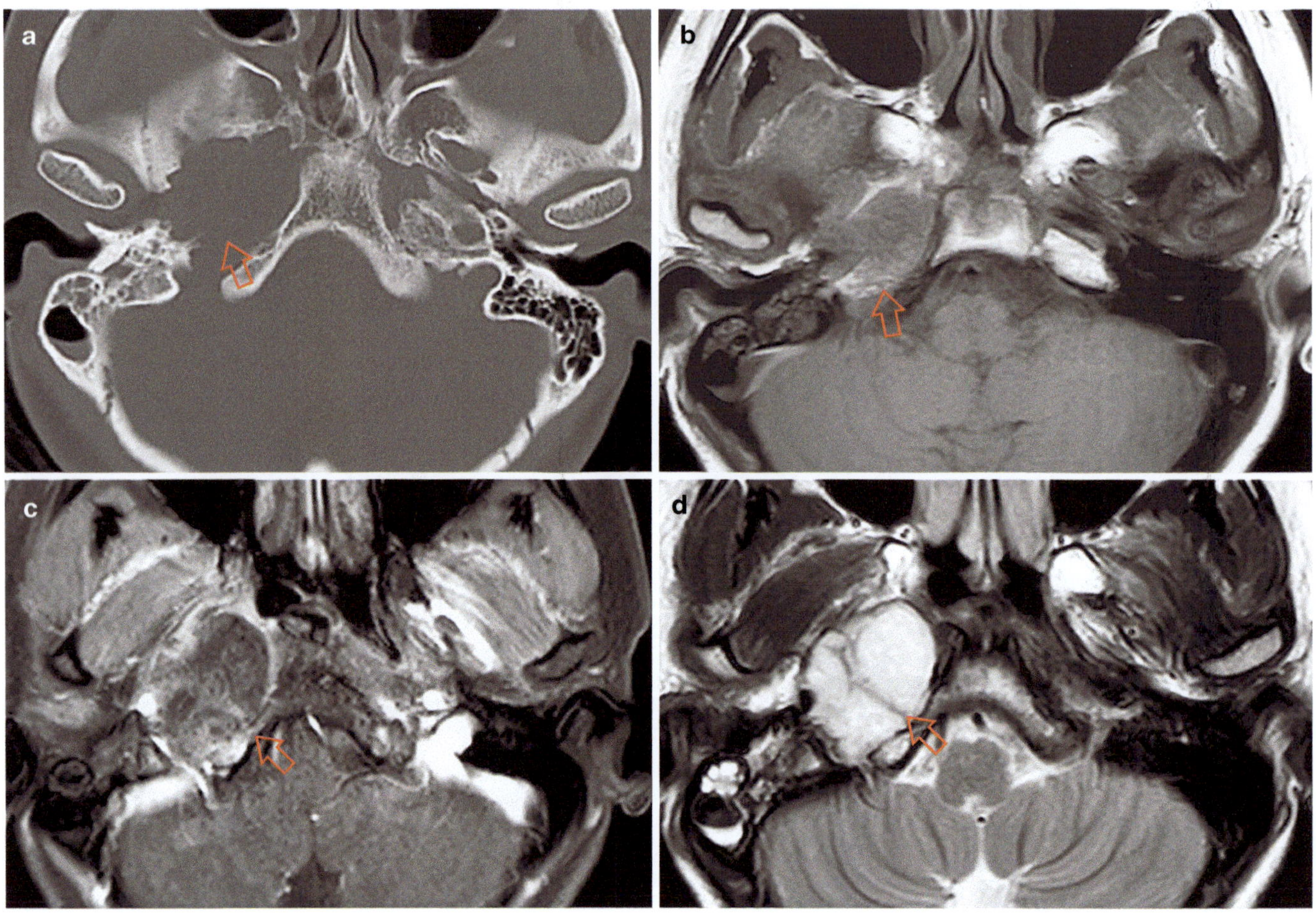

Fig. 9.7 Right nasopharyngeal rhabdomyosarcoma invading petrous apex. (**a**) Axial CT; (**b**) Axial MRI T_1 WI; (**c**) Axial MRI T_1 WI postgadolinium; (**d**) Axial MRI T_2 WI. Female, 29 years old. (**a**) Right skull base bone surrounding foramen lacerum (⇧) was destruction with irregular edge, including sphenoid bone and petrous apex destroyed, petro-occipital fissure enlargement, and replaced by soft tissue; (**b**) Right parapharyngeal space (pterygoid fossa) can be seen equal signal shadow (⇧) with clear boundary. (**c**) Enhanced mass showed margin with mild to moderate uneven hyperintense signal shadow (⇧), center with equal intense signal shadow; (**d**) Even hyperintense signal shadow (⇧) in parapharyngeal space with clear boundary.

Note: Rhabdomyosarcomas comprise the single largest category of soft tissue sarcomas in children and adolescents (Agaram, 2022), but it has a low incidence in the adult population (Ruiz-Mesa et al. 2015) (Fig. 9.7)

9.2 Metastatic Carcinoma of Temporal Bone

See Fig. 9.8.

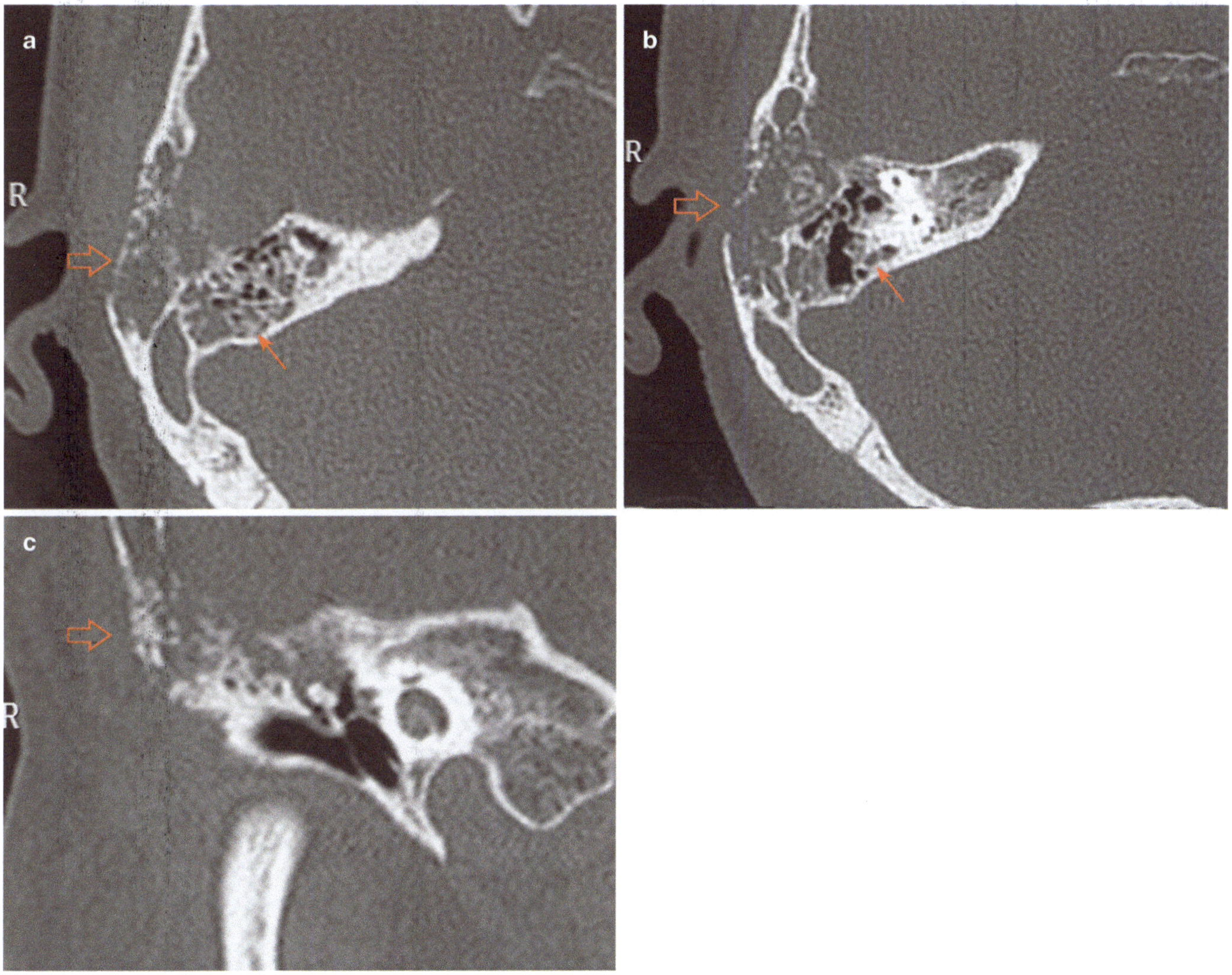

Fig. 9.8 Breast cancer with right temporal bone metastasis. (**a**, **b**) Axial CT; (**c**) Coronal CT. Female, 50 years old, with history of breast cancer. Squamous portion of right temporal bone destruction and absorb (⇧), obstructive change of mastoid cavity (↑).

Note: CT scanning of temporal bone indicated that malignant tumor of temporal bone was waiting to be excluded

Foreign Body in External Auditory Canal and Middle Ear

10

Zilong Yu

Foreign bodies in the external auditory canal are common in children, while foreign bodies in the middle ear are mostly in adults.

10.1 Foreign Body in External Auditory Canal

Foreign bodies in the external auditory canal are common in cotton balls, metal products, plant seeds, insects, powder, etc. They should be removed in time to prevent infection (Figs. 10.1, 10.2, 10.3, and 10.4).

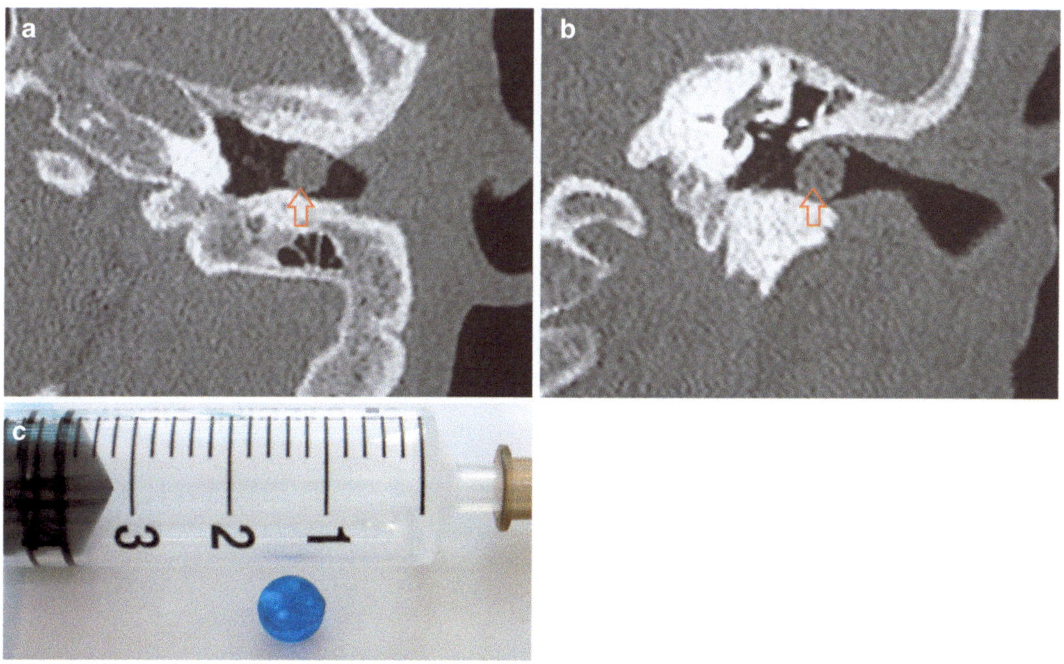

Fig. 10.1 Foreign body in left external auditory canal. (**a**) Axial CT; (**b**) Coronal CT. (**a**, **b**) Circular shadow was showed in middle of external ear canal (⇧); (**c**) Foreign body was plastic bullet

Z. Yu (✉)
Department of Otolaryngology Head and Neck Surgery, Beijing Tongren Hospital, Capital Medical University, Beijing, China

Z. Yu (ed.), *Ear Diseases and CT*, https://doi.org/10.1007/978-981-99-7220-3_10

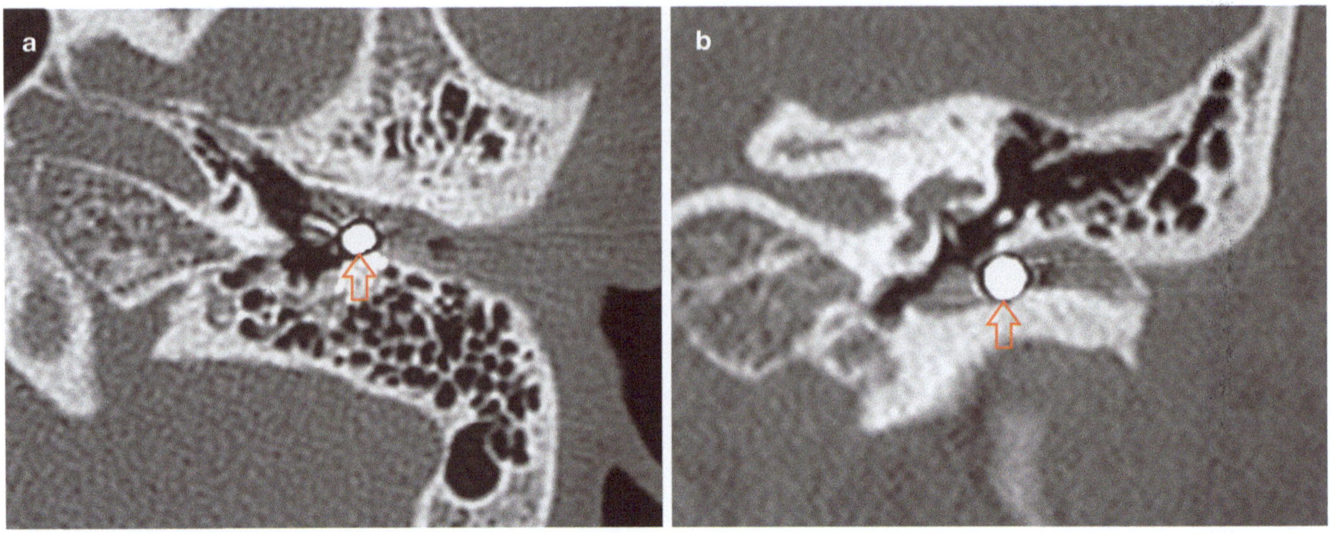

Fig. 10.2 Metal foreign body in left external auditory canal. (**a**) Axial CT; (**b**) Coronal CT. Circular metal foreign body (button battery) was seen in external auditory canal (⇧), inflammation reaction caused soft tissue of external auditory canal swelling

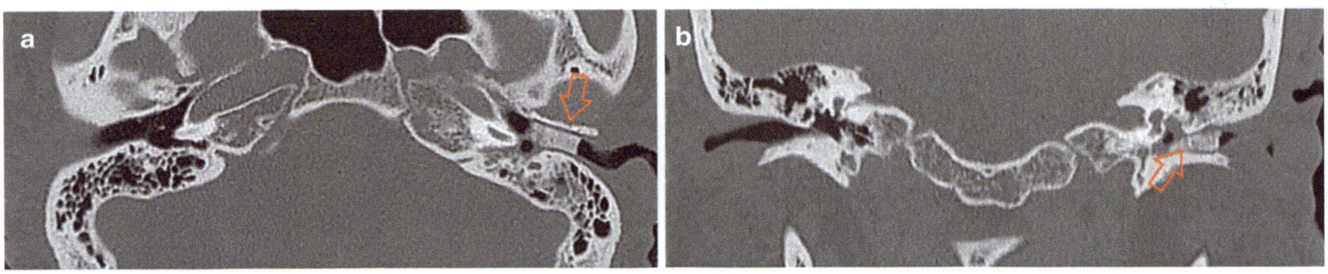

Fig. 10.3 Foreign bodies in left external auditory canal. (**a**) Axial CT; (**b**) Coronal CT. Left external auditory canal was full of minerals (Alum + apatite) (⇧)

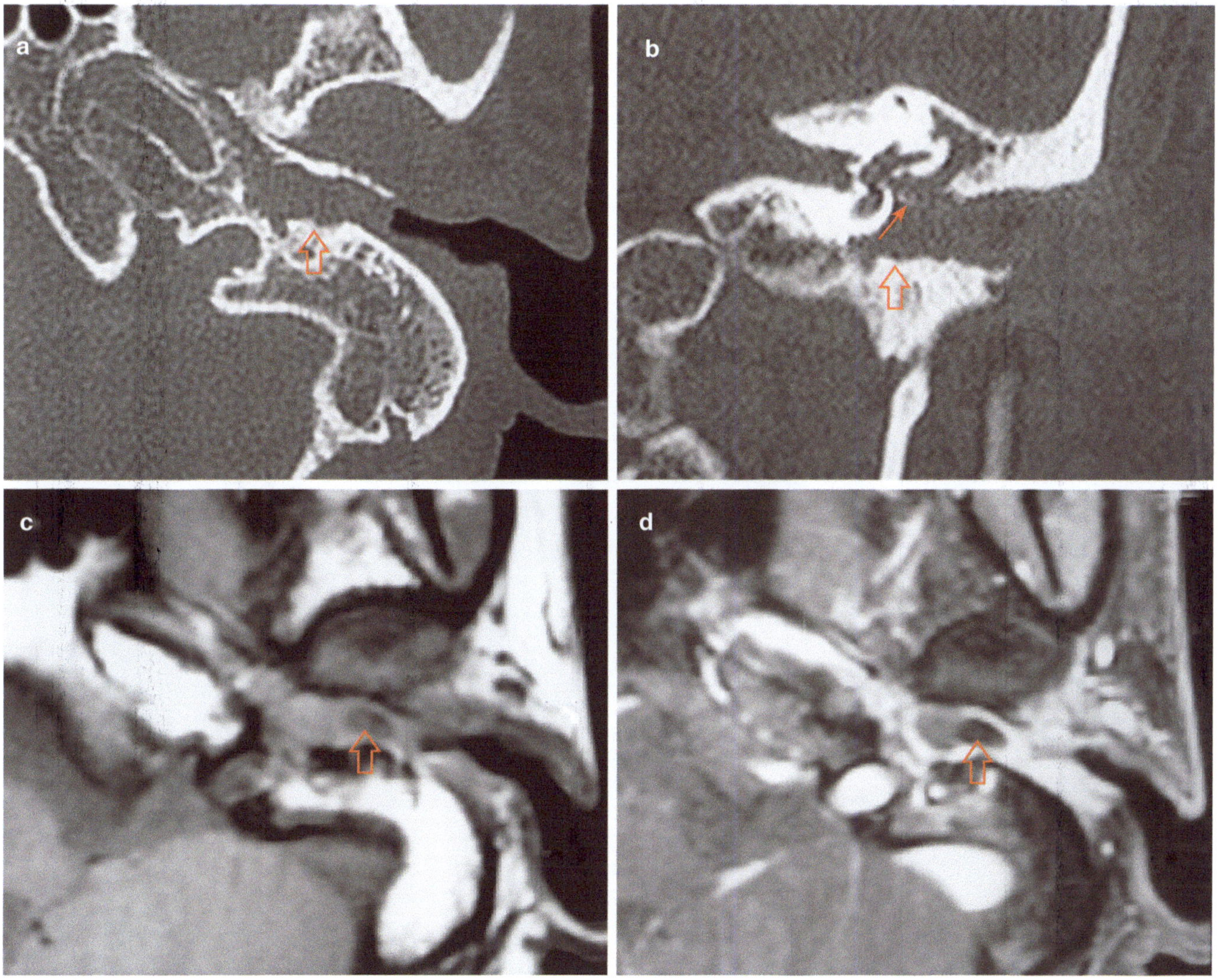

Fig. 10.4 Cholesteatoma of left middle ear with foreign body and granulation in external auditory canal (powder). (**a**) Axial CT; (**b**) Coronal CT; (**c**) Axial MRI T_1WI; (**d**) Axial MRI T_1WI postgadolinium. (**a, b**) Soft tissue shadow (⇧) in middle ear and external auditory canal, faint ossicles (↑), no obvious damage to bone of the external auditory canal; (**c, d**) Hypointense signal shadow (⇧) and surrounding hyperintense signal and central hypointense signal shadow implying cholesteatoma externa

10.2 Foreign Body in Middle Ear

The foreign body in the middle ear usually occurs when the tympanic membrane has been perforated and can also be penetrated into the tympanic cavity by metal sparks and explosive fragments during electric welding (Fig. 10.5).

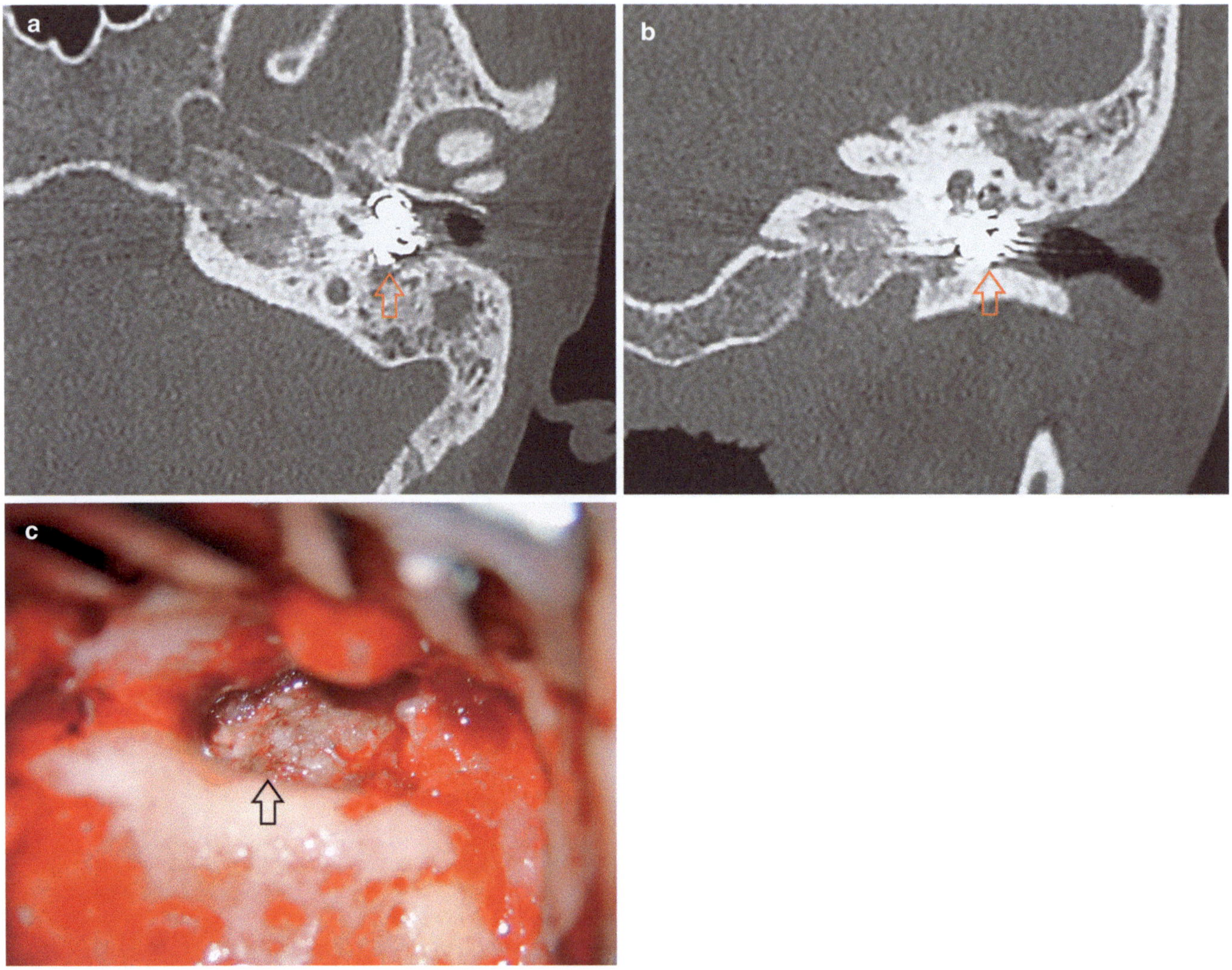

Fig. 10.5 Heavy metal powder in left tympanum. (**a**) Axial CT; (**b**) Coronal CT; (**c**) Intraoperative finding. (**a**, **b**) High density shadow and artifacts are seen in left middle ear cavity (⇧); (**c**) After foreign body removal, ossicles were found to be disappeared, tympanic mucosa necrosis and osteoporosis (⇧)

Otosclerosis

11

Zilong Yu and Bentao Yang

Otosclerosis is a kind of focal lesion originating from the bone labyrinth with unknown etiology, frequently bilateral and affecting women more than men, usually presenting with hearing loss in the second to fourth decades of life (Purohit et al. 2014). It is characterized by the formation of localized, vascular-rich spongy new bone in the capsule of bone labyrinth instead of the original normal bone. On CT, this is appreciated as an area of hypodensity/lucency, and then the new bone becomes ossified and hardened, so it is called otosclerosis. If the lesion extends to the annular ligament, the stapes activity is limited or fixed, progressive conductive hearing loss occurs, this type is called stapedial otosclerosis; If the lesion occurs in the cochlear region, it will cause sensorineural hearing loss, which is called cochlear otosclerosis. If both exist, it will cause mixed hearing loss, which is called mixed otosclerosis.

Otosclerosis can cause conductive, sensorineural, and mixed hearing loss in adults (Figs. 11.1, 11.2, and 11.3)

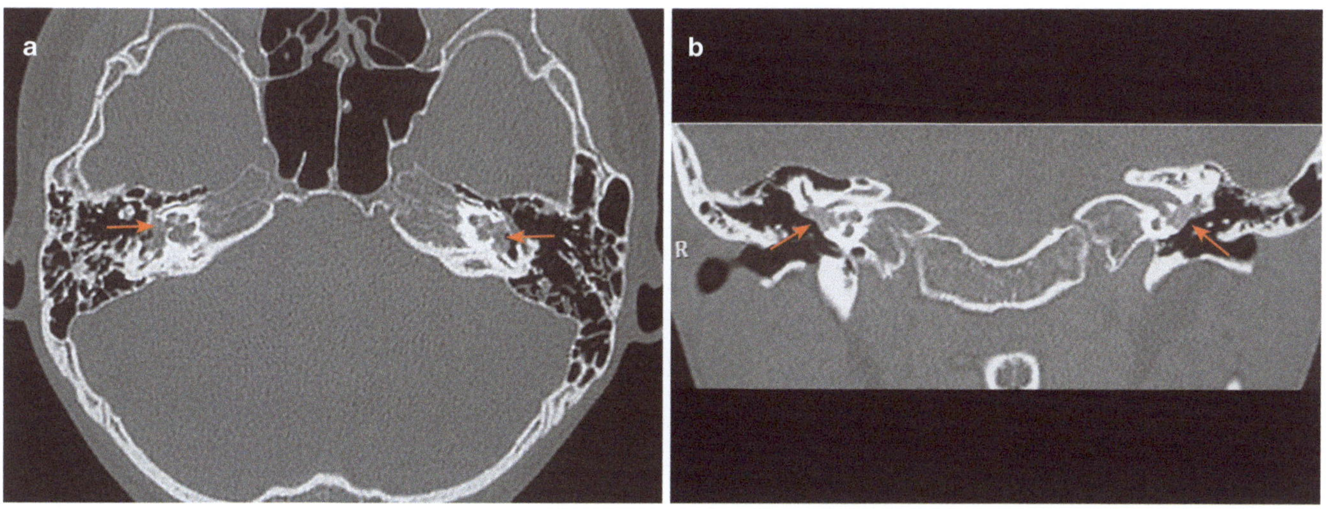

Fig. 11.1 Binaural stapedial (or vestibular window) otosclerosis. (**a**) Axial CT; (**b**) coronal CT. Hypodensity shadows were at fissula ante fenestram in bilateral ears (↑)

Z. Yu (✉)
Department of Otolaryngology Head and Neck Surgery, Beijing Tongren Hospital, Capital Medical University, Beijing, China

B. Yang
Department of Radiology, Beijing Tongren Hospital, Capital Medical University, Beijing, China

Z. Yu (ed.), *Ear Diseases and CT*, https://doi.org/10.1007/978-981-99-7220-3_11

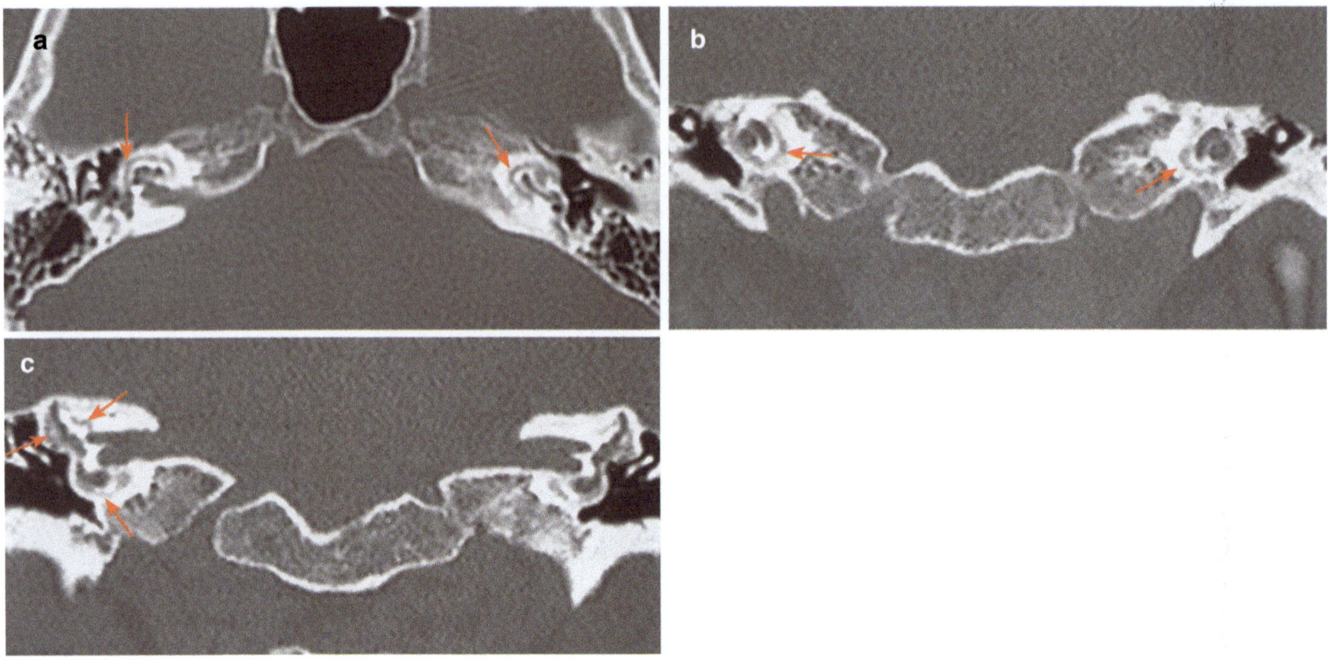

Fig. 11.2 Binaural cochlear otosclerosis. (**a**) Axial CT; (**b**, **c**) Coronal CT. (**a**, **b**) "Lunar halo" hypodensity shadow or double ring sign presented around cochlea (↑); (**c**) Arc-shaped hypodensity shadow shown around semicircular canal and cochlea (↑)

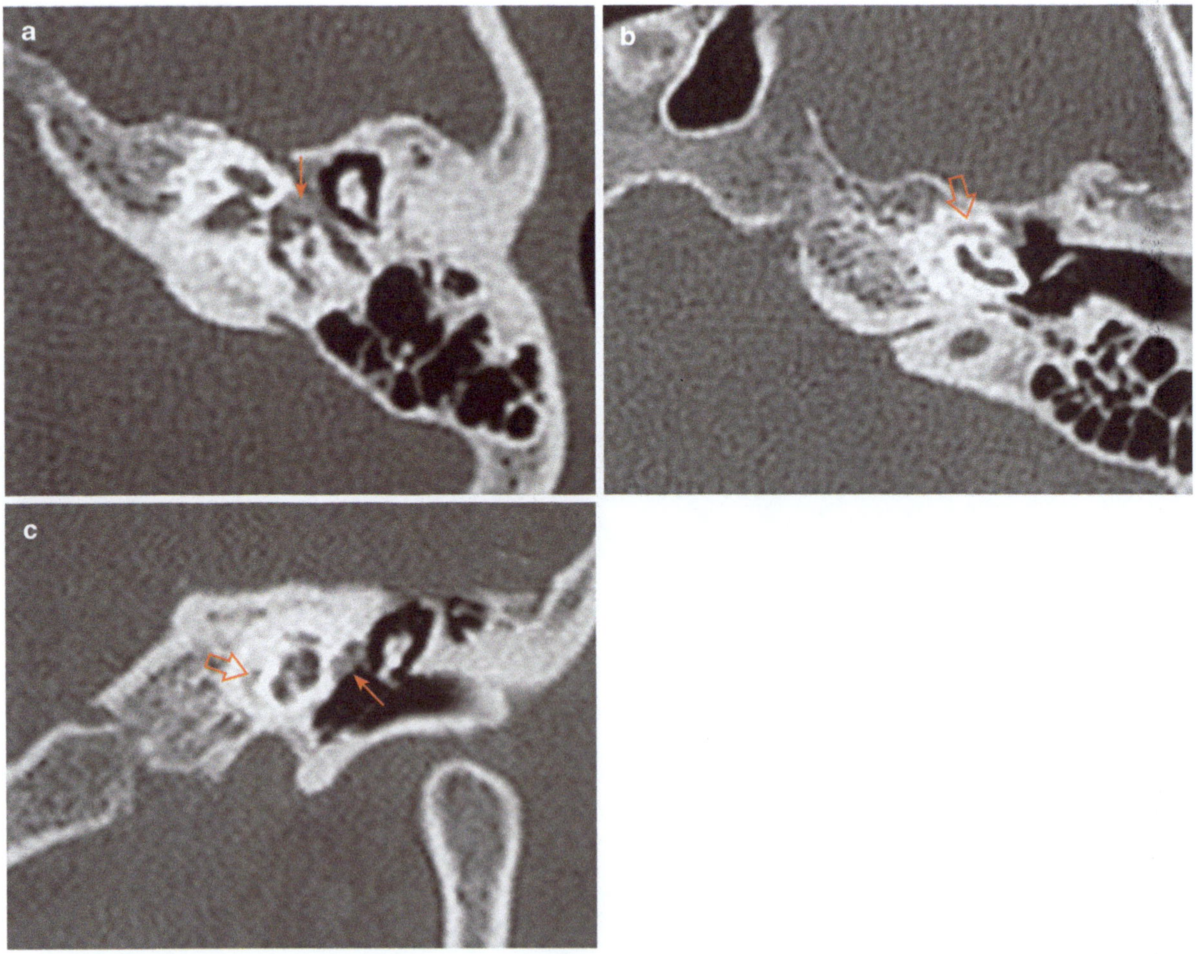

Fig. 11.3 Mixed otosclerosis of left ear. (**a**, **b**) Axial CT; (**c**) Coronal CT. (**a**) Hypodensity shadow was at fissula ante fenestram (↑); (**b**) Arc-shaped hypodensity shadow presented around the cochlea (⇧); (**c**) Hypodensity shadow showed around cochlea (⇧) and in fissula ante fenestram (↑)

Spontaneous Cerebrospinal Fluid Otorrhea

12

Zilong Yu and Bentao Yang

Cerebrospinal fluid (CSF) leaks are extracranial egress of CSF into the adjacent nasal sinus or tympanomastoid cavity due to an osteodural defect involving skull base. They can be due to a multitude of causes including accidental or iatrogenic trauma, congenital malformations (see Figs. 3.22 and 8.1), and spontaneous leaks. Accurate localization of the leak site, underlying causes and appropriate therapy are necessary to avoid associated complications (Hiremath et al. 2019). Spontaneous CSF leaks are those leaks which lack underlying pathologies such as skull base lesions, congenital abnormalities and those with no history of trauma or surgery. It is relatively rare, but is commonly seen in obese, middle-aged women who present with idiopathic intracranial hypertension. Typical imaging findings include prominent arachnoid granulations causing skull base erosions, empty sella, and meningoencephalocele, et al. (Bathla et al. 2016) (Fig. 12.1).

Z. Yu (✉)
Department of Otolaryngology Head and Neck Surgery, Beijing Tongren Hospital, Capital Medical University, Beijing, China

B. Yang
Department of Radiology, Beijing Tongren Hospital, Capital Medical University, Beijing, China

Z. Yu (ed.), *Ear Diseases and CT*, https://doi.org/10.1007/978-981-99-7220-3_12

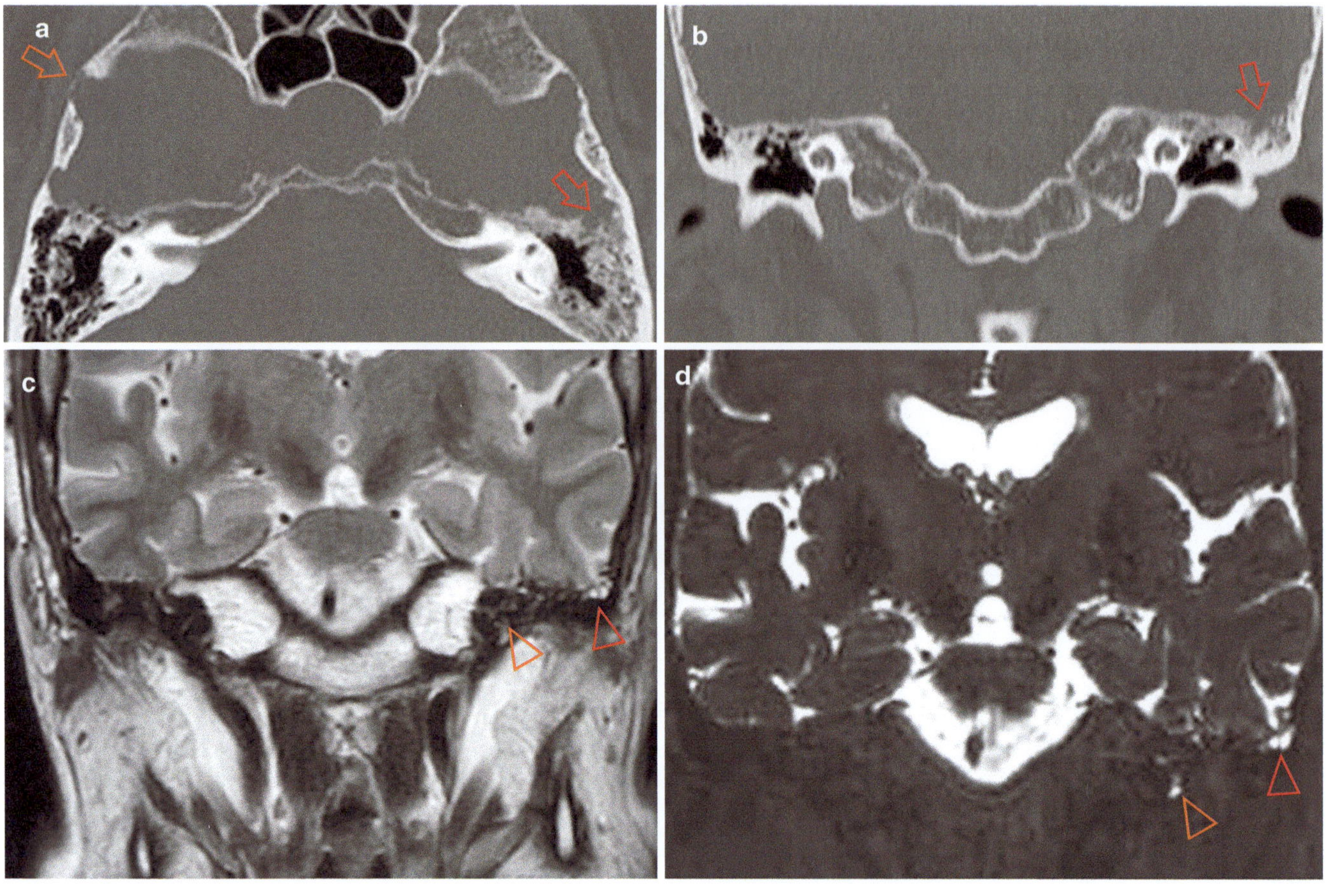

Fig. 12.1 Spontaneous cerebrospinal fluid otorrhea (arachnoid granules) in left ear. (**a**) Axial CT; (**b**) Coronal CT; (**c**) Coronal MRI T_2 WI; (**d**) Coronal MRI hydrography. (**a**, **b**) Greater wing of sphenoid bone (⇧) and petrous portion of temporal bone (⇧) had worm-bitten changes and osteoporosis in bone cortex, and the air cells of tympanic cavity and mastoid process is fuzzy; (**c**) Hyperintense signal shadow was at bone destruction (leakage point) of middle temporal fossa (△), and hypotympanum also had medium signal (△); (**d**) Hyperintense signal at corresponding places(leakage point) (△) and hypotympanum (△)

References

Adad B, Rasgon BM, Ackerson L. Relationship of the facial nerve to the tympanic annulus: a direct anatomic examination. Laryngoscope. 1999;109(8):1189–92.

Agaram NP. Evolving classification of rhabdomyosarcoma. Histopathology. 2022;80(1):98–108.

Agirdir BV, Sindel M, Arslan G, Yildirim FB, Balkan EI, Dinç O. The canal of the posterior ampullar nerve: an important anatomic landmark in the posterior fossa transmeatal approach. Surg Radiol Anat. 2001;23(5):331–4.

Aguilar EA, Yeakly JW, Ghorayeb BY, Hauser M, Cabrera J, Jahrsdoerfer RA. High resolution CT scan of temporal bone fractures: association of facial nerve paralysis with temporal bone fractures. Head Neck Surg. 1987;9(3):162–6.

Akyol Y, Galheigo D, Massimore M, Fatterpekar G. Subarcuate artery and canal: an important anatomic variant. J Comput Assist Tomogr. 2011;35(6):688–9.

Allen CE, Merad M, McClain KL. Langerhans-cell histiocytosis. N Engl J Med. 2018;379(9):856–68.

Aralasmak A, Dincer E, Arslan G, Cevikol C, Karaali K. Posttraumatic labyrinthitis ossificans with perilymphatic fistulization. Diagn Interv Radiol. 2009;15:239–41.

Aslan A, Goktan C, Okumus M, Tarhan S, Unlu H. Morphometric analysis of anatomical relationships of the facial nerve for mastoid surgery. J Laryngol Otol. 2001;115(6):447–9.

Barath K, Huber AM, Stampfli P, Varga Z, Kollias S. Neuroradiology of cholesteatomas. Am J Neuroradiol. 2011;32:221–9.

Bathla G, Moritani T. Imaging of cerebrospinal fluid leak. Semin Ultrasound CT MRI. 2016;37(2):143–9.

Baxter A. Dehiscence of the fallopian canal: an anatomical study. J Laryngol Otol. 1971;85:587–94.

Benson JC, Lane JI. Temporal bone anatomy. Neuroimaging Clin N Am. 2022;32:763–75.

Cannon CR, Jahrsdoerfer RA. Temporal bone fractures. Review of 90 cases. Arch Otolaryngol. 1983;109(5):285–8.

Carey JP, Minor LB, Nager GT. Dehiscence or thinning of bone overlying the superior semicircular canal in a temporal bone survey. Arch Otolaryngol Head Neck Surg. 2000;126:137–47.

Connor SE, Leung R, Natas S. Imaging of the petrous apex: a pictorial review. Br J Radiol. 2008;81:427–35.

Dewan K, Wippold FJ, Lieu JE. Enlarged vestibular aqueduct in pediatric sensorineural hearing loss. Otolaryngol Head Neck Surg. 2009;140:552–8.

Dimopoulos PA, Muren C, Smedby O, Wadin K. Anatomical variations of the tympanic and mastoid portions of the facial nerve canal. Acta Radiol. 1996;37(Suppl 403):49–59.

Eibenberger K, Carey J, Ehtiati T, Trevino C, Dolberg J, Haslwanter T. A novel method of 3D image analysis of high-resolution cone beam CT and multi slice CT for the detection of semicircular canal dehiscence. Otol Neurotol. 2014;35:329–37.

Erixon EH, Wadin K, Rask-Andersen H. Variational anatomy of the human cochlea: implications for cochlear implantation. Otol Neurotol. 2009;30(1):14–22.

Gilberto N, Custódio S, Colaço T, Santos R, Sousa P, Escada P. Middle ear congenital cholesteatoma: systematic review, meta-analysis and insights on its pathogenesis. Eur Arch Otorhinolaryngol. 2020;277(4):987–98.

Guyot-Goubin A, Donadieu J, Barkaoui M, Bellec S, Thomas C, Clavel J. Descriptive epidemiology of childhood Langerhans cell histiocytosis in France, 2000-2004. Pediatr Blood Cancer. 2008;51:71–5.

Hiremath SB, Gautam AA, Sasindran V, Therakathu J, Benjamin G. Cerebrospinal fluid rhinorrhea and otorrhea: a multimodality imaging approach. Diagn Interv Imaging. 2019;100(1):3–15.

Jäger L, Reiser M. CT and MR imaging of the normal and pathological conditions of the facial nerve. Eur J Radiol. 2001;40:133–46.

Juliano AF. Cross sectional imaging of the ear and temporal bone. Head Neck Pathol. 2018;12:302–20.

Kozerska M, Skrzat J. Anatomy of the fundus of the internal acoustic meatus-micro-computed tomography study. Folia Morphol. 2015;74(3):352–8.

Lalwani AK, Jackler RK. Preoperative differentiation between meningioma of the cerebellopontine angle and acoustic neuroma using MRI. Otolaryngol Head Neck Surg. 1993;109(1):88–95.

Lang J. Clinical anatomy of the ear. Wien/New York: Springer; 1992.

Lechner M, Sutton L, Murkin C, Masterson L, O'Flynn P, Wareing MJ, Tatla T, Saeed S. Squamous cell cancer of the temporal bone: a review of the literature. Eur Arch Otorhinolaryngol. 2021;278:2225–8.

LeMay DR, Sun JK, Mendel E, Hinton DR, Giannotta SL. Chondromyxoid fibroma of the temporal bone. Surg Neurol. 1997;48(2):148–52.

Li Y, Li Q, Gong S, Liu H, Yu Z, Zhang L. Multiple osteomas in middle ear. Case Rep Otolaryngol. 2014;2012:685932, 3 pages.

Luntz M, Malatskey S, Braun J. The anatomic relationship between the second genu of the facial nerve and the incus: a high-resolution computed tomography study. Am J Otol. 2000;21(5):686–9.

Maerki J, Riddle ND, Newman J, Husson MA, Lee JYK. Giant cell granuloma of the temporal bone in a mixed martial arts fighter. J Neurol Surg Rep. 2012;73(1):60–3.

Mafee MF, Kumar A, Tahmoressi CN, Levin BC, James CF, Kriz R, Capek V. Direct sagittal CT in the evaluation of temporal bone disease. Am J Roentgenol. 1988;150(6):1403–10.

Mayer TE, Brueckmann H, Siegert R, Witt A, Weerda H. High-resolution CT of the temporal bone in dysplasia of the auricle and external auditory canal. Am J Neuroradiol. 1997;18(1):53–65.

McManus LJ, Wawes PJ, Stringer MD. Surgical anatomy of the chorda tympani: a micro-CT study. Surg Radiol Anat. 2012;34:513–8.

Minor LB. Clinical manifestations of superior semicircular canal dehiscence. Laryngoscope. 2005;115:1717–27.

Minor LB, Solomon D, Zinreich JS, Zee DS. Sound- and/or pressure-induced vertigo due to bone dehiscence of the superior semicircular canal. Arch Otolaryngol Head Neck Surg. 1998;124:249–58.

Nicolay S, De Foer B, Bernaerts A, Dinther JV, Parizel PM. Aberrant internal carotid artery presenting as a retrotympanic vascular mass. Acta Radiol Short Rep. 2014;3(10). eCollection 2014.

Z. Yu (ed.), *Ear Diseases and CT*, https://doi.org/10.1007/978-981-99-7220-3

Ogawa A, Sando I. Spatial occupancy of vessels and facial nerve in the facial canal. Ann Otol Rhinol Laryngol. 1982;91(1 Pt 1):14–9.

Orosz Z, Athanasou NA. Giant cell-containing tumors of bone. Surg Pathol Clin. 2017;10(3):553–73.

Pisaneschi MJ, Langer B. Congenital cholesteatoma and cholesterol granuloma of the temporal bone: role of magnetic resonance imaging. Top Magn Reson Imaging. 2000;11:87–97.

Purohit B, Hermans R, Op de Beeck K. Imaging in otosclerosis: a pictorial review. Insights Imaging. 2014;5:245–52.

Quesnel AM, Santos F. Evaluation and management of facial nerve schwannoma. Otolaryngol Clin North Am. 2018;51(6):1179–92.

Raghavan P, Mukherjee S, Phillips CD. Imaging of the facial nerve. Neuroimaging Clin N Am. 2009;19(3):407–25.

Rajan GP, Leaper MR, Goggin L, Atlas MD, Boeddinghaus R, Eikelboom RK. The effects of superior semicircular canal dehiscence on the labyrinth: does size matter? Otol Neurotol. 2008;29(7):972–5.

Razek AA, Huang BY. Lesions of the petrous apex: classification and findings at CT and MR imaging. Radiographics. 2012;32:151–73.

Ruiz-Mesa C, Goldberg JM, Munoz A, Dumont SN, Trent JC. Rhabdomyosarcoma in adults: new perspectives on therapy. Curr Treat Options Oncol. 2015;16(6):27.

Schart-Moren N, Larsson S, Rask-Andersen H, Li H. Three-dimensional analysis of the fundus of the human internal acoustic canal. Ear Hear. 2018;39(3):563–72.

Schilder AM. Wegener's granulomatosis vasculitis and granuloma. Autoimmun Rev. 2010;9(7):483–7.

Schmalfuss IM. Petrous apex. Neuroimaging Clin N Am. 2009;19:367–91.

Swartz JD, Zwillenberg S, Berger AS. Acquired disruptions of the incudostapedial articulation: diagnosis with CT. Radiology. 1989;171:779–81.

Sweeney AD, Carlson ML, Wanna GB, Bennett ML. Glomus tympanicum tumors. Otolaryngol Clin North Am. 2015;48(2):293–304.

Takahashi H, Sando I. Facial nerve dehiscence: histologic study and computer reconstruction. Ann Otol Rhinol Laryngol. 1992;101:925–30.

Tarhan NC, Yologlu Z, Tutar NU, Coskun M, Agildere AM, Arikan U. Chondromyxoid fibroma of the temporal bone: CT and MRI findings. Eur Radiol. 2000;10:1678–80.

Tringali S, Linthicum FH Jr. Cholesterol granuloma of the petrous apex. Otol Neurotol. 2010;31:1518–9.

Valvassori GE, Mafee MF. Temporal bone. In: Carter BL, editor. Computed tomography of the head and neck. New York: Churchill Livingstone; 1985. p. 171–205.

Viswanatha B. Embryonal rhabdomyosarcoma of the temporal bone. Ear Nose Throat J. 2007;86(4):218, 220–2.

Walcott BP, Nahed BV, Mohyeldin A, Coumans J, Kahle KT, Ferreira MJ. Chordoma: current concepts, management, and future directions. Lancet Oncol. 2012;13(2):e69–76.

Wang Z. Skull base surgery. Shanghai: Shanghai Science and Technology Press; 1994.

Wang Y, Xu L, Guan B, Tian T, Chang L. The study on prognosis in patients with adenoid cystic carcinoma of the external auditory canal. J Int Adv Otol. 2023;19(2):149–54.

Wiatrak BJ, Pensak ML. Rhabdomyosarcoma of the ear and temporal bone. Laryngoscope. 1989;99(11):1188–92.

Yasumura S, Takahashi H, Sando I, Aoki H, Hirsch BE. Facial nerve near the external auditory meatus in man: computer reconstruction study—preliminary report. Laryngoscope. 1993;103(9):1043–7.

Yew A, Zarinkhou G, Spasic M, Trang A, Gopen Q, Yang I. Characteristics and management of superior semicircular canal dehiscence. J Neurol Surg B Skull Base. 2012;73:365–70.

Young K, Arkfeld DV, Ogasawara CT, Squires LD. A systematic review of primary temporal bone mucosal melanoma. Otol Neurotol. 2023;44(3):e118–24.

Yu Z, Han D, Dai H, Zhao S, Zheng Y. Diagnosis of pathological exposure of mastoid portion of facial nerve by CT scanning. Acta Otolaryngologica (Stockh). 2007;127(3):323–7.

Yu Z, Han D, Gong S, Wang Z, Dai H, Zhao S, Zheng Y, Leng T. Facial nerve course in congenital aural atresia-identified by preoperative CT scanning and surgical findings. Acta Otolaryngologica (Stockh). 2008;28(12):11375–80.

Yu Z, Han D, Gong S, Wang Z, Zhang L. The value of scutum erosion in the diagnosis of temporal bone cholesteatoma. Acta Otolaryngologica (Stockh). 2010;130(1):47–51.

Yu Z, Wang Z, Yang B, Han D, Zhang L. The value of pre-operative CT scan of tympanic facial nerve canal in tympanomastoid surgery. Acta Otolaryngologica (Stockh). 2011;131(7):774–8.

Yu Z, Zhang L, Han D. Long-term outcome of ossiculoplasty using autogenous mastoid cortical bone. J Laryngol Otol. 2014;128:866–70.

Yu Z, Zhang L, Han D. Micro-CT of temporal bone. Singapore: Springer; 2021.

MIX
Papier aus verantwortungsvollen Quellen
Paper from responsible sources
FSC® C105338

If you have any concerns about our products,
you can contact us on
ProductSafety@springernature.com

In case Publisher is established outside the EU,
the EU authorized representative is:
Springer Nature Customer Service Center GmbH
Europaplatz 3, 69115 Heidelberg, Germany

Printed by Libri Plureos GmbH
in Hamburg, Germany